Behavioral Approaches to Medicine
Application and Analysis

Behavioral Approaches to Medicine
Application and Analysis

Edited by

J. Regis McNamara
Ohio University
Athens, Ohio

Plenum Press · New York and London

Library of Congress Cataloging in Publication Data

Main entry under title:

Behavioral approaches to medicine.

Includes bibliographical references and index.
1. Medicine and psychology. I. McNamara, J. Regis. [DNLM: 1. Behavioral sciences.
2. Medicine. WB890 B419 (P)]
R726.5.B423   610'.1'9   79-12345
ISBN 0-306-40238-6

© 1979 Plenum Press, New York
A Division of Plenum Publishing Corporation
227 West 17th Street, New York, N.Y. 10011

Printed in the United States of America

To Jane and Regis for their enduring affection and support

and

To Marti and Brian, with love

Contributors

BARRY BLACKWELL, M.D., *Department of Psychiatry, Wright State University School of Medicine, Dayton, Ohio*

EDWARD B. BLANCHARD, PH.D., *Department of Psychology, State University of New York, Albany, New York*

MARGARET A. CHESNEY, PH.D., *Center for Research on Stress and Health, Stanford Research Institute, Menlo Park, California*

RONALD S. DRABMAN, PH.D., *Department of Psychiatry and Human Behavior, University of Mississippi School of Medicine, Jackson, Mississippi*

LEONARD H. EPSTEIN, PH.D., *Western Psychiatric Institute and Clinic, University of Pittsburgh School of Medicine, Pittsburgh, Pennsylvania*

AL. S. FEDORAVICIUS, PH.D., *Psychology Service, Veterans Administration Hospital, Albuquerque, New Mexico*

MICHAEL FEUERSTEIN, PH.D., *Department of Psychology, McGill University, Montreal, Quebec, Canada*

KENNETH A. HOLROYD, PH.D., *Department of Psychology, Ohio University, Athens, Ohio*

FRANCIS J. KEEFE, PH.D., *Department of Psychiatry, Behavioral Physiology Laboratory, Duke University Medical Center, Durham, North Carolina*

MARIE A. MASTRIA, PH.D., *Department of Psychiatry and Human Behavior, University of Mississippi School of Medicine, Jackson, Mississippi*

J. REGIS MCNAMARA, PH.D., *Department of Psychology, Ohio University, Athens, Ohio*

DEBORAH J. OSSIP, PH.D., *Western Psychiatric Institute and Clinic, University of Pittsburgh School of Medicine, Pittsburgh, Pennsylvania*

C. EUGENE WALKER, PH.D., *Division of Pediatric Psychology, University of Oklahoma Medical School, Oklahoma City, Oklahoma*

STEPHEN M. WEISS, PH.D., *Behavioral Medicine Branch, Division of Heart and Vascular Diseases, National Heart, Lung, and Blood Institute, National Institutes of Health, Bethesda, Maryland*

WILLIAM E. WHITEHEAD, PH.D., *Psychophysiology Laboratory, Departments of Psychiatry and Physical Medicine and Rehabilitation, University of Cincinnati, Cincinnati, Ohio*

SUSAN WOOLEY, PH.D., *Department of Psychiatry, University of Cincinnati School of Medicine, Cincinnati, Ohio*

Foreword

BEHAVIORAL MEDICINE: AN IDEA...

As one of the first volumes on behavioral medicine, the authors and editor of this text bear special responsibility for placing the development of this new field in an historical and conceptual perspective with regard to the myriad events currently taking place in biobehavioral approaches to physical health and illness.

Recognizing that the basic concepts embodied in behavioral medicine are at least several thousand years old begs the question of how behavioral medicine offers not only a new perspective but a potentially more productive approach to many of the age-old problems concerning the maintenance of health and the prevention, diagnosis, and treatment of, and rehabilitation from, illness. One must look not only at the historical antecedents of the field but also at the contemporaneous events occurring in related areas on the social and political as well as the biomedical and behavioral levels to fully comprehend the significance of this movement, which has designated itself "behavioral medicine."

The past 40 years have seen the emergence, development, and gradual decline of behavioral medicine's most immediate predecessor, psychosomatic medicine. Recent articles by Engel (1977), Lipowski (1977), Weiner (1977), and Leigh and Reiser (1977), attest to the frustration and concern of leading theorists in psychosomatic medicine concerning the future of this field. In an effort to understand how many of the problems being faced by psychosomatic medicine at this time may relate to the development of behavioral medicine, we might profitably review the theoretical and conceptual underpinnings of each field.

Although efforts to understand mind–body relationships can be found in the literature spanning several thousand years, efforts to systematically develop a body of knowledge relevant to modern medicine can be dated to less than 30 years ago, beginning with the work of Alexander (1950). Through the "specificity" theory, Alexander, using a psychoanalytic framework, postulated unconscious and unresolved conflicts as being responsible for various disease states (e.g., hypertension, ulcers, and asthma). Although efforts were made to develop the area that we today call *psychophysiology* within the psychosomatic medicine movement, the basic roots of the field remained in psychoanalytic theory and practice, with a research methodology primarily ancedotal and observational and its primary emphasis devoted to pathogenesis. Although this field was viewed by many clinicians and researchers in biomedicine with considerable hope and expectation during the 1940s and the 1950s, by the 1960s these expectations were still largely unmet, and the interest of the biomedical community began to fade.

Several concurrent activities, related only by happenstance, were also taking place during this period. No longer were the acute infectious diseases the scourge they had been only a few years before. Even such crippling diseases as polio could now be prevented through immunization. Similar approaches were attempted with major chronic diseases, for example, heart disease, cancer, stroke, and diabetes. The frustration and failure attendant upon these efforts prompted the realization that the virus or bacterium alone—that is, a single-factor approach—did not explain the multifaceted nature of chronic illness. As investigations continued, it became increasingly clear that lifestyle played a major role in the onset and course of many of these illnesses and was intimately related with possible prevention of many chronic diseases.

During this same period, we were entering into what might be termed the age of the consumer, in which people were demanding a more active role in shaping their own destiny. Regulations concerning the protection of human subjects, informed consent, the Freedom of Information and Privacy Acts, and the concerns related to "bioethics" in recent years have focused attention on self-care, self-help, and self-regulation strategies in health as approaches that share a common philosophic base with this movement.

The above approaches also relate directly to the recent emphasis on cost containment in health, which has been prompted by the rapidly escalating health costs in the United States. It is estimated that we will spend close to $160 billion or approximately 12% of our gross national product on health next year. It is further estimated that if we were to double the health expenditures we would probably achieve only a 5–10% improvement in the quality of care. Obviously, these problems cannot be solved by fiscal means alone; by the same token, purely biomedical solutions cannot, by themselves, encompass the multifaceted nature of the problems we are facing in health today.

Given the constellation of facilitating and inhibiting factors described above, we must carefully reexamine our conceptual models in terms of relevance to our current state of knowledge and the current political and social climate relating to health research and practice.

A final, and perhaps the most relevant, factor to consider in attempting to understand the various forces contributing to the emergence of behavioral medicine took place in the late 1960s. Based on the work of Miller and associates (Miller & Dworken, 1977), the term *biofeedback* was coined to characterize the role of the central nervous system in mediating autonomic nervous system functions. This breakthrough, based on a solid theoretical foundation of operant and classical conditioning, provided the long-sought-for tool potentially capable of exploring heretofore unrecognized neural connections in explicating the effect of the environment on peripheral end-organ function. The concept of biofeedback also opened myriad possibilities for ultimately developing self-regulatory systems for both monitoring and modulating physiological function.

This discovery was combined with the realization by the biomedical community that health behavior, compliance with medical regimens, and the nature of the patient–provider relationship were all potent determiners of the ultimate outcome in a health care situation. The presence of thousands of behavioral scientists working in medical schools and other biomedical settings, the development of the concept of health maintenance organizations that would stress prevention as one of their key priorities, and the imminence of some form of national health insurance with stringent cost-containment features were yet additional issues contributing to an environment conducive to the development of a field that would attempt to address this constellation of problems.

The past five years have seen increasing recognition on the part of the biomedical establishment of the potential application of many of the above-described activities to health promotion and disease prevention and control. Behavioral scientists have also become increasingly interested in this area, as they have come to recognize the applicability of their research findings to the problems of biomedicine. This growing realization by both the biomedical and the behavioral communities has been coupled with the recognition of the lack of a unifying theme, a conceptual model that might facilitate their efforts to develop productive collaborative relationships. Parenthetically, it is worthwhile to note here that mere recognition of a commonality of interest has not in the past been sufficient to successfully promote such relationships in most cases where they have been attempted.

The combination of new theory, new technical developments, new understandings, and a different social and political climate, coupled with an inability in the eyes of those most directly concerned to put all of these pieces together in a fashion that would readily blend into an existing structure or model, was the primary impetus bringing together persons of many disciplines to what is now called the Yale Conference on Behavioral Medicine, held in February 1977. During this two-day gathering, distinguished scientists representing eight disciplines agreed upon a single definition (including subareas covered by that definition) that would serve to characterize all of the activities they felt comprised the field of behavioral medicine (Schwartz & Weiss, 1977). This was a landmark conference in several respects, but perhaps the most salient feature noted by all participants was the unanimity and common recognition of purpose that characterized these meetings, in contrast to earlier attempts to achieve such consensus. A good illustration of this sentiment was voiced near the end of the final session of this conference, when one participant expressed the opinion that "this degree of unanimity would have been impossible five years ago." Following a brief silence, another member responded "probably this gathering would not have succeeded even two years ago." The prevailing sentiment was that clearly this was *an idea whose time had come.*

Developments in behavioral medicine accelerated sharply following the Yale Conference. The Yale definition was revised 14 months later during an organizational meeting of the Academy of Behavioral Medicine Research, hosted by the National Academy of Sciences (April 1978). This "second-generation" definition summarized the conceptual development that had taken place in the minds of those most intimately involved with this field over the course of the year, and it more accurately defined the essential and unique characteristic of behavioral medicine, which differentiated it from other previous efforts, to wit:

Yale Conference on Behavioral Medicine, February, 1977

> Behavioral medicine is the field concerned with the development of behavioral science, knowledge, and techniques relevant to the understanding of physical health and illness and the application of this knowledge and these techniques to prevention, diagnosis, treatment, and rehabilitation. Psychosis, neurosis, and substance abuse are included only insofar as they contribute to physical disorders as an endpoint. (Schwartz & Weiss, 1978, p. 249)

Academy of Behavioral Medicine Research, April, 1978

> Behavioral medicine is the interdisciplinary field concerned with the development and integration of behavioral and biomedical science, knowledge and techniques relevant to health and illness and the application of this knowledge and these techniques to prevention, diagnosis, treatment and rehabilitation. (Schwartz & Weiss, 1978, p. 250)

In examining these two definitions, it is readily apparent that the second definition sought to correct the inadvertent implication of mind–body dualism suggested by the first definition and to focus upon the joining of forces of biomedical and behavioral scientists in collaborative efforts to seek solutions to common problems. This emphasis reflected a realization on the part of the academy participants that it was insufficient just to bring behavioral science to bear on biomedical problems; rather, it was essential to encourage and promote joint efforts by biomedical and behavioral scientists working together on common problems. This approach superseded the "parallel" model implied by the earlier definition—that is, behavioral and biomedical scientists working in parallel but separate research activities with only minimal or token consultation with one another—replacing it with an *interactive* model in which "the whole would be greater than the sum of its parts."

It was felt that the combining of the different perspectives on a common problem in such a collaborative fashion would have a synergistic effect that could not be achieved in the absence of this cross-stimulation. Rather than shying away from the perceptual differences among biomedical and behavioral scientists, this model would seek to capitalize upon these differences, making use of the heuristic potential contained therein. This one issue alone has been a source of tremendous intellectual stimulation for both biomedical and behavioral scientists, once they were able to bridge the initial recognition that they did in fact approach common problems from very different perspectives. In this case, a source of traditional divisiveness and mis- or noncommunication has been turned to the advantage of the participants involved. It should be kept in mind that this is not an automatic process, but that taking the time to explore the differences, combined with a recognition that all parties involved need not approach a problem from the same perspective, fosters the necessary climate for capitalizing on these differences. The problem becomes even more challenging when four or six disciplines are approaching a problem common to them all, each from their own particular discipline perspective. This "readiness" on the part of all participants to share in this type of experience is perhaps the greatest conceptual strength of the behavioral medicine model.

Finally, it should be emphasized that we are speaking of a "field of endeavor" rather than a "discipline" of behavioral medicine. Although we speak, in Miller's terms, of "two skills in one skull" (Schwartz & Weiss, 1977), the thrust here is to have the individual fully trained in one discipline but conversant with the language and concepts of the other disciplines involved in behavioral medicine. This approach is particularly relevant to the behavioral scientist, who must come to better understand the concepts and language of biomedicine; conversely, the biomedical scientist must become more familiar with the terms, theories, and concepts of behavioral science. Both biomedical and behavioral scientists must also become more cognizant of the subdisciplines within their own disciplines, as well as the different disciplines within the broad categories of biomedical or behavioral science. While we cannot hope to eliminate all the barriers existing between disciplines, we can at least strive toward reducing these barriers to the point where they do not impede effectiveness, so that the diversity of disciplines serves as a stimulant in our quest for new solutions to old problems.

In summary, just as we find multiple factors involved in the understanding of chronic disease, so we see multiple factors having produced a vehicle that is specifically designed to assess all of the factors involved in chronic disease at the level at which they present themselves. This assessment obviously requires a multidisciplinary approach and, further, the type of collaborative involvement that has not heretofore characterized most of the biobehavioral research on chronic disease. Both federal and private research funding resources increasingly recognize the unique potential of the behavioral medicine model.

The future looks promising for the continued growth and development of behavioral medicine. The ultimate success of this endeavor, however, rests with the creative effort that can be brought to bear on these health problems through the collaborative involvement of researchers and clinicians from *all* relevant disciplines.

STEPHEN M. WEISS

REFERENCES

Alexander, F. *Psychological medicine*. New York: Norton, 1950.

Engel, G. L. The need for a new medical model: A challenge for biomedicine. *Science*, 1977, *196*, 129–136.

Leigh, H., & Reiser, M. F. Major trends in psychosomatic medicine: The psychiatrist's evolving role in medicine. *Annals of Internal Medicine*, 1977, *87*(2), 233–239.

Lipowski, Z. J. Psychosomatic medicine in the seventies: An overview. *American Journal of Psychiatry*, 1977, *134*, 233–244.

Miller, N. E., & Dworkin, B. Critical issues in therapeutic applications of biofeedback. In G. E. Schwartz & J. Beatty (Eds.), *Biofeedback: Theory and research*. New York: Academic Press, 1977.

Schwartz, G. E., & Weiss, S. M. *Proceedings of the Yale Conference on Behavioral Medicine*. DHEW Publication No. (NIH) 78-1424, 1977.

Schwartz, G. E., & Weiss, S. M. Behavioral medicine revisited: An amended definition. *Journal of Behavioral Medicine*, 1978, *1*(3), 249–251.

Weiner, H. *Psychobiology and human disease*. New York: Elsevier North-Holland, 1977.

Preface

The application of behavioral science principles to the understanding and management of emotional problems has been well established in psychiatric practice. More recently, however, the concepts and technologies derived from behavioral psychology have found increasing application in other fields of medicine and health care. Such applications come at a time when some of the biomedical gains in improving health care have been somewhat offset by the introduction and proliferation of environmental hazards, which cannot be entirely managed through biomedical intervention. These hazards that affect health status range from alterations in lifestyle habits such as diet, physical activity, cigarette smoking, and consumption of alcohol to increased exposure to traumatic noise, stress, pollution, and accident resulting from the development of high-speed technology and rapidly changing societal conditions.

For a number of years, experts in the field of health have acknowledged that many factors, coexisting in both the person and the environment, influence the development of and the response to an illness. The role that biophysical stimuli play in this process has been reasonably well established for a large number of disorders. However, the stimuli and mechanisms of learning that influence a person's response along the health–illness continuum has been less clearly established. The role of such psychosocial learning factors is, nonetheless, believed to be important and is currently being examined from a number of different perspectives.

This book presents representative approaches that apply behavioral psychology principles to the field of medicine. The theory and applications presented are diverse with respect to both content and the concepts developed. This variability is not unexpected, given the nascent character of behavioral medicine and the greater elaboration that exists within some areas as opposed to others.

It is hoped that the reader will become better acquainted with the theory, research, and practice existing for the subjects covered and will be better able to appreciate the potential of this new interdisciplinary area. The material presented should be useful to a number of professionals working at the interface of medicine and behavioral psychology. These include psychologists, physicians, nurses, social workers, medical educators, public health administrators, and researchers, as well as graduate and professional students in these disciplines. In addition, those in advanced undergraduate preprofessional or in graduate-oriented programs would find much of value and interest to them throughout the text.

A special note of thanks goes to Eric Stone, who assisted with some aspects of the initial copyediting of the text, and to Dr. Margret Appel for her incisive suggestions on clarifying certain portions of the manuscript.

J. REGIS MCNAMARA

Contents

Chapter 3

THE DEVELOPMENT OF BEHAVIORAL COMPETENCE IN MEDICAL SETTINGS 33

Marie A. Mastria and Ronald S. Drabman

Chapter 6

BIOFEEDBACK: A SELECTIVE REVIEW OF CLINICAL APPLICATIONS IN
BEHAVIORAL MEDICINE 131

Edward B. Blanchard

Chapter 10

BEHAVIORAL MEDICINE IN THE OCCUPATIONAL SETTING 267

Margaret A. Chesney and Michael Feuerstein

1
Behavioral Psychology in Medicine: An Introduction

J. REGIS McNAMÁRA

Ever since the end of World War II, there has been a working professional and scientific relationship between clinical psychology and psychiatry. The understanding and acceptance of psychotherapeutic approaches predicated on behavioral and social learning principles has been a more recent phenomenon, however. Although professional recognition of the legitimacy of behavior therapy practices in psychiatry was given by the American Psychiatric Association in 1973, the development, application, and evaluation of behavior modification procedures in psychiatric settings antedates by several years this professional acknowledgment.

One of the principal historical forces that facilitated the acceptance of behavior therapy within psychiatry was the "discontent explosion" in mental health (Hersch, 1968). This discontent occurred because traditional therapeutic practices were not meeting with much success in resolving very difficult societal and interpersonal problems. This failure to deliver effective services created the opportunity for new intervention strategies, such as behavior therapy, to attempt to ameliorate some of these refractory problems. Beginning in the mid to late 1960s, major works (e.g., Ayllon & Azrin, 1968; Bandura, 1969; Eysenck, 1964; Franks, 1969; Ullmann & Krasner, 1965; Wolpe & Lazarus, 1966) appeared that summarized and highlighted important contributions and gave increased visibility to the potential applications of behavioral techniques.

For the past decade, there has been a rapid acceleration of professional and scientific activity within the field of behavior therapy. This growth is illustrated not only by the number and diversity of topics that have been added to this content area since Krasner's (1971) *Annual Review* article was published, but also by the large number of publications indexed annually under behavior therapy in the journals (Hoon & Lindsley, 1974). Given the meteoric rise of information disseminated about

J. REGIS McNAMARA • Department of Psychology, Ohio University, Athens, Ohio 45701.

behavioral psychology, it was only a matter of time before other disciplines besides psychology became interested in applying behavioral concepts and methods to their areas. Currently, this influence is demonstrated by the large number of fields that report the use of applied behavioral techniques (Kazdin, 1975).

The interpenetration of behavior modification ideas into medicine took place within the larger context of the expansion of all types of behavioral science information in medical school curricula (Wexler, 1976). In order to support this new curricular emphasis, as well as to meet the increasing demands for psychological services, a substantial increase in the number of psychologists employed in medical school settings took place (Lubin, Nathan, & Matarazzo, 1978). Given the fact that psychology constitutes the major discipline involved in research and development within the field of behavior modification, the greater number of psychologists in medical settings provided the opportunity for the dissemination and application of behavior-analytic and intervention approaches to both mentally and physically based health disorders.

Behavior therapists were not the only group that was becoming more involved in the health field, however. The whole field of psychology devoted more attention to understanding the relationship between psychological variables and health status. As a result of this type of scrutiny, there was an increased realization that service and research contributions to the field of health could be made by psychology and other nontraditional medical disciplines (APA Task Force, 1976). Also, at a professional level, more and more psychologists were identifying themselves as health service providers (Gottfredson & Dyer, 1978).

The potential usefulness of psychological interventions also became particularly apparent within certain health contexts. For instance, it was found that short-term counseling drastically reduced the subsequent utilization of the health care system by individuals who mistakenly believed that their subjective distress was caused by an organic problem (Cummings & Follette, 1976). It was also recognized that the provision of psychotherapy as an adjunct to medical treatment could benefit some patients who were coping with a chronic disease or an acute illness (Olbrisch, 1977). The movement of behavioral ideas and practitioners into the health care field thus took place within the context of a more generalized shift of psychological attention to this whole area.

BEHAVIORAL SCIENCE CONTRIBUTIONS TO HEALTH CARE

The potent influence that a person's environment and lifestyle exert on both the development of and the response to disease has been recognized for many years by epidemiologists. However, the success of medical investigators in the early part of the 20th century in both identifying and developing treatments for infectious agents responsible for disease encouraged an approach that concentrated on the causative role that germs play in illness. This conceptual framework de-emphasized or completely negated the role of behavioral and environmental variables in influencing a disease process. An operating assumption derived from such an orientation was "that illness is a thing in itself, essentially unrelated to the patient's personality, his bodily constitution or his mode of life" (Dubos, 1965, p. 319).

Renewed interest in the contribution of human behavior to medicine is now occurring for several reasons. First, the germ theory model is being incorporated into larger theories of health and sickness that include behavioral and environmental events and processes (Wadsworth, 1974). Single- and multiple-element conceptual models have been proposed that relate in an interacting way a person's behavior to his/her status along a health–illness continuum. A single-element model, such as "biosocial resonation," stresses the importance of interlinked clusters of social and physiological communication networks (Moss, 1974). More complex models of psychosocially mediated illness attempt to identify the factors and describe the mechanisms accounting for disease. For example, Kagan and Levi's (1974) model examines how psychosocial stimuli and the psychobiological program combine to determine the psychological and physiological reaction mechanisms of the person. Under the proper circumstances, these reactions can lead to precursors of disease and to disease itself. Additional interacting variables and a cybernetic control system influence the continuance or cessation of the disease process.

The identification and management of psychosocial stimuli and the processes that govern them thus make possible a new type of "behavioral epidemiology" (Epstein & LaPorte, 1978). In this approach, behaviors are identified that are considered risk factors and that contribute to the development and prevalence of a disorder. After these factors have been identified, behavioral intervention strategies are implemented that attenuate or eliminate their impact. For instance, a behavioral prescription for the management of cardiovascular health would be likely to include the following:

1. Adjustment of eating habits to reduce intake of saturated fat, cholesterol, sugar, and salt
2. Restriction of caloric intake to attain and maintain optimal body weight
3. Establishment of regular physical activity to improve physical condition and avoid overweight
4. Avoidance of cigarette smoking
5. Acquisition of relaxation and stress-management skills conducive to a relaxed and unhurried pattern of behavior
6. Adherence to regimens of self-medication if necessary for the control of hypertension and hyperlipidemia (McAlister, Farquhar, Thoresen, & Maccoby, 1976, p. 46)

Each recommendation, in turn, requires that a behavior modification strategy be developed in order to produce the type and level of behavior change specified in the prescription.

Of particular concern in this area is the relationship of psychological stress and the behavior patterns associated with such stress to the development and exacerbation of various medical disorders. Recent evidence suggests that psychological stress is linked in a complex interactive way with the onset of heart and neoplastic disorders (Glass, 1977; Hurst, Jenkins, & Rose, 1976). One of the variables that influence this interaction is the behavior pattern known as Type A (Friedman &

Rosenman, 1974). The Type A behavior pattern is characterized by such factors as: competitive striving for achievement, a sense of time urgency with self-imposed deadlines, and aggressiveness.

It appears that Type A individuals are their own worst enemies in subjecting themselves to a style of life with which a high degree of risk for cardiovascular disease is associated. Only recently have well-articulated behavior therapy programs been developed that train patients to identify stress indicators and then teach them to eliminate inappropriate stress reactions from their behavior patterns. Initial results from a behavior therapy program called "Cardiac Stress Management Training" (CSMT) (Suinn, 1975) indicate that it can be helpful to postmyocardial patients in altering a number of risk factors for infarction (Suinn, Brock, & Edie, 1975). A promising future application of CSMT would be its prophylactic use on identified groups of nonpatient Type A individuals to prevent the disease and disability attendent on cardiovascular illness.

Preventive medicine is one of the areas in which the application of behavioral principles may make its most important contribution to medical practice (Pomerleau, Bass, & Crown, 1975). Part of the reason is that the present health care system, which is largely treatment- rather than prevention-oriented, is not very cost-effective (Abelson, 1976). Furthermore, it is unlikely that a substantial improvement in health can be obtained through greater expenditures for the treatment of disease. If an enhancement of health status is to be achieved, then a structural change in the health system is needed. This change could be accomplished by emphasizing the preventive aspects of medicine. Such a system would attempt to promote the health-related habits of all citizens and improve the quality of the environment in which they live and work (Kristein, Arnold, & Wynder, 1977).

Such a preventive system could use behavioral techniques at either a primary or secondary level. Intervention at the primary prevention level entails environmental modification that diminishes the probability that susceptible individuals will develop a risk factor. Several in-progress studies on primary prevention have focused their attention on modifying the health habits of children in school and workers in their places of employment (Kristein *et al.*, 1977). In secondary prevention, an attempt is made to advance health or to prevent further disease or disability subsequent to the detection of an illness or precursors of it. Behavioral intervention techniques in the area of secondary prevention include such procedures as a program that increases parents' use of seat belts with their children in order to prevent or diminish the injury resulting from a possible automobile accident, as well as the use of a lottery to ensure screening and treatment initiation for hypertensive individuals (Epstein & Martin, 1977).

A variety of behavioral techniques have also been developed to treat numerous physical disorders (Knapp & Peterson, 1976). These procedures range from contingency management strategies to control epileptic seizures (Balaschak, 1976) to the operant modification of chronic pain (Fordyce, 1976). Probably one of the more widespread applications of behavioral technology to medicine has been in the area of biofeedback. Ever since Birk's (1973) juxtaposition of the terms *biofeedback* and *behavioral medicine*, many individuals—both in and outside the fields of medicine and psychology—have thought that the two were synonymous. A number of factors seem to account for this confusion. Biofeedback made important early contributions in the area of neuromuscular reeducation. These initial demonstrations generated great optimism about the potential for biofeedback's application to other physical disorders. Although biofeedback is no panacea, it does make a treatment contribution, either directly or in combination with other procedures, to the management of a number of health problems (see Blanchard's chapter). Given this type of success, biofeedback will continue to occupy a role of principal importance in behavioral medicine for years to come.

BEHAVIORAL MEDICINE: THE CONVERGENCE OF BEHAVIORAL PSYCHOLOGY AND MEDICINE

The paths of medicine and behavioral psychology have now merged in the area of behavioral medicine. The confluence of several historical trends as well as more recent developments has facilitated this occurrence. The field of behavior therapy has increasingly expanded the scope of its technology and merged its procedures with other areas like medicine to create a new era of "synergistic" interventions (McNamara, in press). When combined, such procedures provide an incremental benefit that is greater in magnitude than each is capable of producing individually. For instance, oral medication must be ingested before it can become effective. Yet many individuals refuse to take medication as prescribed, even though this refusal may mean life-threatening consequences for them (Blackwell, 1976). These compliance problems lend themselves to behavior management techniques, which not only impact on drug adherence but may also improve patients' motivation for further involvement in their treatment program (Zifferblatt, 1975).

More emphasis is now afforded to the role that human behavior occupies in medical practice. A principal reason is the renewed interest in "reuniting technical medicine with human medicine" (Wexler, 1976, p. 276). With the person and his/her behavior reestablished as an important part of the medical equation, attempts have been made to incorporate social factors into physical diagnosis (McWhinney, 1972) and again link mind with body in holistic treatment endeavors (Pelletier, 1977).

Several more recent events have highlighted the formal development of behavioral medicine. The first noteworthy occurrence was the convening of a conference at Yale University in February 1977. At the conference, invited participants addressed emerging issues in behavioral medicine and proposed a preliminary definition of the field (Schwartz & Weiss, 1978).

The second milestone was achieved with the appearance of the first edition of the *Journal of Behavioral Medicine* in 1978. This new journal has served as a major vehicle for disseminating research focused on this area. Both of these events heralded the birth of a new area of research and application for medicine and the behavioral sciences. These events, coupled with the recent formation of the Society of Behavioral Medicine and the addition of Division 38 on Health Psychology to the American Psychological Association, have contributed to a strong base of support for this interdisciplinary interest area.

Although born, the field is still in its infancy and struggles with such basic growth problems as formulating a more acceptable definition of the field and determining the disciplinary and content boundaries for research and application within it. Given the interdisciplinary focus of behavioral medicine, behavioral science approaches will be but one of many social and biomedical systems used to study and solve problems in the field. The extent to which interdisciplinary cooperation and understanding can be achieved will in large measure determine the success of the field of behavioral medicine in resolving health-related problems.

FUTURE ISSUES AND DIRECTIONS

The behavioral science areas that are likely to be emphasized in behavioral medicine in the near future are somewhat more discernible than those that will evolve as the field progresses. It is assumed that those areas in which preliminary work has already been done will continue to expand apace with the level of activity and discovery within them. For instance, Jenkins (1972) has identified four frontiers of psychosomatic research in which the behavioral sciences can make a significant contribution. These include etiological studies, research on the behavioral concomitants of physiological dysfunction, investigations to identify factors that lead individuals to adopt a "sick role" and then seek medical care, and studies that track the long- and short-term response to illness. Another area in which there is likely to be increased activity is secondary prevention. Most of the behavioral attention to secondary prevention is currently directed toward cardiovascular disease. In the future, however, behavioral technologies will be used to limit or reduce exposure to carcinogens, thus assisting in the prevention of cancer (Fox, 1978; Fox & Goldsmith, 1976).

Greater opportunity for the improvement of direct patient care should materialize consequent to the development of more reliable and extensive behavior modification procedures. As this improvement occurs, it should affect the organization and delivery of medical services. At present, behavior modification procedures are prinicipally utilized within medical settings either within the confines of specialized treatment programs for a particular problem, such as psychosomatic illness (e.g., Wooley & Blackwell, 1975), or in a special center for behavioral medicine that offers broad-based treatment programs for a variety of mental and physical disorders (Weiss, 1978). In the future, accompanying behavioral psychology's expansion in both of these settings there will be a broader incorporation of behavioral principles in the total operation of the hospital environment using systems derived from ecobehavioral psychology (Rogers-Warren & Warren, 1977).

The actual influence that behavioral psychology will have on medicine will depend on factors coexisting within and outside the field of behavioral medicine. Externally, the availability of monies, settings, and personnel to support basic and applied research and development will influence the magnitude of the results achieved. However, given the interdisciplinary character of behavioral medicine, it should be possible to attract sufficient financial and professional support to refine and extend existing accomplishments.

Internally, issues relevant to education and training appear important. A fundamental issue that needs to be addressed deals with identifying the most effective interdisciplinary training methods by which to educate disciplinary scientists and practitioners. Disciplinary curricular changes, postdisciplinary continuing education, and/or the development of new interdisciplinary training programs are all options that need to be explored. Even prior to training, however, basic decisions will have to be made regarding disciplinary representation in the training and the emphasis it is to be given.

These and many other issues relevant to the role of the behavioral sciences in behavioral medicine are now being considered by the newly formed scientific and professional organization, the Academy of Behavioral Medicine Research (Baldwin, 1978). This group, working in conjunction with other interested scientists and practitioners in health-related areas, will attempt to resolve these issues and encourage the growth and development of behavioral medicine as a field.

REFERENCES

Abelson, P. H. Cost-effective health care. *Science*, 1976, *192*, 619.

Ayllon, T., & Azrin, N. H. *The token economy: A motivational system for therapy and rehabilitation.* New York: Appleton-Century-Crofts, 1968.

APA Task Force on Health Research. Contribution of psychology to health research. *American Psychologist*, 1976, *36*, 263–274.

Balaschak, B. A. Teacher implemented behavior modification in a case of organically based epilepsy. *Journal of Consulting and Clinical Psychology*, 1976, *44*, 218–223.

Baldwin, D. Health behavior researchers create a new professional organization. *APA Monitor*, 1978, *9*(8), 4, 16.

Bandura, A. *Principles of behavior modification.* New York: Holt, Rinehart, & Winston, 1969.

Birk, L. (Ed.). *Biofeedback: Behavioral medicine.* New York: Grune & Stratton, 1973.

Blackwell, B. Treatment adherence. *British Journal of Psychiatry*, 1976, *129*, 513–531.

Cummings, N. A., & Follette, W. T. Brief psychotherapy and medical utilization: An eight-year follow-up. In H. Dorken & Associates, *The professional psychologist today: New developments in law, health insurance, and health practice.* San Francisco: Jossey-Bass, 1976.

Dubos, R. *Man adapting.* New Haven, Conn.: Yale University Press, 1965.

Epstein, L. H., & LaPorte, R. E. Behavioral epidemiology. *The Behavior Therapist*, 1978, *1*(1), 3–5.

Epstein, L. H., & Martin, J. E. Behavioral medicine. *Association for Advancement of Behavior Therapy Newsletter*, 1977, *4*, 5–6.

Eysenck, H. J. *Experiments in behavior therapy.* Oxford, England: Pergamon, 1964.

Fordyce, W. F. *Behavioral methods for chronic pain and illness.* St. Louis: Mosby, 1976.

Fox, B. H. Premorbid psychological factors as related to cancer incidence. *Journal of Behavioral Medicine*, 1978, *1*, 45–133.

Fox, B. H., & Goldsmith, J. R. Behavioral issues in the prevention of cancer. *Preventive Medicine*, 1976, *5*, 106–121.

Franks, C. M. (Ed.). *Behavior therapy: Appraisal and status.* New York: McGraw-Hill, 1969.

Friedman, M., & Rosenman, R. H. *Type A behavior and your heart.* New York: Knopf, 1974.

Glass, D. C. Stress, behavior patterns and coronary disease. *American Scientist*, 1977, *65*, 177–187.

Gottfredson, G. D., & Dyer, S. E. Health service in psychology. *American Psychologist*, 1978, *33*, 314–338.

Hersch, C. The discontent explosion in mental health. *American Psychologist*, 1968, *23*, 497–506.

Hoon, P. W., & Lindsley, O. R. A comparison of behavior and traditional publication activity. *American Psychologist*, 1974, *29*, 694–697.

Hurst, M. W., Jenkins, C. D., & Rose, R. M. The relation of psychological stress to onset of medical illness. In *Annual review of medicine*. Palo Alto, Calif.: Annual Reviews, Inc., 1976.

Jenkins, C. D. Social and epidemiologic factors in psychosomatic disease. *Psychiatric Annals*, 1972, *1*(2), 8–21.

Kagan, A. R., & Levi, L. Health and environment—Psychological stimuli: A review. *Social Science and Medicine*, 1974, *8*, 225–241.

Kazdin, A. E. The impact of applied behavior analysis on diverse areas of research. *Journal of Applied Behavior Analysis*, 1975, *8*, 213–229.

Knapp, T. J., & Peterson, L. W. Behavior management in medical and nursing practice. In W. E. Craighead, A. E. Kazdin, & M. J. Mahoney (Eds.), *Behavior modification: Principles, issues, and application*. New York: Houghton-Mifflin, 1976.

Krasner, L. Behavior therapy. In *Annual review of psychology*. Palo Alto, Calif.: Annual Reviews, 1971.

Kristein, M. M., Arnold, C. B., & Wynder, E. L. Health economics and preventive care. *Science*, 1977, *195*, 457–462.

Lubin, B., Nathan, R. G., & Matarazzo, J. D. Psychologists in medical education: 1976. *American Psychologist*, 1978, *33*, 339–343.

McAlister, A. L., Farquhar, J. W., Thoresen, C. E., & Maccoby, N. Behavioral science applied to cardiovascular health: Progress and research needs in the modification of risk taking habits in adult populations. *Health Education Monographs*, 1976, *4*(1), 45–74.

McNamara, J. R. Behavior therapy in the seventies: Some changes and current issues. *Psychotherapy: Theory, Research and Practice*, in press.

McWhinney, I. R. Beyond diagnosis: An approach to the integration of behavioral science and clinical medicine. *New England Journal of Medicine*, 1972, *287*, 384–387.

Moss, G. E. Biosocial resonation: A conceptual model of links between social behavior and physical illness. *International Journal of Psychiatry in Medicine*, 1974, *5*, 401–410.

Olbrisch, M. E. Psychotherapeutic interventions in physical health: Effectiveness and economic efficiency. *American Psychologist*, 1977, *32*, 761–777.

Pelletier, K. R. *Mind as healer, mind as slayer*. New York: Dell, 1977.

Pomerleau, O., Bass, F., & Crown, V. Role of behavior modification in preventive medicine. *New England Journal of Medicine*, 1975, *292*, 1277–1282.

Rogers-Warren, A., & Warren, S. F. (Eds.). *Ecological perspectives in behavior analysis*. Baltimore: University Park Press, 1977.

Schwartz, G. E., & Weiss, S. M. Yale Conference on behavioral medicine: A proposed definition and statement of goals. *Journal of Behavioral Medicine*, 1978, *1*, 3–12.

Suinn, R. M. The cardiac stress management program for type A patients. *Cardiac Rehabilitation*, 1975, *5*, 13–15.

Suinn, R. M., Brock, L., & Edie, C. A. Behavior therapy for type A patients. *American Journal of Cardiology*, 1975, *36*, 269–270.

Ullmann, L. P., & Krasner, L. *Case studies in behavior modification*, New York: Holt, Rinehart & Winston, 1965.

Wadsworth, M. Health and sickness: The choice of treatment. *Journal of Psychosomatic Research*, 1974, *18*, 271–276.

Weiss, S. M. News and developments in behavioral medicine. *Journal of Behavioral Medicine*, 1978, *1*, 135–139.

Wexler, M. The behavioral sciences in medical education. *American Psychologist*, 1976, *31*, 275–283.

Wolpe, J., & Lazarus, A. A. *Behavior therapy techniques: A guide to the treatment of neurosis*. Oxford, England: Pergamon, 1966.

Wooley, S. C., & Blackwell, B. A behavioral probe into social contingencies on a psychosomatic ward. *Journal of Applied Behavior Analysis*, 1975, *8*, 337–339.

Zifferblatt, S. M. Increasing patient compliance through the applied analysis of behavior. *Preventive Medicine*, 1975, *4*, 173–182.

2
Health Care Delivery:
A Behavioral Perspective

LEONARD H. EPSTEIN AND DEBORAH J. OSSIP

INTRODUCTION

The Task Force on Health Research of the American Psychological Association (APA) has recently discussed the uses and potential for psychological techniques in health care (APA Task Force on Health Research, 1976). The authors report that psychological techniques and procedures have been used in the psychobiological aspects of health, including stress, psychosomatics, health and biological cycles on behavior; health care delivery; and attitudes related to health and health care. The relative proportion of the 311 published articles surveyed in these areas are psychobiological aspects of health, 66%; health care delivery, 18%; and health and health care attitudes, 16%. The authors suggest that the application of psychology to health is just beginning and that the opportunities are numerous.

The overwhelming majority of psychological and medical articles on health deal with attempts not only to understand the causes of various diseases but also to develop treatments for these diseases. Certainly, the health of the general populace could not improve or be maintained if research in the prevention or treatment of disease or disability were not emphasized. However, the full impact of treatment on clinical problems can be expected only if our health care systems are designed to provide widespread, efficient, and correct use of contemporary medical technology. However, health care is not now being delivered in an organized or systematic fashion. A more integrated and orderly health care network could be developed in accordance with research that suggests optimal ways to bring people into the system and to keep them there while high-quality medical care is provided to them. Cur-

LEONARD H. EPSTEIN AND DEBORAH J. OSSIP • Western Psychiatric Institute and Clinic, University of Pittsburgh School of Medicine, Pittsburgh, Pennsylvania 15261.

rently, however, the APA Task Force on Health Research (1976) suggests that the majority of health care specialists and facilities still operate relatively independently. Thus, the coordination and integration of health care services becomes a goal not readily achieved under the present system.

Problems in health care delivery are at least partly attributable to the fact that the costs for medical care are not determined by the factors of supply and demand for quality medical services. The increasing use of third-party payments has reduced the concern of the patient about the actual cost of medical care. Also, the average patient does not have the intellectual, financial, or motivational capacity to compare critically the relative effectiveness of services provided by several health care facilities. Certainly, when life-threatening or irreversible procedures, such as surgery, are indicated, patients are advised to shop around. However, after soliciting the opinion of two or even three physicians, it is unclear how the patient comes to make his/her eventual decision. It is likely that the decision is not based totally on the comparative data presented by each physician regarding the likelihood of the accuracy of the diagnosis and the probability of success of the treatment, but rather on whether the patient is impressed by the therapist and on anecdotal stories conveyed to the patient. Thus, as the use of third-party payments increases, and patients have continued difficulty in determining the relative cost–benefit of comparative medical services, the relative cost of medical care continues to increase, without a concomitant increase in the quality of the services delivered.

This chapter is designed to present a review of the use of behavioral procedures to improve the utilization of health care services, with the goal of developing a behavioral technology of health care delivery (Epstein & Cinciripini, 1977). Behavioral procedures are well suited to improving health care delivery, as many of the problems encountered in delivery of services may be conceptualized in terms of behavior. Two models that relate health to specific behavioral and psychological factors that may influence engaging in health behaviors are presented in the following section. A review of the models that relate behavior to health may be useful in developing intervention strategies to improve health by modifying health behaviors. In addition, the models indicate the potential importance of understanding and controlling behavior in providing realistic health care. It should be emphasized that the relationships between health and behavior suggested in this chapter, and in these two models, are not designed to describe how psychological factors influence health or how behavioral problems are often observed in concurrence with medical problems. These topics are best discussed in chapters on psychosomatic medicine or psychobiology. Rather, these articles suggest that, in order to provide proper health care for physical disorder and disability, an understanding of health and illness behavior is necessary. Further, the modifications of certain health and illness behaviors may be useful in improving the health of the general populace.

Kasl and Cobb (1966) list three general ways in which health-related behavior can be conceptualized: health behavior, illness behavior, and sick-role behavior. Health behaviors are those behaviors engaged in while the person perceives him/herself as healthy, in order to prevent disease or to discover asymptomatic disease. Illness behaviors are those behaviors of a person when he/she feels ill, and sick-role behaviors are observed when the person defines him/herself as being ill.

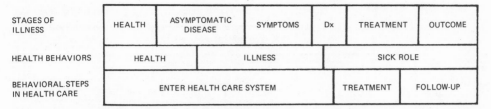

Figure 1. The relationship between the progression of disease and health behaviors. Dx in the Stages of Illness refers to diagnosis of the disorder. (Adapted from Kasl & Cobb, 1966.)

This schema corresponds to the sequences of stages that relate to the development of health behavior in most diseases. The relationship between behavioral stages in health care delivery and the stages of disease can be observed in Figure 1, which is adapted from a figure by Kasl and Cobb (1966). Within Kasl and Cobb's behavioral schema presented in the middle line of Figure 1, this chapter covers some components of health, illness, and sick-role behavior. The primary focus is on illness and sick-role behaviors, with some discussion of health behavior, primarily involving entrance into the health care system.

Two of the major models of behavior and health care, the health belief model (Rosenstock, 1966) and the behavioral framework for the study of human disease models (Fabrega, 1974), are presented next.

HEALTH AND BEHAVIOR

Health Beliefs Model

The health beliefs model was formulated by Rosenstock (1966) to relate patient expectations and perceptions, along with various environmental cues, to predict the likelihood of patients' engaging in health or illness behaviors. Becker and Maimon (1975) related the health beliefs model to expectancy theory. Basically, the underlying assumption is that predictions for many of the health behaviors involved in preventive medicine may be a function of the threat of a particular disease. The formal model contains three major elements. First is the patient's subjective *readiness* to initiate preventive health behaviors, which includes the perceived susceptibility to and seriousness of the disease. Second, the individual evaluates the *feasibility* and the effectiveness of the recommended health behavior, which may be a function of demographic and sociopsychological variables, as well as the physical, psychological, and financial-response cost involved. Third, stimuli that initiate *action* must be present. The source of the stimuli may be such external factors as media presentations, advice from friends, or personal experiences with illness, or such internal factors as the perception of abnormal bodily responses.

Becker and Maimon (1975) have expanded the health beliefs model to include compliance to recommended therapeutic regimens. The initial statement of their model is presented in Figure 2.

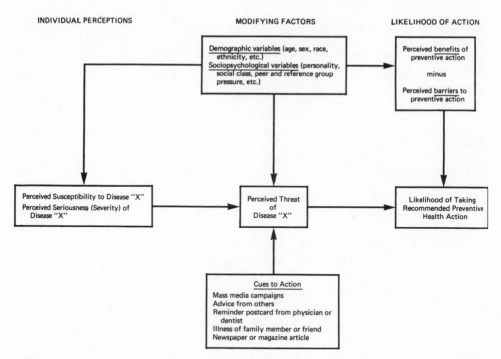

Figure 2. Hypothesized model for predicting and explaining compliance behavior. (From Becker & Maiman, 1975. Copyright 1975 by J. B. Lippincott Co. Reprinted by permission.)

The Becker and Maimon model involves describing the perceptual and motivational variables that may affect treatment compliance. It is sufficiently broad to encompass all behavioral components that will be covered in this chapter. However, it does not clearly develop the importance of the measurement or modification of behavior in disease. Rather, the major emphasis is on subjective factors. The importance of these factors in influencing behavior cannot be overemphasized. However, the subsequent model of illness behavior presented by Fabrega (Fabrega, 1974; Fabrega & Van Egeren, 1976) is more explicit in relating health behaviors to overt, measurable behavior.

Behavioral Framework for the Study of Human Disease

Fabrega (1974) has written extensively on behavior and the health care system. He has noted three ways in which diseases are manifested in behavior. First, disease tends to interfere with the execution of certain behaviors. As Fabrega and Van Egeren (1976) stated, the analysis of the interference with behavior by a disease in combination with the social group demands can be used to assess the cost of the disease. Second, diseases tend to influence a person's social roles, which include, but are not limited to, occupational, familial, recreational, and religious roles. The execution of behaviors in these roles may be disrupted by a disease. Third, diseases may have effects on psychological (cognitive) components. The cognitive effects may be consolidated in four areas: psychological discomfort, emotional violations, moral discreditations, and physical integrity. Fabrega and Van Egeren suggested that a taxonomy of the effects of disease on these varied behaviors could be developed. The organization of disease according to behavior may result in commonalities among behaviors for several disparate diseases. However, the behavioral similarities in disease clusters that develop may provide useful information that would be important in the management of behavior in these diseases.

Fabrega (1974) has developed a nine-stage model of patients' medical decision-making that involves the effects of disease on behavior. In Stage 1, *illness recognition* and *labeling* occur. During this stage, subject definitions of illness are formulated on the basis of internal or external sources of information. The behavioral changes produced by a disease can be seen as deviations from normal behavior, and self-observations of these changes may serve to stimulate health or illness behaviors. In Stage 2, the patient assesses the *illness disvalues*, which are quantified in units of disvalue partly on the basis of behavioral disruption produced by the disease. Stage 3 involves the development of *treatment plans*, and in Stage 4, the patient attempts an *assessment of treatment plans* to determine the probability of the treatment's changing units of disvalue. The computations of the potential *treatment benefits* are then subjectively derived in Stage 5, and the *treatment costs* are considered in Stage 6. The *net benefit or utility* of a treatment plan is developed in Stage 7 by weighing treatment benefits against cost of treatment. In Step 8, the patient makes a *selection of treatment plan*, eventually reevaluates his/her condition in Step 9, and is now *set up for recycling* back to Stage 1.

The model presents a logical series of stages that a patient may go through, from detecting that something is wrong to initiating treatment. The model does not deal extensively with the factors involved in compliance with treatment regimens. However, the model is notable because of the use of behavior as a major dependent variable in assessing the *costs* of disease and the benefits of treatment.

In the remaining sections of the chapter, illustrative studies relevant to the use of behavioral procedures in health care delivery are presented. The conceptualization of the behavioral steps related to health care that are discussed in this chapter are presented in Figure 3.

This figure depicts the behavioral steps involved in health care delivery, beginning with the entrance into the health care system and concluding with follow-up. The steps and problems presented in this figure will serve as the basis for the next three sections of the chapter: entering the health care system, treatment, and follow-up. As the conceptualization of behavioral principles in health care delivery becomes more detailed, steps may be identified and reconceptualized to improve the current flow diagram.

The scope of the area is too great to allow complete reviews of the literature for each topic area. However, it is expected that the reader will be able to get the flavor of the clinical and research trends in the areas that are discussed. The first section involves detailed procedures to ensure the proper entry of a patient into the health care system.

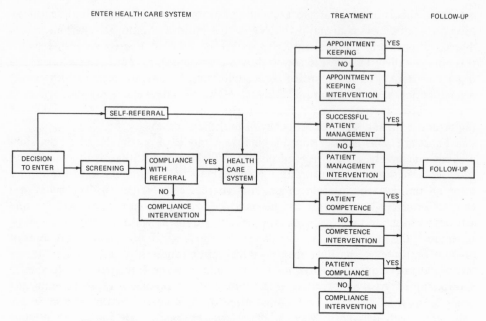

Figure 3.   Flow diagram of behavioral steps in health care delivery.

ENTERING THE HEALTH CARE SYSTEM

Entry into the health care system typically occurs when a person becomes aware of a given dysfunction and subsequently seeks treatment from a health care facility. Entry may be on the basis of a self-referral, or it may be mediated by a screening process conducted by an outside screening program and/or by the person him/herself.

Screening and Health Monitoring

Mass screening programs are available for detecting such disorders as breast cancer, cervical cancer, hypertension, and diabetes. However, the utility of these programs is a direct function of the number and types of people who use these services. A key problem has been the limited use of screening programs by people regarded as being at high risk. For example, diagnostic X-ray screening programs, used particularly for the early identification of tuberculosis, were prevalent in the 1950s. Hochbaum (1956) interviewed 1,200 randomly selected persons over 25 years of age and found that 17% (204 people) had never had X rays. Of the subjects who had X rays, only 42% had been X rayed voluntarily, in a preventive fashion, without any symptoms. Other reasons given for having an X ray examination were symptoms, social pressure, or job requirements and to check for diseases other than tuberculosis. Although subsequent concerns regarding the negative effects of X rays decreased the importance of this particular diagnostic procedure, there is considerable evidence that people continue to respond to other screening programs in a manner similar to their response to X rays in the mid-1950s. More recently, Fink, Shapiro, and Lewison (1968) arranged a screening program for breast cancer for women at risk (aged 40–64). These investigators reported that over one-third did not attend, despite repeated individual contacts. Of the women who did participate, 65% attended after receiving one notice of the program, 17% after a second letter or a phone contact, and the remaining 18% required additional phone contacts. Over 4,000 of the original sample of 11,500 were not seen at all.

One of the few studies involving attempts to manipulate attendance at a health screening program was conducted by Kirscht, Haefner, and Eveland (1975). Three alternative approaches were compared: a control condition that simply stated that the services were available; a threat condition that emphasized the possibility that one may be sick and not know it, as well as the negative aspects of being sick; and a positive condition that stated how easy it is to be checked up and how this checkup could lead to continued good health. Over 1,000 persons served in the control group, which was selected from eligible persons in the community who had not been seen in the facility for over a year. The experimental subjects (132 in the threat condition and 86 in the positive condition) were obtained from subjects already attending other clinics in the hospital. Consequently, there was some difference in the sampling procedures for control and experimental groups; however, the experimental groups could be compared. The positive condition proved to be best in terms of the percentage of people making appointments (36.0), as compared to the control (32.1) and threat (27.7) conditions. Also, a higher percentage of people kept appointments in the positive condition (90) than subjects in the control or threat condition (59.8 and 69.4, respectively). These results suggest that positive procedures may be the most effective in encouraging attendance at screening programs.

While screening programs are popular, they have not been notably successful, and there are a number of drawbacks to screenings. First, they may be costly to the sponsoring agency. Second, their effectiveness in reaching the high-risk population is often limited. Third, attendance at a screening program at relatively infrequent intervals is often misused as a technique that people employ to monitor their health as a substitute for a periodic checkup. However, these periodic assessments provide the person with nonsystematic or incomplete information as to the state of his/her health. A new alternative and/or supplement to at least some types of periodic screenings or checkups is the relatively continuous *self*-monitoring of health parameters. Often, risk factors can be assessed from such measures of fitness and health as pulse rate, blood pressure, weight, smoking, skin lesions, breast nodes, the 12-minute fitness test, postexercise heart rate, and the Harvard Step Test. These factors may be easily recorded by a person with little training. Knapp and Peterson (1976) have discussed the potential of self-monitoring in assessing health, and Goldstein, Stein, Smolen, and Perlini (1976) have provided hospital physicians with daily health indicators of ambulatory patients using self-monitoring. The advantages of self-monitoring as a basic component of self-care, a revolutionary approach to the delivery of medical care (Levin, 1976), are evident. One advantage of self-monitoring is the relatively continuous measurement of health indices, which, in many cases, can provide more accurate estimates of changes in health or illness than periodic screening in an artificial setting such as a clinic. A second advantage is the potential for the feedback produced by monitoring to selectively modify engaging in unhealthy behaviors. This dual utility of a self-monitoring approach to preventive health may be discussed in terms of the health goals outlined by Breslow and Somers (1977). Breslow and Somers presented a "Lifetime Health Monitoring Program" in which they outlined a series of age-group specific preventive health procedures. Ten age groups have been identified, based on changing lifestyles, health needs, and health problems over the course of a life span. These groups include pregnancy and perinatal period, infancy (first year), preschool (1–5 years), school age (6–11 years), adolescence 12–17 years), young adulthood (18–24 years), young middle age (25–39 years), older middle age (40–59 years), elderly (60–74 years), and old age (75+ years). For each age group, Breslow and Somers have specified relevent health goals and professional services that they suggest can be easily incorporated into existing medical treatment procedures. The potential for self-monitoring in this program is twofold. First, self-monitoring can be used to assess risk factors specific to the various age groups (e.g., self-examination of breasts, testes, skin, etc., during young middle age), and second, self-monitoring can be employed to determine the degree to which age-appropriate health goals, established to facilitate preventive health, have been met.

Screening Referral Compliance

Following the identification of a health problem, through external or self-screening procedures, the next step is to take appropriate action to alleviate the problem. Often, this involves complying with referrals by screening agencies to other health care services.

Several studies have investigated parents' compliance to postscreening follow-up recommendations for their children. Cauffman, Peterson, and Emrick (1967) attempted to find the percentage of parents who followed up on school requests to obtain medical or dental care for their children in Los Angeles County. The data indicate that approximately 50% of the children were seen for medical checkups after the parents were notified of their child's condition. Gabrielson, Levin, and Ellison (1967) found much better compliance in New Haven, Connecticut, and Scarborough, Canada, with follow-up rates of 70% in both cities. Clearly, there are differences in rates in parental compliance, which may be related to such sources of variation as suggested by Cauffman *et al.* (1967), which include the socioeconomic, educational, and job levels of the parents, as well as the age of the parents. A prototypical investigation on effecting follow-up care for children identified in screening programs was recently reported by Reiss, Piotrowski, and Bailey (1976). The authors attempted to develop a cost-effective procedure for getting low-income rural parents to obtain follow-up care for children identified as requiring dental health care after a screening program. Three procedures were compared, the first two based in part on the work of Cauffman *et al.* (1967), who reported that repeated contacts were superior to only one contact in influencing referral outcome. The first procedure used by Reiss *et al.* (1976) was a one-prompt, or note-only, procedure,

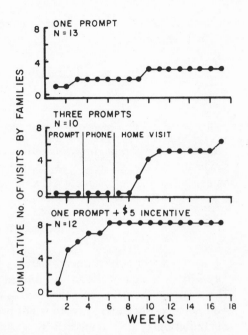

Figure 4. Percentage of families making initial visit and cumulative number of families making initial visits across weeks in each of the three treatment conditions. (From Reiss, Piotrowski, & Bailey, 1976. Copyright 1976 by the Society for the Experimental Analysis of Behavior. Reprinted by permission.)

where the parents received one notification of the need for their child to receive dental care. The second procedure was a three-prompt condition, using a note, a telephone call, and a home visit. The third procedure used an incentive, in which one written prompt was sent and the parents were provided with a "dental coupon" worth five dollars if they obtained follow-up care for their child. The results, presented in Figure 4 in terms of families' making either one visit (top graph) or cumulative visits (bottom graph), showed the equivalent effects of the three-prompt and incentive conditions on the frequency of dental care, both of which conditions were superior to the control condition. Cost–benefit data, relating treatment effectiveness to the cost of treatment, play a key role in evaluating the three procedures. The one-prompt condition was the cheapest, costing $.88 per participating student. However, this procedure proved to be the least effective. The effective incentive and three-prompt conditions cost $6.21 and $19.75, respectively, per participating student. The expense of the latter was due, in large part, to the costs of individual time in making the phone calls and home visits, which exceeded the cost of simply paying people for going to the dentist. Thus, the incentive procedure appeared to be the most cost-beneficial. Additionally, follow-up data indicated that the families in the incentive condition made more visits and completed dental care significantly more often than the subjects in the other two groups.

Finnerty, Shaw, and Himmelsback (1973) assessed several additional factors in their report of success in reducing the percentage of hypertensive patients who failed to keep their screening referral appointment. Their interventions included personal contact, home visits, and scheduling of the appointment 24–48 hours after the screening. The authors reported that 50% of the identified hypertensive persons did not attend their first verification visit. The use of personal contacts and home visits decreased the percentage of nonattenders to 29%, and subsequent faster scheduling of appointments further decreased the percentage of no-shows to less than 5% after the first screening.

TREATMENT

Once a person has contacted the appropriate health care agency, treatment procedures may begin. Implementation of treatment, however, may be impeded by problems in several areas. These areas include appointment keeping, patient management, patient competence, and patient compliance with treatment regimens.

Appointment Keeping

Not keeping appointments can be detrimental to treatment efforts in several ways. First, the client cannot be treated unless he/she shows up for appointments. The treatment benefits for patients who attend irregularly are likely to be minimal. Additionally, when an ill person is not provided with proper medical care, the larger community may be endangered by a communicable disease. Finally, the treatment facility must absorb the cost of arranging for a staff member to see a client who does not attend, thereby possibly increasing the charges for other patients.

Various intervention strategies have been implemented in the attempt to modify appointment-keeping behaviors. As with much of the literature on health care delivery, there are a number of methodological problems with many of the studies on appointment keeping, such as a lack of sufficient controls and varying definitions of appointment keeping. Nevertheless, the findings suggest that intervention can significantly reduce nonattendance.

Intervention has been attempted on several levels. One commonly used strategy has been to provide prompts to the client to show up for the appointment. The prompts have generally been in the form of written reminders, telephone contacts, and/or personal visits. Nazarian, Mechaber, Charney, and Coulter (1974) investigated the effect of a mailed reminder on appointment keeping. A postcard reminder, mailed one week prior to the appointment, resulted in a keep rate of 64%, which significantly differed from a keep rate of 48% for the control group. Barkin and Duncan (1975), however, were unable to replicate these results. Although their data showed a similar trend (broken appointment rate: 25% in control group; 19% in experimental group), these differences did not reach significance. This discrepancy in the findings of the two studies may be accounted for by differences in populations, in types of clinics, and in initial keep rates.

Turner and Vernon (1976) evaluated a second type of prompt procedure for increasing the attendance of clients at the initial intake interview. The prompt simply involved calling the client one to three days before the scheduled appointment. As depicted in Figure 5, the procedure was implemented in an ABAB withdrawal design, with baseline, prompts, baseline, and prompts conditions. Results over 18 months showed changes in percentage of no-shows from 32% (A_1) to 11%

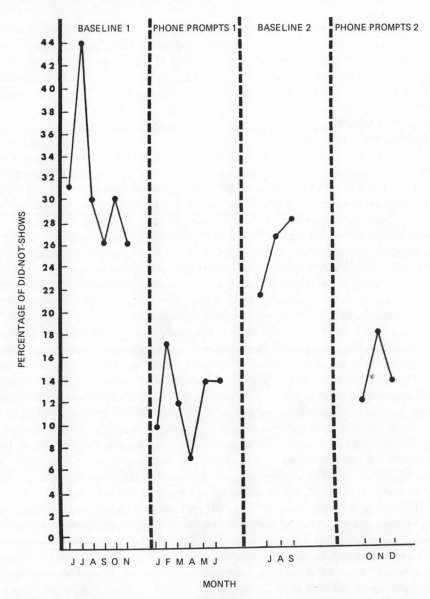

Figure 5.   Percentage of those not attending appointments under baseline and prompt conditions. (From Turner & Vernon, 1976. Copyright 1976 by the Society for the Experimental Analysis of Behavior. Reprinted by permission.)

(B_1), back to 25% (A_2), and then decreasing to 14% (B_2) over the four phases. Thus, attendance was markedly better when the prompt procedure was in effect.

A second type of intervention strategy has involved varying some aspects of the actual clinic procedure. In addition to assessing procedures for influencing compliance with screening, Finnerty *et al.* (1973) assessed attendance at treatment.

Hypertensive patients were randomly assigned to one of three groups: a "stepped-up" care group (Group A), who were provided intensive, more individualized care; a usual medical care group, who received reminders of their appointments one day in advance (Group B); and a usual medical care group, who received no reminders (Group C). At the time of publication, 84% of the patients in group A had remained in treatment, as compared to 33% in Group B and 17% in Group C. Thus, Finnerty *et al.* underscored the benefits of increasingly personalized medical care in addition to an appointment reminder.

Tracy (1977) attempted to assess various strategies of patient evaluation that might affect attendance at subsequent treatment sessions. During intake, patient problems were defined and treatment goals determined according to either the traditional problem descriptions used in the mental health center or a new behavioral analysis report. In addition to the differences in content of the two reports, the behavioral analysis report was designed so that the client's problem behavior, adaptive behaviors, treatment goals, and disposition were discussed with the client. The results indicate that significantly more clients returned for treatment when behavior analysis, rather than the traditional evaluation, was used, independent of the training level of the interviewer. Further, significantly more clients remained in treatment when the behavioral analysis report was initially used.

Rockart and Hofmann (1969) observed physicians' and patients' behavior under different scheduling systems in an outpatient medical setting. The clinics studied used one of three types of scheduling systems: block unassigned (patient given a block appointment time and seen by the first available physician), block assigned (block appointment time, but with a specific physician), or individual unassigned (patient given a specific appointment time, but not assigned a specific physician). No clinics using the fourth possible system (i.e., individual assigned) were available for study. Rockart and Hofmann's findings show the individual-unassigned system to be clearly superior to the other two methods in reducing patients' no-show rate. Interestingly, in the block-assigned and the individual-unassigned groups, both patients *and* physicians tended to arrive early for scheduled appointments. Rockart and Hofman speculated that the use of personalized scheduling systems may motivate both patients and therapists to improve the implementation of health care services.

A third intervention strategy was discussed by Reiss *et al.* (1976) to increase compliance with dental screening referral. As previously described, the authors found that paying patients for attending a first dental visit was cost-effective as well as successful in increasing attendance. Further, they reported that these patients continued to have a higher follow-up visit rate than nonpaid control patients, even though the monetary incentive was not continued beyond the first visit. Thus, it appears that providing incentives may be useful in increasing appointment making and that the effectiveness of this approach might be further increased by providing additional incentives during the entire course of treatment.

A fourth approach, developed to decrease dropout rate in obesity treatment, is contracting. This procedure involves requiring the subjects to leave a monetary deposit with the experimenter at the onset of the study, with refund of the deposit contingent on regular attendance. Hagen, Foreyt, and Durham (1976) reported that requiring a monetary deposit significantly reduced attrition in subjects' attendance in a weight loss program. Fourteen subjects were assigned to one of three groups, a $20, a $5, or no-deposit group. Attrition at the end of the six-week treatment was 1, 6, and 9 subjects, respectively, suggesting that the size of the deposit may have been important in decreasing attrition. This appears to be an effective approach, and adaptation of the contracting procedure for use in other health care settings may prove useful in reducing nonattendance rates.

Patient Management

Patient management problems arise when the patient engages in behaviors that make the implementation of treatment difficult. This section deals with patient management in relation to dental, surgical, and needle fears.

Management of Fear and Avoidance Behaviors

Many people are fearful of obtaining medical care. Types of fears vary from fear of pain (Friedson & Feldman, 1958), to fear of separation from loved ones and fear of loss of control (Melamed, 1977). An unfortunate consequence of fear is that it may result in a person's not seeking needed care. Further, should such a person be seen for treatment, fear-related disruptive behaviors may impede effective health care delivery. Two common fears—dental fears and surgery fears—along with intervention strategies, are discussed here. Additionally, a technique effectively used in treating a specific needle phobia in a hemodialysis patient is mentioned.

Dental Fears. Friedson and Feldman (1958) reported that 51% of the population may not obtain regular dental care. Of these, 9% list fear as the primary obstacle to seeking care. Extrapolating from these figures, Gale and Ayer (1969) stated that for about 5% of the American population, or 10 million people, fear of dental care is sufficiently anxiety-provoking that treatment is avoided, even though nontreatment may result in severe pain. Based on behavioral principles, two common procedures to reduce fear, desensitization and modeling, have been implemented in attempts to reduce dental fear.

Machen and Johnson (1974) conducted a study examining the effects of a modified desensitization procedure and modeling on the dental behavior of children. The desensitization procedure involved gradual presentation of a hierarchy of anxiety-provoking items by a therapist who encouraged verbal interaction between the children and him/herself. Children in the modeling condition viewed a film of a child exhibiting positive behavior during the dental treatment and being positively reinforced by the dentist for appropriate behaviors. The control group subjects had no fear-reducing interventions. Behavioral ratings were made of children at each of three subsequent dental appointments. Ratings ranged from definitely negative (e.g., refusal of treatment, overt resistance, and extreme fear) to definitely positive (e.g., good rapport with operator and no sign of fear). Significant differences were found between experimental and control subjects, with the former exhibiting fewer negative behaviors during the second and third visits. No significant differences were found between the two treatment groups.

The most extensive work on modeling and dental fear behaviors has been conducted by Melamed and associates (Melamed, Hawes, Heiby, & Glick, 1975; Melamed, Weinstein, Hawes, & Katin-Borland, 1975). Through a multidimensional assessment of behavioral, subjective, and physiological responses, they have demonstrated that viewing a filmed modeling of appropriate dental behavior reduces anxiety-related disruptive behaviors. Melamed, Weinstein *et al.* (1975) assigned matched groups of inner-city children to one of two groups, an experimental group (film modeling) or a control group (drawing task). The children were seen during three visits to a pedodontic clinic. The first two visits involved dental examinations only; the last visit was for restorative treatment, including a local anesthetic injection. Immediately before the third visit, children were asked either to draw or to view a videotape. The tape showed a 4-year-old black child successfully coping with his anxiety during dental restorative treatment. The child was verbally reinforced by the dentist for cooperative behavior and was given a prize at the end of treatment. Data collected for each child included a maternal anxiety scale, completed by the mother; a fear survey schedule, read to and completed by the child; and behavioral ratings of disruptive behaviors and of anxiety.

Results showed significant differences in frequency of disruptive behaviors for experimental and control groups during the third, restorative session. Experimental subjects, who observed the model, maintained an initial low level of disruptive behavior during restoration, despite the added stress of this treatment, whereas control subjects showed a drastic increase in disruptive behaviors.

Additionally, behavioral observations of anxiety supported the effectiveness of viewing the film. Interestingly, no differences between the experimental and control groups were found in scores of the self-report Fear-Survey Schedule, and no significant correlation was found between self-report of anxiety and actual behavior during treatment.

The experimental procedures were replicated in a second, more carefully controlled study (Melamed, Hawes *et al.*, 1975), in which an additional control group observed a film of a peer in a non-dental-related situation. One additional measure, the palmar sweat index, was obtained at various points during the study. The results for disruptive behaviors and rated anxiety for experimental and control subjects were similar to those presented by Melamed, Weinstein, Hawes, & Katin-Borland (1975). However, the palmar sweat index data were only suggestive, as the experimental group tended toward lower arousal from pre- to posttreatment, but significant differences were not obtained.

The results from these studies show that modeling is useful in reducing fear-related uncooperative behaviors. The use of a filmed model appears to be an improvement over other previous studies using live models (e.g., Adelson & Goldfried, 1970), in that the film is easily shown, and the modeling procedure is not dependent on the availability of an appropriate live model. The variability of the results across measures highlights the importance of the multimodal approach to assessing fear.

Surgery Fears. Hospitalization and surgery are stressful, anxiety-provoking events, particularly to the young child. It is generally agreed that some sort of prehospitalization and/or presurgery preparation is beneficial; however, the exact nature of this preparation has not been formulated. Melamed (1977) stated that studies attempting to investigate the effects of various preparatory techniques have yielded ambiguous findings, often because of methodological problems inherent in the studies. Melamed described a series of three well-controlled studies that she and her associates conducted in order to identify and manipulate variables relevant to effective, fear-reducing, presurgical preparation of children. Melamed's previously discussed work with filmed modeling in facilitating appropriate dental behavior provided a technology that could be readily adapted for use with surgery fear.

The first study assessed the effectiveness of watching a filmed peer model cope with anxieties experienced during hospitalization that involved surgery. As measured by self-reported medical fears, palmar sweating activity, and behavioral observations, the results showed significant reductions in anxiety in the experimental subjects who viewed the film just prior to hospitalization. The results for self-reported medical fears are presented in Figure 6. Palmar sweating increased for experimental subjects immediately after viewing the film, but decreased during the pre- and postoperative periods. The control subjects, who viewed a non-hospital-related film,

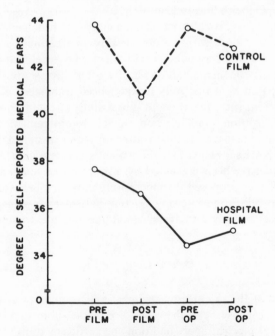

Figure 6. Degree of self-reported medical fears for the experimental and control groups across the four measurement periods. (From Melamed, 1977. Copyright 1977 by Pergamon Press. Reprinted by permission.)

showed the opposite pattern. Differences between experimental and control subjects on all the above measures were maintained at the 3–4-week posthospitalization examination.

The second experiment investigated differences in time and type of preparation according to the age of the child. Children being admitted to the hospital for the first time were randomly assigned to one of four treatment conditions, which varied the day on which the children viewed the film (day of admission versus 5–9 days prior to admission) and the amount of staff preparation of the child (minimal versus standard).

The results showed no significant effect of degree of staff preparation in reducing preoperative anxiety. The data indicated age differences related to time of viewing of film, with older children (age 7 and older) benefiting more from the prehospitalization preparation, and younger children (below 7 years) showing greatest reductions in anxiety following preparation on the day of hospital admission.

A final study in this series examined the relationship between prehospital coping styles and in-hospital behaviors. Parents were given questionnaires assessing strategies typically employed by them in dealing with their child's encountering a fearful situation. It was found that parental reinforcement for approaching new situations, combined with modeling and reassurance, was positively related to the child's effective coping with hospitalization.

Needle Fears. The particular patient management problems encountered may be specific to the conditions surrounding the type of treatment administered. Katz (1974) described the case of a young renal patient who developed a phobic reaction to the use of a needle in hemodialysis shortly after having his first treatment, in which he was prepared by a relatively inexperienced technician. Katz reported that this adverse reaction was quickly and successfully treated through the use of systematic desensitization, fading, and social reinforcement techniques. The desensitization component was achieved after only one session. Despite the success of this treatment, Katz suggested that the patient's extreme negative reaction to the hemodialysis might have been prevented by a more effective handling of his initial treatment. Katz further proposed the incorporation of such behavioral techniques as desensitization and relaxation into any existing patient care plans, in order to help patients deal more effectively with aversive, but unavoidable, treatment procedures.

Patient Competence

The execution of the therapeutic regimen is dependent on at least two factors: that the requested response be in the repertoire of the subject and that the environmental and personal motivational conditions be sufficient to produce and maintain the response. The issue of behavioral compliance to instructional requests can be discussed only after it has been established that the person has the behavior in his/her repertoire. Thus, an analysis of behavioral competence may be very important in some cases where the patient is noncompliant. Behavioral competence involves the analysis of the behaviors required to implement a treatment. Zifferblatt (1975) suggested the importance of both behavioral competence and motivational issues in compliance.

Noncompliance with physician requests has long been considered a function of poor motivation or poor willpower, particularly for health-habit problems such as obesity, smoking, and exercise. The role of competence in the execution of health-habit change instruction has received relatively little attention, though in a preliminary evaluation of two behavioral weight-control programs, Epstein and Martin (1977) suggested that clients often are poor self-monitors of eating behavior. Variations in the degree of self-monitoring skill is important since research by Romanczyk (1974; Romanczyk, Tracey, Wilson & Thorpe, 1973) suggests self-monitoring to be a major, if not *the* major, factor in successful weight loss.

In many cases, deficits in behavioral competence are easy to observe, particularly those that relate to the incorrect use of equipment. Renne and Creer (1976) reported that numerous asthmatic children have difficulties in using a medication dispenser for the self-administration of bronchodilator medications. Three responses that the authors suggested interfere with correct equipment use were targeted; they included eye fixation on the equipment, facial posture to ensure that the child's mouth is around the mouthpiece and that medication is brought into the lungs, and diaphragmatic breathing to produce the best distribution of medication into the lungs. Contingencies to modify these three targets were arranged in a multiple-baseline fashion. The results for four children indicated that the general effectiveness of equipment use increased from 41% to 82% after treatment. The authors then reported a second study in which nurses were trained to teach two additional youngsters correct use of the equipment by modifying the three target responses.

Patient Compliance

A second problem in treatment implementation is compliance, which involves getting patients to implement treatments as prescribed. The targeting of compliance is based on the assumption that competence is not a problem. The primary compliance problem that has been studied is medicine compliance. Medicine noncompliance has been a serious problem in treatment, as estimates of noncompliance suggest that about one-third of the patient sample (Davis, 1966) are noncompliers, with some estimates as high as 92% (Marston, 1970). In addition to the effects of noncompliance on treatment, research efforts to compare alternative treatments for varied diseases on outpatients can not be correctly evaluated unless the patients correctly take their medicine.

Zifferblatt (1975) has outlined the applications of behavioral technology to medicine compliance, and several studies have recently been carried out showing the positive effects of behavioral procedures. Two of these studies have been on Antabuse intake, which is used to inhibit alcohol use. Haynes (1973) designed a program for individuals with habitual arrests for public intoxication. The contingencies were arranged so that a person could either enter a year of Antabuse treatment or go to jail for 90 days. If the person chose Antabuse, he/she had to come to the probation office twice a week to take his/her Antabuse. After a maximum of two violations, the people were then returned to jail. The results showed that almost one-half of the chronic offenders were still on Antabuse after one year, and the arrest rate for the sample had dropped from 3.8 to 0.3 arrests per year. Bigelow, Strickler, Liebson, and Griffiths (1976) developed a response-cost procedure for Antabuse intake. Twenty male problem drinkers were requested to place a deposit of from $100 to $150 at the clinic, and $5–$10 were sacrificed for every failure to make a scheduled appointment. Patients were to come daily for the first two weeks, and then on every other day. The results indicated that the patients were abstinent for 95% of the treatment days over the initial contract (at least three months) days. Of these patients, 95% were abstinent for at least two months, while 40% were abstinent for at least six months. Of these patients, 80% were abstinent for longer periods as compared with abstinence during the three years preceding treatment.

An approach to compliance based primarily on stimulus control procedures was presented by Azrin and Powell (1969). They developed a portable apparatus that signaled when medication was to be taken, thus providing a prompt for the medication ingestion response. The tone signal stayed on until medication was removed from the apparatus. The device was used with six normal subjects, who were instructed to take a pill with no active pharmacological agents every half hour during the workday. The percentage of pills missed with the use of the medication dispenser (3%) was significantly less than the percentages missed with the use of a pill container (16%) or of an alarm timer (11%) that signaled when to take the pill but was not functionally linked to the behavior of pill ingestion.

Epstein and Masek (1978) compared several behavioral procedures in the modification of vitamin C intake in college students. The subjects were informed that they were participating in a study of the effects of vitamin C in preventing the common cold, and each deposited nine dollars before the study began. The use of vitamin C in this way serves as an analog to medication use for prevention or for asymptomatic disorders. After a three-week baseline period to determine which subjects were noncompliant, the subjects were randomly assigned to one for four groups: a no-treatment control group; a self-monitoring group, in which the subjects recorded the time of pill ingestion; a taste group, in which the subjects were provided with pills flavored neutral, orange, or quinine to increase their saliency (Zifferblatt, 1975); and a self-monitoring plus taste group. The results after three weeks indicated that the self-monitoring groups were significantly superior to the control or taste group. During the final phase, one-half of the subjects in each group were exposed to a response-cost condition. This condition was implemented by making the return of one dollar each week contingent on a criterion level of compliance. The results over the final three weeks showed improvements in groups containing subjects who experienced response cost, independent of prior history. In addition, the self-monitoring plus taste subjects were equivalent to the subjects who received the response cost. One final aspect of the study was the measurement procedures. In each week's supply of pills, the subjects were provided with three pills that contained phenazopyridine in a prearranged sequence. Phenazopyridine is a urinary tract analgesic that colors urine bright orange. The subjects were requested to record each occasion on which they noticed the urine discolorations, and the compliance with the four-times-per-day medication regimen could be established by comparing when the subjects reported urine discolorations to the time a phenazopyridine pill was presented in the prearranged schedule. This procedure was useful in that it reduced the necessity of laboratory or pill count assessment of compliance, which often may not reflect on-going medicine intake. The results of the compliance for subjects in the four groups is presented in Figure 7.

Compliance problems are certainly not limited to medicine compliance. Behavioral procedures have been used to improve compliance with treatment regimens in several other areas. Malament, Dunn, and Davis (1975) developed an avoidance learning procedure to prevent the development of pressure sores in paralyzed persons in wheelchairs. This procedure was necessary since many paralyzed patients do not follow instructions to do wheelchair pushups to relieve pressure on their ischia. The authors programmed a Sidman avoidance schedule by using an auditory alarm that was presented if the patient did not perform a four-second pushup each 10 minutes. After stable, low rates of pushups were established for four of the five subjects screened, the contingency was initiated for two of the subjects, with increases in wheelchair pushups maintained after termination of the contingency. The other two patients were discharged before treatment could be implemented.

A medical problem with serious health consequences was presented by Barnes (1976). The author worked with a hemodialysis patient who had severe physiological complications due in part to fluid overload. A token program was set up with a

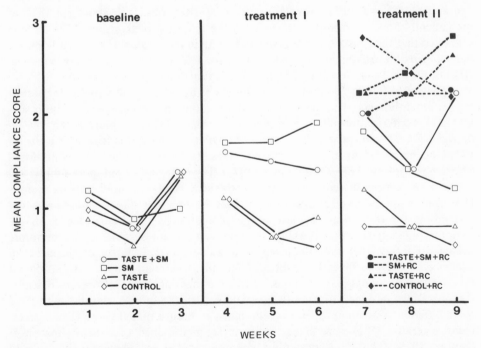

Figure 7. Mean compliance score for subjects in all groups during baseline and the two treatment phases. (From Epstein & Masek, 1978. Copyright 1978 by the Society for the Experimental Analysis of Behavior. Reprinted by permission.)

small amount of water intake, a maximum of 800 cc/day, available as a reinforcer for appropriate dietary restrictions. Water and salt with meals, as well as snacks, were prohibited. Points were also earned for less than a two-pound daily weight gain. The results showed a decrease in weight gain as well as large decreases in standing blood pressures, with positive effects being noted up to the six-month follow-up.

FOLLOW-UP

The process of follow-up to medical care has recently begun to interest medical personnel (Brook, Appel, Avery, Orman, & Stevenson, 1971) as well as behavioral therapists (Stokes & Baer, 1977). Follow-up to medical care is important for numerous reasons, including a most basic reason: to develop end result data to establish the quality of medical care (Brook *et al.*, 1971). Brook *et al.* reviewed the process and outcome variables related to the inpatient care of 403 patients in a major intercity teaching hospital, Baltimore City Hospitals. The patient's status six months after discharge was used as an end point to quantify the quality of inpatient care. In general, the results were quite disappointing, with 28% of the patients showing an equal or a decreased capacity to function after treatment. The outcome, assessed according to their previous symptoms, changes in degree of major activity, and ambulation, was consistent across all three categories, with about one-third of the patients showing no improvement from the initiation of treatment. The authors suggested that the cause of the negative follow-up in most cases was patient noncompliance with the treatment protocol, with only a small percentage (approximately 10%) of the total sample not getting better as a function of inadequate care.

The use of follow-up measures also functions as a dependent variable for assessing treatment effects. This procedure is quite common and has recently been suggested as a criterion for publication in a major behavior therapy journal, the *Journal of Behavior Therapy and Experimental Psychiatry*. The difficulties in the use of follow-up measures to evaluate treatment results have previously been discussed (Epstein & McCoy, 1975; Goldiamond, 1975). The issue can be put quite simply: if a symptom is reduced or removed after Treatment X is administered, and six months later the symptom has returned, this is not to say that Treatment X was not responsible for the initial decrease in symptomatology. The reappearance of the symptom suggests that the effects of the treatment are not durable or, in other more behavioral terms, that the conditions responsible for the control of the problem behavior were not sufficiently modified. Clinically, treatment procedures that do not produce lasting results may often not be the treatment of choice. However, logically, the operations designed to modify a behavior (i.e., treatment) may be considered quite different from those operations designed to ensure that the effects of a treatment generalize (Stokes & Baer, 1977) or are maintained over time (Epstein & McCoy, 1975). Thus, it is becoming common practice in behavioral literature to separate the procedures as well as the effects of treatment from follow-up (Stokes & Baer, 1977).

There are a variety of procedures that may be used to ensure that the effects of treatment generalize over time, producing an absence of symptoms when problem behaviors are measured sometime after formal treatment has terminated. Stokes and Baer (1977) listed nine categories of techniques. The one component common to all successful maintenance procedures may be a continuation of some therapeutic procedures in the absence of personal therapeutic contact. While this continuation is not sufficient for treatment success, as the actual procedures suggested may be inappropriate, the continuation is a necessary component of all follow-up strategies. Two procedures that may assist in the implementation of a maintenance treatment procedure have been suggested in the clinical literature, and they both involve substance abuse problems: obesity and smoking. These problems serve as a good model for follow-up procedures, as the short-term effects of treatment have been easily obtained, but the long-term effects of these procedures have been negative.

Hall, Hall, Borden, and Hanson (1975) assessed the effects of various follow-up strategies on continued weight loss in obese patients. After all patients received a common self-management treatment, subjects were randomly assigned to no-contact, self-monitoring only, or booster sessions. The results in terms of weight reduction indexes suggested continued monitoring to be the best follow-up approach. When patients receiving booster sessions were then subdivided according to whether their booster was administered by the same therapist who delivered treatment, the effects for patients of same-therapist boosters were equivalent to effects by continued self-monitoring. These results suggest that self-monitoring was the treatment of choice, as it was more cost-beneficial than repeated boosters, particularly because of the possible deleterious effects produced when the therapists were changed during follow-up. The motivating conditions that are necessary to maintain engaging in the skills learned during treatment may be provided in another way. Dubren (1977) evaluated the effects of recorded phone messages on short-term maintenance of nonsmoking. The author provided about one-half of the subjects who participated in a TV stop-smoking clinic with a phone number they could call to hear a recorded message that reinforced them for not smoking. The results suggested that fewer persons having access to the recorded message began to smoke again than subjects not provided access to the message. The importance of this procedure is that it represents a simple and cost-beneficial procedure for delivering therapeutic contact in similar fashion to booster sessions. Further, it can be used to maintain motivating conditions for adhering to the skills learned during treatment. Both of the above procedures share one popular conception of maintenance: follow-up strategies are designed to maintain the motivation to engage in the skills learned during treatment, and no new skills are learned during follow-up.

SUMMARY

This chapter was designed to acquaint the reader with the use of behavioral procedures in the health care delivery process. This is a new area for behavioral technology, but an area that appears particularly well suited to the implementation of behavioral procedures, since much of health care delivery depends on the client's emitting certain health- or illness-specific behaviors.

In addition to the applicability of conceptualizing health care delivery in terms of specific behaviors, health care delivery holds particular promise as an area of research because of its extreme significance in medical care. After all, independent of the development of new treatment modalities, the effectiveness of treatment approaches can be realized only if the treatments can be correctly delivered to those in need.

ACKNOWLEDGMENTS

Appreciation is expressed to Pete Fabrega for shaping many of the authors' ideas on health care delivery and to Lynn Bunch, Nancy Manown, and especially Sharon Johnston for secretarial services.

REFERENCES

Adelson, R., & Goldfried, M. R. Modeling and the fearful child patient. *Journal of Dentistry for Children*, 1970, *37*, 34–47.

APA Task Force on Health Research. Contributions of Psychology to Health Research: Patterns, problems, and potentials. *American Psychologist*, 1976, *31*, 263–274.

Azrin, N. H., & Powell, J. Behavioral engineering: The use of response priming to improve prescribed self-medications. *Journal of Applied Behavior Analysis*, 1969, *2*, 39–42.

Barkin, R. M., & Duncan, R. Broken appointments: Questions, not answers. *Pediatrics*, 1975, *55*, 747–748.

Barnes, M. R. Token economy control of fluid overload in a patient receiving hemodialysis. *Journal of Behavior Therapy and Experimental Psychiatry*, 1976, *7*, 305–306.

Becker, M. H., & Maiman, L. A. Sociobehavioral determinants of compliance with health and medical care recommendations. *Medical Care*, 1975, *13*, 10–24.

Bigelow, G., Strickler, D., Liebson, I., & Griffiths, R. Maintaining disulfiran ingestion among outpatient alcoholics: A security deposit contingency contracting procedure. *Behaviour Research and Therapy*, 1976, *14*, 378–381.

Breslow, L., & Somers, A. R. The lifetime health-monitoring program: A practical approach to preventive medicine. *The New England Journal of Medicine*, 1977, *296*, 601–608.

Brook, R. H., Appel, F. A., Avery, C., Orman, M., & Stevenson, R. L. Effectiveness of inpatient follow-up care. *The New England Journal of Medicine*, 1971, *285*, 1509–1514.

Cauffman, J. G., Peterson, E. L., & Emrick, J. A. Medical care of school children: Factors influencing outcome of referral from a school health program. *Journal of Public Health*, 1967, *57*, 60–73.

Davis, M. S. Variations in patient's compliance with doctor's orders: Analysis of congruence between survey responses and results of empirical investigations. *Journal of Medical Education*, 1966 *41*, 1037–1048.

Dubren, R. Self-reinforcement by recorded telephone messages to maintain nonsmoking behavior. *Journal of Consulting and Clinical Psychology*, 1977, *45*, 358–360.

Epstein, L. H., & Cinciripini, P. M. Behavioral Medicine III: Health Care Delivery. *Association for Advancement of Behavior Therapy Newsletter*, 1977, *4*, 7–9.

Epstein, L. H., & Martin, J. E. Compliance and side effects of weight regulation groups. *Behavior Modification*, 1977, *1*, 551–558.

Epstein, L. H., & Masek, B. J. Behavioral control of medicine compliance. *Journal of Applied Behavior Analysis*, 1978, *11*, 1–10.

Epstein, L. H., & McCoy, J. F. Issues in smoking control. *Addictive Behaviors*, 1975, *1*, 65–72.

Fabrega, H., Jr. *Disease and social behavior: An interdisciplinary perspective*. Cambridge, Mass.: M.I.T. Press, 1974.

Fabrega, H., Jr., & Van Egeren, L. A behavioral framework for the study of human disease. *Annals of Internal Medicine*, 1976, *84*, 200–208.

Fink, R., Shapiro, S., & Lewison, J. The reluctant participant in a breast cancer screening program. *Public Health Reports*, 1968, *83*, 479–489.

Finnerty, F. A., Shaw, L. W., & Himmelsback, C. K. Hypertension in the inner city: II. Detection and follow-up. *Circulation*, 1973, *47*, 76–78.

Friedson, E., & Feldman, J. J. The public looks at dental care. *The Journal of the American Dental Association*, 1958, *57*, 325–335.

Gabrielson, I. W., Levin, L. S., & Ellison, M. D. Factors affecting school health follow-up. *Journal of Public Health*, 1967, *57*, 49–73.

Gale, E. G., & Ayer, W. A. Treatment of dental phobias. *The Journal of the American Dental Association*, 1969, *78*, 1304–1307.

Goldiamond, I. Toward a constructional approach to social problems: Ethical and constitutional issues raised by applied behavior analysis. In C. M. Franks & G. T. Wilson, (Eds.), *Annual Review of Behavior Therapy Theory and Practice*. New York: Brunner/Mazel, 1975.

Goldstein, M. K., Stein, G. H., Smolen, D. M., & Perlini, W. S. Biobehavioral monitoring: A method for remote health measurement. *Archives of Physical Medicine and Rehabilitation*, 1976, *57*, 253–258.

Hagen, R. L., Foreyt, J. P., & Durham, T. W. The dropout problem: Reducing attrition in obesity research. *Behavior Therapy*, 1976, *7*, 463–471.

Hall, S. M., Hall, R. G., Borden, B. L., & Hanson, R. W. Follow-up strategies in the behavioral treatment of overweight. *Behaviour Research and Therapy*, 1975, *13*, 167–172.

Haynes, S. N. Contingency management in a municipally-administered Antabuse program for alcoholics. *Journal of Behavior Therapy and Experimental Psychiatry*, 1973, *4*, 31–32.

Hochbaum, G. M. Why people seek diagnostic X-rays. *Public Health Reports*, 1956, *71*, 377–380.

Kasl, S. V., & Cobb, S. Health behavior, illness behavior, and sick role behavior. *Archives of Environmental Health*, 1966, *12*, 246–266.

Katz, R. C. Single session recovery from a hemodialysis phobia: A case study. *Journal of Behavior Therapy and Experimental Psychiatry*, 1974, *5*, 205–206.

Kirscht, J. P., Haefner, D. P., & Eveland, J. D. Public response to various written appeals to participate in health screening. *Public Health Reports*, 1975, *90*, 539–543.

Knapp, T. J., & Peterson, L. W. Behavior management in medical and nursing practice. In. W. E. Craighead, A. E. Kazdin, & M. J. Mahoney (Eds.), *Behavior modification: Principles, issues, and applications*. Boston: Houghton Mifflin, 1976.

Levin, L. S. Self-care: An international perspective. *Social Policy*, 1976, *7*, 70–75.

Machen, J. B., & Johnson, R. Desensitization, model learning, and the dental behavior of children. *Journal of Dental Research*, 1974, *53*, 83–87.

Malament, I. B., Dunn, M. E., & Davis, R. Pressure sores: An operant conditioning approach to prevention. *Archives of Physical Medicine Rehabilitation*, 1975, *56*, 161–165.

Marston, M. Compliance with medical regimens: A review of the literature. *Nursing Research*, 1970, *19*, 312–323.

Melamed, B. G. Psychological preparation for hospitalization. In S. Rachman (Ed.), *Contributions to Medical Psychology*. New York: Pergamon, 1977.

Melamed, B. G., Hawes, R. R., Heiby, E., & Glick, J. Use of filmed modeling to reduce uncooperative behavior of children during dental treatment. *Journal of Dental Research*, 1975, *54*, 797–801.

Malamed, B. G., Weinstein, D., Hawes, R., & Katin-Borland, M. Reduction of fear related dental management problems with use of filmed modeling. *Journal of the American Dental Association*, 1975, *90*, 822–826.

Nazarian, L. F., Mechaber, F., Charney, E., & Coutler, M. P. Effects of a mailed appointment reminder on appointment keeping. *Pediatrics*, 1974, *53*, 349–352.

Reiss, M. L., Piotrowski, W. D., & Bailey, J. S. Behavioral community psychology: Encouraging low-income parents to seek dental care for their children. *Journal of Applied Behavior Analysis*, 1976, *9*, 387–397.

Renne, C. M., & Creer, T. L. Training children with asthma to use inhalation therapy equipment. *Journal of Applied Behavior Analysis*, 1976, *9*, 1–11.

Rockart, J. F., & Hoffman, P. B. Physician and patient behavior under different scheduling systems in a hospital outpatient department. *Medical Care*, 1969, *7*, 463–470.

Romanczyk, R. G. Self-monitoring in the treatment of obesity: Parameters of reactivity. *Behavior Therapy*, 1974, *5*, 531–540.

Romanczyk, R. G., Tracey, D. A., Wilson, G. T., & Thorpe, G. L. Behavioral techniques in the treatment of obesity: A comparative analysis. *Behaviour Research and Therapy*, 1973, *11*, 629–640.

Rosenstock, I. M. Why people use health services. *Milbank Memorial Fund Quarterly*, 1966, *44*, 94–127.

Stokes, T. F., & Baer, D. M. An implicit technology of generalization. *Journal of Applied Behavior Analysis*, 1977, *10*, 349–368.

Tracy, J. J. Impact of intake procedures upon client attrition in a community mental health center. *Journal of Consulting and Clinical Psychology*, 1977, *45*, 192–195.

Turner, A. J., & Vernon, J. C. Prompts to increase attendance in a community mental health center. *Journal of Applied Behavior Analysis*, 1976, *9*, 141–145.

Zifferblatt, S. M. Increasing patient compliance through the applied analysis of behavior. *Preventive Medicine*, 1975, *4*, 173–182.

3

The Development of Behavioral Competence in Medical Settings

MARIE A. MASTRIA AND RONALD S. DRABMAN

The art and science of medicine have advanced greatly over the past several decades. Its technology is sophisticated and often awe-inspiring. Faulty body parts can be mended or replaced at costs that are not prohibitive. Prevention and rehabilitation are at the point where certain illnesses are almost nonexistent.

Psychology, however, has not had a major impact on patient care. Before the recent introduction of behavioral techniques into medicine, psychology was deemed useful only in explaining and treating emotional disorders, that is, those neuroses or psychoses that caused one to behave differently from others and for which no identifiable physical antecedent had been found. For the most part, medicine and psychology went their separate ways. One exception was in psychosomatics, the branch of psychology that treats illnesses regarded as having their basis in emotional disturbances (ulcers, colitis, migraine headaches, etc.). The patient was still considered emotionally disturbed, but the disturbance was thought to be manifested through a physical disorder. Treatment consisted mainly of uncovering the hostilities, anger, and neurotic thinking underlying the physical disorder.

Psychosomatic medicine is still with us and serves a distinct purpose. Yet, its practitioners have not been able to bridge the gap between psychology and medicine. Only specific disorders, specific personality types, and specific treatments are seen as the domain of psychosomatic medicine. One would not, for example, consult a specialist in psychosomatic medicine for a compliance problem (unless, perhaps, it was seen as a suicidal gesture). This inability to meld the two fields causes problems in the delivery of health care and in the training given health care providers.

Care delivery is frequently impeded because the primary emphasis is on medical technology, to the exclusion of other factors such as the psychosocial aspects of ill-

MARIE A. MASTRIA AND RONALD S. DRABMAN • Department of Psychiatry and Human Behavior, University of Mississippi School of Medicine, Jackson, Mississippi 39206.

ness and its treatment. Research on these topics has not advanced as far as in other areas of medicine because adequate research models have been lacking. Since the advent of behavioral psychology, however, research models have been developed that offer new means of measuring change in behavior (Davidson & Costello, 1969). For example, the single-case study allows clinical research to be carried on more easily. Designs such as multiple baseline across behaviors enable the clinician to use a single patient to determine the effectiveness of a treatment modality. All that remains is the integration of these designs into the mainstream of the medical setting.

As these new research designs have proved effective, clinical researchers have begun to expand the kinds of problems attacked and the populations considered appropriate for treatment. Today, there is a trend toward implementing the principles and techniques of psychology, especially behavioral psychology, in such diverse problem areas as compliance with therapeutic regimens (Sackett & Haynes, 1976), substance abuse (Miller & Mastria, 1977; Stuart, 1971), the prevention and treatment of disorders such as asthma (Renne & Creer, 1976), hypertension (Patel, 1976), and pain (Bonica, 1975; Fordyce, 1976).

Clinicians have long known that the patient's attitude could either facilitate or impede recovery. Establishing an appropriate doctor–patient relationship, conveying the right set to the patient, and prescribing placebos are well-recognized adjuncts to treatment. These strategies are partially based on various psychological principles. It is the intent of behavioral medicine to systematize and expand this influence. Blanchard (1977) called behavioral medicine "an idea whose time has come" (p. 2).

The utility of behavioral techniques in medicine has been demonstrated (Fordyce, 1976; Ince, 1976; Sackett & Haynes, 1976). Health providers have reported the use of behavioral procedures to enhance techniques peculiar to their profession. For example, Aiken (1970) found that teaching becomes more effective when nurses assist surgical patients through the use of such behavioral techniques as allowing the patient to master information in stepwise fashion and shaping the use of medical procedures. Nurses may also assist more directly in alleviating the patient's preoperative and postoperative fears through relaxation training and systematic desensitization (LeBow, 1976).

Roberts, Dinsdale, Matthews, and Cole (1969) described the implementation by medical and nursing staff of a behavioral program to teach self-care skills to a 35-year-old hemicorporectomized male. Inadequate self-care led to recurrent and persistent decubitus ulcers, which were life-threatening. The problem could not be solved by a traditional medical approach, but the rehabilitation team was able to implement an effective program to teach self-care through the use of education, systematic training, and appropriate rewards.

THE HEALTH PROFESSION/BEHAVIORIST

Education and retraining are integral aspects of health provision. Behavioral medicine offers principles and procedures both for health providers who wish a comprehensive understanding of illness and for those who wish to use their particular knowledge and skill in a more effective and efficient manner (see, e.g., Guze, Matarazzo, & Saslow, 1953).

In the following pages, we discuss issues in training behavioral practitioners (many of whom owe primary allegiance to other disciplines) and present some models for training. Our primary focus is on the nonpsychiatric physician, the nurse, and the psychologist. However, implicit in our discussion is the development of behavioral competence among other groups, such as physical and occupational therapists and dentists. Throughout this chapter, we endeavor to use studies and examples that have relevance for health care providers in a variety of disciplines.

The Physician as Behavioral Practitioner

Brown (1969) has stated that "the practice of medicine is 50 or 60% psychological and sociological" (p. 965). Brady (1971) described a dissatisfaction among nonpsychiatric physicians with traditional dynamic psychotherapy. However, he suggested that medicine's need for psychological theory and technique may be met by behavior therapy because, like many aspects of medicine, behavior therapy is empirical in nature. Its format fits well with medical interventions: goals are accurately stated, treatment outcome may be assessed, and supervised paraprofessionals may be used to carry out most treatment.

Behavioral medicine provides the physician with alternatives or adjuncts to medication and other medical interventions (Maxmen, 1976). A good example is the treatment of chronic pain. The alleviation of pain is one of the major motivating factors in medicine. Pain patients have been difficult patients for neurologists, orthopedic surgeons, nurses, and physical and occupational therapists. Treatment is long, complicated, and expensive and often fails. Patients may "doctor-shop" in the hope of finding some relief. Too often, they undergo numerous surgical interventions, become addicted to pain medications, and experience changes in personality. Lately, pain programs have been implemented to eliminate or decrease chronic pain primarily through the use of behavioral techniques (Bonica, 1975; Fordyce, 1976; Melzack & Chapman, 1973).

Historically, pain has been considered a medical problem and has been treated by physiological interventions. If no organic reason could be found for a patient's pain, it was likely to be labeled psychogenic and the patient was referred for psychotherapy. It is now generally accepted that pain has both psychological and physiological components, and, therefore, psychological interventions are frequently implemented for its alleviation (Bonica, 1975; Fordyce, 1976). Reinforcement of nonpain behavior, shaping of appropriate behaviors, distraction procedures, and relaxation training are among the behavioral treatments used to modify pain response. Particular mention should be made of treatment to control the undue taking of pain medications. For example, pharmacists give patients a "cocktail" composed of masked pain medications. The amount of medication is slowly lowered with no adverse effect to the patients, for, at the same time, control or avoidance techniques are being learned. Also, since the cocktail is given on schedule rather than as requested (prn), the pairing of pain relief with medication no longer occurs.

Although the use of behavioral intervention with pain is probably the most significant marriage of behavioral psychology with medicine, there are also others. The treatment of childhood illnesses (Renne & Creer, 1976) and of substance abuses (Bigelow, Strickler, Liebson, & Griffiths, 1976), screening for diseases (Fink, Shapiro, & Lewison, 1968), and the development of compliance with medical regimens (Sackett & Haynes, 1976) are among the others. Behavioral medicine, the combination of behavioral techniques and medicine, accomplishes what is surely difficult or impossible to accomplish with any one of the components alone. Later, we discuss models of training that bring the knowledge and skills needed to carry out such work into the hands of the nonpsychiatric physician.

The Nurse as Behavioral Practitioner

The association of nursing with behavioral techniques is not new. As early as 1959, Ayllon and Michael presented the concept of the psychiatric nurse as a behavioral engineer. As behavior therapy extends into the general hospital, it is natural, then, that the nonpsychiatric nurse be targeted as a user of these techniques. Since the nurse has the greatest amount of contact with the patient, she/he is also in a natural position to have the greatest impact on the care and education given to the patient.

Behavioral medicine offers the nurse an alternative to the traditional nursing concept of "noncontingent forms of caring (e.g., tender loving care)" (LeBow, 1976, p. 146), a concept that is much like the "unconditional positive regard" of traditional psychotherapy. LeBow, however, sees this very concept as the major stumbling block to the acceptance of behavioral techniques. Nurses must be won over to the idea that "noncontingent caring" is not best for the patient. Nurses can make a contribution to patient treatment (Wiley, 1973), patient education (Grout & Watkins, 1971), shortening or eliminating the hospital stay (Barnard, 1968), and prevention (Pasternack, 1974). The consequent expanding of the nurse's role would give nursing more autonomy and recognition as an independent profession (LeBow, 1976), and it would support the new trend toward greater professionalism of which the nurse–practitioner and nurse–midwife are a part.

The Psychologist as a Behavioral Practitioner in the
Medical Setting

Behavioral medicine offers the psychologist the opportunity to act as a trainer of other professionals and to serve as a consultant and a primary care giver. As behavioral medicine develops, more psychologists will take leadership roles. As is true of other professionals, however, psychologists are still in the early stages of developing models for training practitioners of behavioral medicine. Of particular importance is the development of a training model that will provide the psychologist working in behavioral medicine with the medical knowledge necessary to function effectively in a medical setting (Mastria & Hosford, 1976).

Other Behaviorally Competent Practitioners

As we stated earlier, behavioral medicine is just beginning to define itself and therefore is accessible to broad use in the medical setting. The basic model, which we present later, is useful to a wide range of technical groups, for example, dentists; physical, occupational, and recreational therapists; and speech and hearing specialists. Behavioral interventions have been applied to both prevention and direct care in many areas of medicine, and we expect that more uses will be reported as the area develops.

ISSUES IN TRAINING

Several issues must be considered in developing a behavioral training program for use in the medical setting. A listing of important considerations follows:

1. Resistance
   a. Professional resistance
   b. Patient resistance
2. Ethics
3. Comprehensive approach to patient care
4. Cost–benefit
5. Effectiveness
6. Patient considerations
   a. Patient education
   b. Patient choice
   c. Patient participation
   d. Patient control
   e. Patient compliance
7. Rationale for inclusion of
   a. Learning theory
   b. Behavior therapy
   c. Research training
8. Content
9. Training models
10. Guidelines to teaching

Resistance

Professional Resistance

Professional resistance to the use of behavioral techniques appears to be influenced by several factors. There is often a provincialism among trainees, who may discount education that is out of the mainstream of their training. Some feel that unless a technique is part of the work for which one has been trained, it is a waste of time and interferes with one's "real" work. Health providers and instructors have contributed to this resistance by minimizing the role of behavior in health and disease, because they either fail to understand the relationship or have had no effective means of dealing with it. It appears that the resistance is based on unfamiliarity, bad experiences with irrelevant dynamic therapies, lack of trained behavioral instructors, and the poor integration of the behavioral curriculum with the general health care program (Brown, 1969; Hooper & Roberts, 1968; Moss & Boren, 1974; Stern, 1975).

Professional resistance can be broken down by discussing the problems that are of particular concern in health care delivery and by demonstrating how behavioral techniques may be used with the basic medical techniques. Of course, as more practitioners are trained and become teachers, these appropriate role models will alleviate much of the trainee resistance.

Patient Resistance

Patient resistance to behavioral intervention may occur because of faulty information or a lack of understanding. For example, patients may view the use of behavior modification as an attempt at manipulation or as an indication that they have been diagnosed as emotionally ill. Noncompliance can be traced to a lack of motivation or a lack of willingness or ability to fit the recommended regimen into the individual's daily routine.

It is necessary, therefore, to anticipate such concerns and to educate patients as to the utility of behavior therapy. In a later section, we discuss techniques of allaying patients' concerns.

Ethics

Professional influence and behavioral techniques offer powerful and effective tools for changing behavior. The development and application of appropriate professional standards and safeguards are of major concern to practitioners of behavior therapy. Organizations such as the Association for the Advancement of Behavior Therapy (AABT) continually discuss current ethical issues and the guidance that should be offered to those using behavior therapy. At one time, ethical issues consisted of confidentiality, competency, and sanctions against monetary and sexual exploitation. Although these issues are still extremely important, professionals must now also deal with (1) the effect of behavior therapy on society; (2) control of the professional individual and groups; (3) the use of certain behavioral techniques such as aversive control; and (4) the appropriate manner in which to carry out human research (Kanfer & Phillips, 1970).

In training programs, issues such as the above may be presented and discussed in order to develop ethical and moral attitudes among trainees. The case presentation approach used by the American Psychological Association (1953) in its development of ethical standards for its members is an effective means of addressing these problems with the trainees.

The Comprehensive Approach to Patient Care

Among the complaints registered by both patients and health care providers is the failure of providers to meet the emotional and educational needs of patients (Maxmen, 1976; Wittkower & Dudek, 1973), as well as their failure to attend to the social, environmental, and behavioral components of health problems (Katz & Zlutnick, 1975). This failure is mainly the result of overspecialization: the psychiatrist and the psychologist are expected to deal with emotional and behavioral problems, social workers are expected to deal with family and environmental problems, nurses with the strictly defined aspects of nursing-related health problems, and physicians with another limited area of the health problem.

Incorporating behavioral theory and techniques into the training program of health providers allows trainees to view the patient as a whole person once more. The interaction of physical disorder, environment, patient behavior, and medical treatment can be assessed and used to best advantage.

In presenting their concept of the comprehensive approach to medicine, Guze, Matarazzo, and Saslow (1953) stated:

> An approach to the problem of disease that is comprehensive clearly requires a description of it from several points of reference. . . . (1) What factor in the environment (or life situation) of this patient are operating to promote disability? (2) What factors in the individual's heredity and past experience are pertinent to the explanation of his sickness? (3) What are the changes in the function and structure of the various parts of his body which actually result in symptoms, signs, and ultimately serious disability or death? . . . (4) In what way do these changes contribute to subsequent behavior responses of the organism, and what is the nature of these responses?
>
> . . . By dealing with relevant factors in other areas, or in the same area, which may also be contributing to the disability, but which are more amenable to change, we may also alter the entire balance in favor of more successful adaptation. (pp. 128–129)

An example of the new comprehensive approach to patient care is demonstrated by Borkovec (1977) in the treatment of certain types of insomnia. Other examples of behavioral interventions used either instead of or in conjunction with medical treatment are presented by Andrews (1964) in retraining neuromusculature in a hemiplegic; Ratliff and Stein (1968) in neurodermatitis; Shumway and Powers (1973) in obesity; Zlutnick, Mayville, and Moffat (1975) in seizure disorders; and Fordyce (1976) in chronic pain.

Cost–Benefit

An investigation by Schwartz and White (1977) illustrates how behavioral approaches can contribute to more cost-effective service. This behavioral intervention aimed at increasing the number of patients who kept their clinic appointments. Patients receiving social reinforcement, such as prompt service and full and understandable explanations of their disorder (e.g., treatment, expected drug reactions, course of the disease, and prognosis), returned for their appointments more regularly than did a control group.

Cost–benefit also needs to be viewed from the perspective of both the practitioner and the patient. For the practitioner, sufficient time should be allotted during the training program for the acquisition of usable behavioral skills. As a result of being more adequately trained in this area, the practitioner can develop health care programs that have the potential for better cost containment.

Effectiveness

Some trainees may feel that elaborate behavioral interventions produce change that is small, short-lived, or insignificant in the resolution of the problem. These concerns are valid, of course, but research shows that, properly carried out, change produced by behavioral intervention is durable and significant (Kanfer & Phillips, 1970).

Criticisms regarding the ineffectiveness of behavioral interventions are negated by such studies as those by Horner (1971). Horner used a 10-step operant program to train a young spina bifida child to walk with crutches. A 50-day follow-up check showed that the child was walking in 100% of the provided opportunities. Horner's method is a clear demonstration of the significant contributions that can be made in rehabilitation and other branches of health care.

Patient Considerations

Patient Education

Education is an important component of the prevention and treatment of disease and disorders. Various interest groups such as the American Cancer Society, the President's Committee on Physical Fitness, and the American Heart Association have based major prevention campaigns on education of the public concerning the effects of smoking, diet, and exercise on health and stressing the importance of early detection of physical disorders. Part of the treatment of diabetes, spinal cord injury, obesity, and hypertension consists of educating patients in medical and personal self-care.

Patient education can take various forms. The distribution of appropriate medical literature to the patient, placement in special training programs, and information dissemination during the clinical interviews are important facets of patient education with which the trainee should be familiar. In addition, the trainee should be instructed on how to determine the differential effectiveness of various patient education programs.

Patient Choice

An important issue in medicine today is the right of the patient to some choice in treatment. Hopefully, knowledge provided to the patient is used as one component in the decision-making process. In assisting the patient, the practitioner may take him/her through the problem-solving process, provide information, act the role of the devil's advocate, and weigh the pros and cons of the available alternatives.

Patient Participation

In probably no other treatment approach is the patient's participation more sought than in behavior therapy. Not only does a motivated patient cooperate more, but a patient who understands the treatment and its goals can contribute much in evaluating progress and suggesting modifications.

The behavioral medicine trainee is taught to use patient participation to its greatest advantage. One way this is done is by asking patients to keep behavioral records. The behavioral record may be used to monitor such things as the target behavior and its intensity, what the patient did to increase or decrease it, and how often the treatment technique was used. The information obtained from such a record can assist both the patient and the practitioner to a better understanding and planning of further treatment.

Patient Control

Behaviorists are developing self-control techniques as a means of facilitating treatment and prolonged its effects (Mahoney & Thoresen, 1974). This is particularly appropriate to behavioral medicine, for it allows the patient to take charge of some of his/her treatment, thus freeing the health care providers from unnecessary tasks. Professionals are more likely to use such techniques when there is a maximum benefit with minimum output or intrusion on other duties.

Patient Compliance

All the patient considerations we have just discussed must be regarded as components of patient compliance. A major aspect of compliance concerns patients' adherence to medical regimens. A problem frequently noted in medicine is that patients will take a medication only during the acute phase of an illness. To be beneficial, however, a full course of some medications must be taken. Although physicians are aware of this problem, aside from attempts to instruct the patient at the time the medication is prescribed, they have had little at their disposal to offset this nonadherence. Behavioral techniques have developed a number of provocative remedies (Cole & Emmanuel, 1971; Dixon, Stradling, & Wooton, 1957; Linkewich, Catalano, & Flack, 1974).

Rather than assuming that the patient is able to comply with the prescribed regimen, Zifferblatt (1975) suggested testing for and developing the behavioral skills that are lacking. He also suggested rearranging factors in the environment so that compliance becomes more likely. Scheduling medicine intake to coincide with the patient's daily tasks (meals, for example) is one effective environmental manipulation.

Such environmental manipulations need not be complicated or costly. Epstein and Masek (1978) showed that patient self-monitoring and a response cost procedure were more effective means of enhancing compliance with vitamin C intake on a four-times-a-day regimen than were pill flavoring or a control condition. It is easy to transpose this piece of clinical research to a hospital or clinic: when a regimen (medication, exercise, or other program) is prescribed, the practitioner need only request the patient to record *when* compliance occurs. This information is then supplied to the practitioner on the patient's next visit. This procedure could be standardized by the use of recording forms printed on the back of the appointment card given out by most medical and dental clinics. Such a behavioral technique could easily find its way into the training of every health care provider.

Although recording various sources of information (e.g., temperature, blood pressure, medication records) is part of inpatient care, outpatient care has not relied on such continuous systematic recordings because of the problems associated with obtaining that information. These difficulties can be overcome if patients are invited to collaborate in their own treatment. This data collection method was tested by Goldstein, Stein, Smolen, and Perlini (1976) and was found to be eminently workable. Their population consisted of 37 outpatients with Laennec's cirrhosis. Such patients are considered unreliable and noncompliant and consequently receive little or no outpatient care. The patients in this study were requested to make self-observations (weight, ethanol intake, movement index by pedometer readings, hours worked, ounces of liquid other than ethanol, abdominal girth) and report them daily by telephone into a recording system that gave no feedback to the patient. Spouses were used as reliability checks, and the recordings covered a period of six months. The authors reported that 11,144 requests for data met with 90.4% compliance. They concluded that patients can easily be taught to monitor medical data effectively.

Thus, the application of behavioral medicine techniques by a wide range of health professionals is appropriate because in many instances, they provide efficient and effective means of utilizing the sophisticated medical technology now available. Their use is appropriate in both primary and secondary prevention as well as in treatment of the sick (Epstein & Cincirpini, 1977). In addition, they assist the professional in examining his/her own methods of providing care and of improving interaction with patients.

Rationale for Teaching Behavior Therapy

Many students enter professional training having had some exposure to behavior therapy in undergraduate psychology courses. During graduate training, however, students generally become involved with the skills and theory of only their own profession. They are receptive to other techniques, if those procedures are presented as being more effective and beneficial than those of their own profession. Therefore, more thought needs to be given to the more effective presentation of behavioral theory and technique in a relevant and integrated manner during a professional's training.

Behavior therapy frequently assists in making medical treatment more effective and efficient. It can mean a briefer, less costly regimen, which, given the current cost of medical treatment, must be consideration for any health professional as well as for any patient. Surely, the rationale as to *why* to teach health providers to be competent behavioral practioners is sound. The question of what to teach and how to teach are more difficult ones to answer. Below we explore these questions and offer some suggestions.

Content

If behavior therapy is to become an integral part of patient care services in the general medical setting, it must offer a system of theory and techniques that is practical and that will help meet the general goals of more efficient and more effective patient care. The role of the health care provider defines much of the content needed for training the behaviorally competent practitioner (Kanfer & Phillips, 1970). The trend in medicine toward a "patient-centered (or more properly, a person-centered) curricula with the object of reuniting technical medicine with human medicine" (Wexler, 1976, p. 276) is an elegant call for the incorporation of behavior therapy into the training of physicians, nurses, psychologists, and other providers of health care.

Attempts to change the role of the health care provider have been ineffective in the past, largely because of behavioral scientists' inability to train students to apply a relevant, useful, workable technology. Additionally, psychological theory, although intrinsically interesting, has contributed little to the overall goals of training. Even when psychologically derived treatment techniques were applied to psychotic and mentally retarded populations, there was a tendency to view the treatments and the theories supporting them as appropriate only to those populations. Students could not transfer the diagnosis and treatment of the psychiatrically ill patient to the general patient population (Earley, 1969; Scheflen, 1958). Psychodynamics did not meet the day-to-day needs of the nonpsychiatric staff, other than by providing the criteria for diagnosing a patient and by setting the guidelines for psychiatric consultation (Gelfand, 1972; Levene, Breger, & Patterson, 1972; Lewis, Schriver, & MacDonald, 1969; Lidz & Edelson, 1970).

This dilemma began to resolve itself when behavior therapy widened its patient population to include those with behavioral or adjustment problems. Theory and technique began to be used in unique ways. Diagnosis (or, more properly, problem analysis) and treatment became both useful and more meaningful to health care providers (Burnet, 1969; Clark, Evans, & Hamerlynck, 1972; Usdin, 1973). Behavioral medicine, although relatively new, is completing the process of expanding psychological theory and technique to the nonpsychiatric hospital (Epstein & Cincirpini, 1977; Ince, 1976; Mahoney & Thoresen, 1974).

Programs are now in existence that provide this training to some extent (Agras, 1971; Benassi & Lanson, 1972; Cameron & Schmauk, 1977; Davidson, Goldfried, & Krasner, 1970; LeBow, 1976). Yen (1971) reported that 84% of psychology doctoral programs offered courses in behavioral therapy. Brady's (1973) survey of medical school offerings presents a bleaker picture: only 4% of the schools had a required course in behavior therapy; however, 68% offered elective courses. LeBow (1976) reported that a growing number of courses and practica were being offered to students training for the various branches of nursing. Except for graduate programs of psychology, behavioral principles and procedures are too often taught in less than optimum conditions. Furthermore, nowhere is the application of these principles and procedures to medical disease and disorder taught adequately. Yet, these established programs do serve as guides to what is and is not necessary to the training of behavioral medicine practitioners.

As in any other skills, different degrees of behavioral competence may be attained. Not every professional desires or needs high levels of knowledge or skill in order to use behavioral principles and procedures to advantage. It is important that content and competency be developed not solely from a theoretical or provincial framework, but from the goals that the user wishes to meet (Brown, 1969).

However, to be a competent behavioral practitioner demands certain basic knowledge and skills. The ability to analyze behavior and develop treatment programs calls for an understanding of the principles of experimental psychology upon which behavior therapy is based. This knowledge allows for the development of more than a mere implementation of a technology. With this basic training, the behavioral practitioner can continue to learn through reading, workshops, and practical experience.

Because of the vast amount of knowledge that must be imparted by various disciplines, it is well worth considering the real importance of information before incorporating it into a training program. Also, theory and skill should complement each other. Wexler (1976) described a structure for teaching behavioral techniques that is being followed by many schools throughout the country. It consists of a major or basic core and an elective group. As one moves through to the elective group, one becomes more proficient as a behavioral specialist. The proficiency or expertise may be developed in a particular area as, for example, assessment procedures or a certain type of behavioral intervention. This seems to be an economical way of developing behavioral practitioners.

Although there is currently no agreement on what should be offered in the three tracks, consideration should be given to the *alloted teaching time*, the *overall structure of the professional school*, and the *goals of teaching* (Wexler, 1970). It is expected that a greater amount of teaching time would be allotted to the development of the techniques that will be used most frequently by the practitioner, will facilitate his/her work, and will help to advance the profession or to contribute to the overall care and treatment of the patient. Wexler suggested a cost–benefit ratio to determine inclusion.

The structure of the profession and the particular training program will also influence what is offered in behavior therapy. Learning principles, the application of the experimental analysis of behavior, and simple treatment techniques are most appropriate in the basic training courses. In specialized or advanced programs, more complicated treatments or in-depth training would be expected.

The goals of training will reflect the interests and the biases of those teaching as well as the assumptions of the trainee on how to best utilize his/her education. Nurses, with frequent access to patients and their families, might benefit from training in such techniques as modeling, parent training, contingency contracting with families, and reinforcement procedures (Hahn & Dolan, 1970; Hecht, 1970; Putt, 1970).

The behaviorally competent health professional must be able to *observe* events (behavioral, environmental, physiological), *analyze* them into their components, and *conceptualize their relevance within a behavioral framework*. Clinical data must be identified, collected, and interpreted in a manner that facilitates the development of a meaningful treatment program for the patient. For example, Bigelow, Strickler, Liebson, and Griffiths (1976) used response cost to increase Antabuse intake compliance with 20 outpatient alcoholic males. A compliance check was done by supplying each patient with packs of sequential pills, some of which contained an additive that caused the urine to become orange. The patients recorded the time of urine color change, and this color change was assessed against a scheduled program upon clinic visits. In this instance, behavioral and pharmacological procedures complemented one another.

TRAINING MODELS

Certain training procedures, information, and problems are important in behavioral medicine. A listing of these elements is presented in Table 1. In the spirit of empiricism, we present these items as a tentative listing that can be modified in accordance with training needs and the results of comparative outcome research on training methods.

Basic Core

Learning Theory

Behavior therapy developed out of the application of learning principles to the analysis and treatment of behavioral disorders (Brady, 1972). These basic learning principles form the core of training of the behaviorally competent practitioner.

Out of respondent conditioning research have come the concepts of *conditioned stimulus, unconditioned stimulus, conditioned response, extinction, generalization, gradients of generalization,* and *discrimination* (Birk, 1974).

While respondent conditioning deals with elicited responses, operant conditioning concerns itself with emitted behaviors and is therefore of special importance to the behavior of humans. Animal and human research in operant conditioning has provided principles that help us understand how behavior is acquired, maintained,

Table 1.   Outline of Training Topics

Basic core
  1. Learning theory
    a. Respondent conditioning
        Conditioned stimulus
        Unconditioned stimulus
        Conditioned response
        Extinction
        Generalization, gradients of generalization
        Discrimination
    b. Operant conditioning
        Reinforcement
        Punishment
        Schedules of reinforcement
        Stimulus control
  2. Behavior therapy
    a. Assessment and evaluation
        Observational techniques
        Recording of data
        Behavioral interview
        Functional analysis of behavior
        Targeting behaviors
        Use of schedules and scales
        Measurement of change
    b. Treatment
        Token economies
        Reinforcement
        Punishment
        Premack principles
        Response cost
        Systematic relaxation
        Self-observation
        Self-control techniques
        Fading procedures
        Follow-up
  3. Research
    a. Critical use of literature
    b. Use of single-case designs
Advanced training
  Above topics are studied in greater depth or in a specialized
  manner.

---

and modified. *Reinforcement, punishment, schedules of reinforcement*, and *stimulus control* are some of the principles about which the trainee should become knowledgeable. Excellent books (Bandura, 1969; Franks, 1969; Kanfer & Phillips, 1970; Meichenbaum, 1977; Ullman & Krasner, 1965) are available that clearly explain these principles and demonstrate their applicability to treatment.

    The goals of teaching learning theory should be to assist the students in understanding and applying treatment and to enable them to read the technical literature in a critical manner.

Behavior Therapy

It is quite necessary that the trainee understand the theoretical difference between traditional psychotherapy and behavior therapy. In dealing with general health providers, one often hears of attempts to understand the psychological components of the physical disorders they treat. These attempts usually take the form of describing these components in traditional terms (denial, death wish, need for insight, willingness to change, etc.). Unfortunately, these labels and the resulting treatment are seldom useful. The student must learn to conceptualize problems in a behavioral manner before she/he can be an effective behavioral practitioner.

It is also important that the integration between assessment and treatment be fully understood. *Assessment* is an active process that is conducted throughout the course of behavior therapy; it is not simply confined to the initial stage. Some of the data that influence the assessment are the patient's *behavioral repertoire* (the behavioral manifestations of the physical disease or disorder, for example, speech dysfluencies in a stroke patient); *reinforcement history* (what is reinforcing and thus maintaining the problem behavior, for example, nurses and family members responding inappropriately to the pointing and grunting requests of the dysfluent patient); the importance of *controlling stimuli* in the patient's physical and social environment (the individuals and conditions that elicit positive and negative responses pertaining to the presenting problem); and the *limitations* within which patient and health providers must operate (the physical, sociological, moral, psychological limitations, for example, course of illness and treatment available) (Kanfer & Saslow, 1965).

Behavioral assessment is a crucial part of behavior therapy. Behavioral analysis was developed in reaction to and as an alternative to conventional psychiatric diagnosis. Behaviorists consider conventional diagnosis unreliable, inconsistent, inaccurate in predicting appropriate treatment and diagnosis, and premature when one considers the state of knowledge of normal and abnormal human behavior (Kanfer & Saslow, 1965; Zigler & Phillips, 1961). Furthermore, under traditional diagnosis, behavioral manifestations of physical disease and disorders are forced to fit categories of abnormal behavior, which proved undesirable in two ways. First, in labeling the behavior of a physically ill individual as neurotic or psychotic, it excluded from study and treatment the interactional effects of physical disease and disorders on a wide range of human behavior. Second, it left a large group of health providers to their own devices in explaining and "treating" problems associated with physical disease.

The experimental analysis of behavior is the fundamental evaluative device of the behavioral practitioner. The effectiveness of the treatment program rests on the accuracy and completeness of the analysis. The analysis, in turn, is dependent on the accurate observation and reporting of previously defined target behaviors. Like the approach to the treatment of physical problems, the behavioral approach, in limiting itself to the presenting problem, is often able to assess and treat in a straightforward manner.

Training medically oriented personnel in behavioral assessment is in keeping with their previous medical education, which used diagnosis as a step in the provision of treatment. Therefore, training in behavioral data collection can be associated easily with medical data collection (e.g., temperature, blood pressure, chemistry levels). The behavioral focus on antecedent and consequent behaviors would be well understood by trainees who look for medical signs in a similar manner.

Behavioral data collection differs from traditional approaches both in scope and in assignment of importance. That is, where as psychiatric diagnosis depends chiefly on interview and past history, behavioral assessment also includes structured and unstructured observations with family, friends, and staff members; physical and psychological testing; and the use of schedules and rating scales. However, the behavioral approach assigns more importance to information that is observable and able to be measured and replicated. As in general medicine, unless one can observe a phenomenon, one cannot measure change and so be sure of what is being treated. Also, unless a phenomenon occurs more than once, treatment is not meaningful.

The basic core of training should allow for didactic and practical experience in several methods of collecting data. It should include the *behavioral interview*, which attempts a determination of the behavioral *excesses*, *deficits*, and *assets* pertinent to the presenting problem. It should also include training in methods of *observing* and *rating* behavior, the use of *reliability checks*, *targeting behaviors*, simple *schedules*, and *tests*, as well as the use of *physical*, *psychological*, and *sociological* data.

Students may feel overwhelmed by the seemingly vast amount of information required for a behavioral analysis. Their fears should be allayed by the fact that such an analysis leads naturally into specification of treatment techniques. For instance, an individual who, upon assessment, shows pain in some situations but not in others is in need of treatment in only certain situations. Behavioral assessment may also indicate that the patient unknowingly uses pain-reducing procedures only within certain given contexts. Treatment, then, may consist of extending to other situations the procedures already defined in assessment. In this way, assessment not only defines the problem but suggests treatment that is essentially nonintrusive for the individual, because it is already being used, albeit in too limited a manner.

Behavioral assessment and therapy have only recently been extrapolated to the medical setting. Their continued use is limited only by the practitioner's ability and willingness to implement them.

Treatment

Inclusion of *treatment techniques* in a basic training program should be based on ease of applicability and broad potential for use. The appropriate use of some techniques requires broader, more sophisticated training. Certain techniques are becoming standard in behavior therapy, and their inclusion is essential. These include simple *reinforcement* programs, punishment techniques such as *time-out procedures*, *self-monitoring*, which is as much a treatment as an assessment procedure (Blanchard, 1975), *token economy systems*, *self-control techniques*, *progressive relaxation*, *stress innoculation*, *thought stopping*, *response cost*, *modeling*, *practice* and *feedback*, and *systematic training to criteria*. Training should include methods of selecting treatment techniques based on the goals and objectives that have been defined for therapy (Agras, 1972; Wolpe, 1969; Yates, 1970).

The student should be given practical training in the use of these techniques. This training should include use not only in controlled situations but also in the clinical setting under supervision. Such training allows the student to gain confidence in the real-life setting, where all variables cannot be controlled.

Earlier, we discussed resistance to behavior therapy that is based on the mistaken view that the patient's rights are abused through behavioral manipulation. The current trend toward the use of self-control techniques speaks to this objection (Mahoney & Thoresen, 1974). Here, the patient is initially made partner in his/her own treatment and is even provided with the knowledge and skills needed for self-treatment (Mastria, Robertson, & Sanders, 1977). This approach not only avoids the problem of abuse of the patient's rights but, in a more positive vein, it frees the health provider's time after initial assessment and training of the patient. The health provider then acts as a consultant and troubleshooter for the patient.

Of course, not all patients and problems lend themselves to the use of this method, but, given appropriate training, we are beginning to see more applications than were once expected. For example, children and individuals with limited resources and skills have been trained in self-control techniques with good results (Mahoney & Thoresen, 1974).

The proper use of referral mechanisms is another important part of treatment. When and to whom to refer for treatment of which the primary practitioner does not feel capable are an important and often neglected part of training. How the patient is prepared, how the consultee and the consultant work together, and how treatment is designed to fit into the overall program are all considerations in the referral process.

Follow-Up

It has been found that systematic *follow-up* treatment sessions are important in prolonging the use and the effect of behavioral techniques taught to patients. Spacing appointments gradually farther apart allows the patient to assume greater responsibility for his/her own treatment and allows the therapist to judge the patient's ability to continue changes independently of therapeutic contact. Trainees should be taught how to use follow-up sessions for giving patients more responsibility and for booster treatments.

Research

Behavior therapy is fundamentally distinguishable from other therapeutic efforts by one mark only: *The application of the experimental method to the understanding and modification of abnormalities of behavior.* There can be little doubt that, if this aim is lost sight of, behavior therapy will rapidly degenerate into just another "school" impervious to and resentful of criticism. The present writer hopes that this will not happen, but is by no means sure that it can be avoided. (Yates, 1970, p. 420).

Yates has offered the major rationale for including research as an integral part of the training of the behaviorally competent health provider. Behavior therapy *is* the experimental method. Its assessment calls for the measurement of change, not only in the laboratory setting but also clinically as a check on the effectiveness and efficiency of treatment. If research methodology is not presented adequately, the training program has missed one of its major purposes. We believe this is especially so in the newly developing field of behavioral medicine. Research methodology allows one to understand the development of treatment techniques, to assess the appropriateness of their application to a problem, and to help promote the use of behavior therapy in new areas. Such training also gives a broader perspective to the health provider. It allows for greater understanding of behavior therapy, greater competence as a behaviorist, and greater freedom to attempt treatments that are clinically sound but as yet untried.

As in the areas of assessment and treatment, different levels of competence may be attained. Not everyone wishes or needs to be fully versed in research methodology. Again, the amount of training required is dependent upon ultimate use.

On a basic level, it is extremely important that the trainee learn to use the *literature* correctly. That is, he/she must be able to read studies critically in order to determine those that are methodologically sound. The student must be shown the importance of such critical reading, for after formal training, he/she must look to the journals for guidance in the use of treatment techniques, both old and new.

The understanding and use of research designs is another important aspect of training. The *single-case design* is the fundamental approach suitable both to the researcher and to the clinician. It is appropriate to any patient and any disorder that presents itself. "It enables him [the practitioner] to deal with the client as an individual rather than as a member of a class, while at the same time providing for a rigorous rather than an intuitive approach" (Yates, 1976, p. 303).

Training components should include identification of appropriate measures (self-report, behavioral, psychological); procedures for carrying out single-case research (taking baseline, length of phases, evaluation of irreversible procedures); and use of various designs (Hersen & Barlow, 1976).

Demonstration and practical experience are the primary vehicles for the teaching of research skills. The use of animals to demonstrate the various principles and procedures allows trainees to view clearly what is occurring. Practical experience with children and adults, however, seems more economical and in keeping with the goal of direct relevancy in training. Experience in research also helps the trainee to become more astute in reading technical reports.

To summarize, there are certain areas that must be covered in a training program such as the one we describe. They are principles of learning theory, behavioral assessment and therapy, and application of research techniques. We have presented what we believe to be the minimum basic knowledge and skill needed to define a health care practitioner as behaviorally competent.

Advanced Training

After attaining competence in the basic core, some health providers will wish to reach greater proficiency in a particular area of behavior therapy. Special and elective training will meet the needs of such individuals.

Advanced training allows the trainee to spend an intensive period of time on one area of treatment or research. Elective courses enable the trainee to round out the basic training program with work in areas of a particular field or specialty. Just as traditional psychotherapy has offered diagnostic consultation and specialized treatment, so it is appropriate to offer these in the behavioral framework. Psychiatric diagnosis becomes behavioral assessment, consultation may be broadened to include training of patients and staff, and specialized treatment may consist of clinics for the treatment of disorders such as pain, sleep disturbances, anxiety associated with surgery or dental treatment, substance abuse, and rehabilitation of stroke and spinal cord injuries or the use of particular techniques such as systematic desensitization, self-control techniques, and biofeedback.

Advanced training and electives in laboratory and clinical research may center on any of the three areas: learning theory, behavioral assessment and treatment techniques, or research methodology. Given the recent applications of behavior therapy to medicine, there is a great need for research in all of these areas. Behavioral medicine lends itself nicely to certain research areas. These especially include compliance with medical regimens, the prevention of disease and disorders, behavioral pharmacology, the application of behavioral techniques to the modification of physiological functioning, clinical comparison of behavioral techniques and alternative treatments, and comparison of the effects of different behavioral techniques on the same problem (Brady, 1972).

Guidelines to Teaching

The behavioral approach lends itself to various training models. Of major consideration in the development of training models are the goals and objectives for which particular behaviors are taught. These will change somewhat according to the professional group being insructed and the setting to which the training will be applied. However, certain objectives will remain constant. One of these is the development of the appropriate need, attitude, and willingness to use the behavioral approach together with the primary skills (for example, nursing skills) of the practitioners. This goal can be reached in two ways. First, it can be addressed directly, using lectures and demonstrations to illustrate the applicability of behavior therapy to physical disease and disorders. Second, it can permeate the entire structure of the training program. Teaching students how behavior therapy is made to fit in as unobtrusively as possible, how it allows the health provider to be more effective and efficient in his/her major work, and how it promotes better patient care will cause trainees to develop a positive attitude and a willingness to continue its use.

The guidelines (Table 2) for teaching behavioral medicine are predicated on the use to which the practitioner will put his/her new training. The guiding questions

Table 2.   Guidelines to Teaching Behavioral Medicine

1. Setting
   a. What patient population is available?
   b. Does training originate from a separate department or division, is it incorporated into other departments, or is a dual approach used?
2. Trainees
   a. Will professional groups be taught together or separately?
   b. Are the trainees in professional school, in-service training, or continuing education?
3. Faculty
   a. What is/are the primary discipline(s) of the behavioral faculty?
   b. Is there a professional balance among the faculty?
4. Time allotment
   a. Does the training material meet the criteria for inclusion: efficiency, effectiveness, and utility?
   b. Is the course integrated into the overall curriculum?
5. Training techniques
   a. Is evaluation built into the training program?
   b. Are various procedures, including behavioral tests, used in evaluation?
6. Evaluation
   a. Is evaluation built into the training program?
   b. Are various procedures, including behavioral tests, used in evaluation?

are: What does the health provider do? How can he/she do it better? What should he/she know? (Agras, 1971; Armstrong & Bakker, 1976; Wexler, 1976). Each health care provider group is trained to offer a particular type of service. Therefore, while the behavioral principles and skills will be the same, they may be used in diverse ways, depending on the needs of the practitioner. An illustration is the case of a child brought to the hospital under emergency conditions. Fearful of the new environment, unfamiliar faces, and painful bodily sensations, the child cries and refuses to cooperate in the physical examination. The parents, distressed by the situation and feeling powerless to help, react much as their child, crying, distracted, and giving little useful information. The nurse may use his/her behavioral skills to assess the parents' and child's behavior and apply interventions aimed at calming them, allowing them to be more cooperative, and thus enabling them to receive better care. The physician might use the same behavioral process in a slightly different channel but to the same end, that of better care. The nurse and the physician might act as models of calmness for the parents to emulate; the parents can then help calm their child, in turn acting as models. Other techniques are also appropriate, such as shaping and reinforcing appropriate behavior, time out for inappropriate behavior, and the use of information, trial runs, and distraction procedures before performing a painful test.

Other considerations in developing training models for behavioral medicine include (1) the setting in which it is taught; (2) the group composition of the trainees;

(3) the faculty responsible for training; (4) the time allotment; (5) the training techniques used; and (6) evaluation procedures (Table 2).

Setting

The general training hospital offers opportunities for the application of learning principles and behavioral techniques for use with a great number of diseases and disorders. Within the hospital, training may originate from a department or division separate from other departments, may be incorporated into other departments, or may use a combination of both. There are positive and negative aspects in each. A separate department or division allows for greater autonomy but also gives an artificial separation of behavior therapy from the areas with which it seeks to become involved.

Incorporation into various departments allows behavior therapy to be seen as a necessary adjunct to the delivery of the primary service of a particular department. However, there is a real danger that it may be taught in a diluted manner and by instructors who are not thoroughly knowledgeable about the area.

Trainees

Programs may be arranged to train professional groups individually or together. Although groups trained individually (nursing groups, psychology groups, dental groups, etc.) may be allowed more time to develop ways in which behavior therapy can best be utilized to advance their particular work, they do lose the opportunity to develop an understanding of the work of other professional groups, to explore various ways of working together, and to exchange knowledge and information. Training programs in behavioral medicine may offer a unique opportunity to accomplish the goals of interdisciplinary education.

Brief mention must also be made of professionals who wish to learn these techniques through in-service or continuing education courses. This group poses an especially rewarding challenge because their motivation is often based on an awareness that their jobs could be made more fruitful if they had the means to deliver better care. They usually come into training with a wealth of situations that may be useful in explaining and demonstrating behavior theory and practice. A training model for this group is presented later.

Faculty

Although increasing numbers of psychiatrists and social workers are receiving behavioral training, at this time most professionally trained behaviorists are psychologists. Psychologists are also evident in leadership roles in the field of behavioral medicine. Therefore, psychologists will likely constitute the bulk of faculty members in this training field. However, since their training is not medical (although most of them have obtained formal and informal training in certain aspects of medicine), it is important that the training staff be composed of members of other disciplines who have also received some behavioral training. Additional personnel might include a nurse and a physician (a family practitioner or an internist would be a good choice for a generalist). Other appropriate specialists might be dentists, dieticians, speech therapists, and physical therapists.

Time Allotment

The amount of information and skills presented in professional programs is becoming greater each year. Consequently, schools are beginning to realize that beyond basic core courses, electives and specialty courses must be offered. Information and skills presented in electives such as behavioral medicine must be chosen carefully in order to utilize time allowances most effectively.

Brown's (1969) dilemma, making social sciences more visible to the beginning student of health care, is no less important to the advancement of behavioral medicine. By allotting time throughout the course of the student's training, it is more likely that behavior therapy will be seen as an integral and necessary part of training rather than as an addition.

Training Techniques

A combination of procedures is needed to present the three areas (learning theory, behavioral assessment and therapy, and research). Lectures, readings, seminars, and discussion groups are good ways to present didactic material. Demonstrations, audiovisual techniques, projects, supervised practice, and the mentor system, which is especially popular in medical schools, allow trainees to observe and gain experience in using behavioral assessment and treatment.

Of course, the use of behavioral techniques to teach behavior therapy is urged because (1) it is functional; (2) it allows students to gain the patient's perspective; and (3) it helps students develop the appropriate attitudes toward the use of behavior therapy. Armstrong and Bakker (1976) described the use of behavioral techniques in teaching a six-week course at the first-year level in medical school. It was an ambitious course that used a three-step program to develop the behavior change strategy that these authors termed "PRI/TTA" (Pinpoint, Record, Intervent/Try, Try, Again)" (p. 759). They reported positive results in accomplishing their teaching goals. It is hoped that a follow-up report will be done to determine the extent to which these students have used their training in patient care.

Evaluation

Program assessment is necessary for upgrading the training program, and a combination of procedures will give more complete information. The following suggestions are offered: first, *paper* and *pencil* or *oral tests* may be used to determine if students have grasped the facts and information presented; second, *behavioral tests* may determine if students can actually use the assessment and therapy techniques that were taught; third, *student feedback* concerning various aspects of the course will provide invaluable information; fourth, *patient feedback* concerning students' handling of various aspects of the presenting problem should provide information not readily available otherwise; fifth, to complete the evaluation, *follow-up assessment* after varying time periods may be used to determine (a) what techniques continue to be used in practice; (b) which aspects of training students found especially useful and which ones proved of lesser value; and (c) suggestions for inclusion in future courses.

The criticism of "irrelevance" that has been leveled at much of psychology and psychiatry in the medical setting may be bypassed if we continue to be sensitive to the needs of practitioners and the realities of their circumstances. Course evaluation provides one way of accomplishing this goal.

Below we describe models for training health providers to be behaviorally competent. We have attempted to develop these models along the lines of existing programs, on the assumption that what is more familiar has a greater likelihood of being put to use. We have also, however, attempted to tailor the models to the behavioral mold, since the program should be the best advertisement for the use of behavior therapy in the medical setting.

MODELS FOR TRAINING

Model I

The first model is a basic one that may be incorporated into the training program of the specialty school (e.g., nursing, dental, and medical schools). Trainees would be students already enrolled in the specialty school. The goal of this model is to make training an integral part of the overall training program.

4–6 Hours
A. Learning Theory

Procedure: Lectures, reading, demonstrations of basic learning theory.
Goals: Students are given an understanding of the rationale behind the behavioral techniques that they will later learn to use.
Content: Basic principles of respondent and operant conditioning.
Evaluation: By written and oral tests.

35– 45 Hours
B. Behavior Therapy

1 Hour:
    1. Overview of Section
       Ethical considerations; the practitioner–patient relationship.
       Behavior therapy in the general medical setting.
Procedure: Lectures, small-group discussion.
Goals: To assist students in developing correct attitude and to "think behaviorally."

Content: Description of section and examples of its utility. Ethical concerns,
              including patient rights, question of control, humane treatment.
Evaluation: Through oral probes during discussion.

4 Hours:
    2. Assessment
Procedure: Lectures, readings, demonstrations, practice.
Goals: To develop skills in behavioral assessment.
Content: Experimental analysis of behavior; data collection; analysis of
              antecedent and consequent behaviors; observing, recording measure-
              ment; graphing behavior; reliability; validity.
Evaluation: By having trainees carry out and criticize several assessments.

30– 40 Hours:
    3. Behavioral Treatment Techniques
Procedure: Clinical practice, mentor system, staffings, readings.
Goal: To develop skills in behavioral treatment techniques; gain experience
              in using techniques with general medicine patients; be able to evaluate
              effectiveness of treatment.
Content: Use of reinforcement, punishment (as time out), progressive relaxa-
              tion, thought stopping, response cost, contingency contracting, model-
              ing, fading, and shaping procedures in the following areas: compliance
              with medical regimens; pain and the negative affects such as anxiety
              and depression as they affect the course of physical disease and
              disorders (Wexler, 1976); treatment of children; substance abuse such
              as obesity, alcoholism, smoking; sexual dysfunctions; inpatient and
              outpatient setting is desirable.
Evaluation: By observing and behavioral ratings of trainees, critique of written
              treatment plans and progress notes.

8–10 Hours
C. *Clinical Evaluation and Research*

Procedure: Lectures, reading, demonstrations, practica.
Goals: To learn to read the literature in a critical manner; use single-case
              designs; and evaluate clinical treatment.
Content: Use of multiple-baseline, reversal designs; review and critique of litera-
              ture.
Evaluation: Trainees will critique studies; carry out clinical research.

5–10 Hours
D. *Related Core Topics*

Procedure: Lectures, reading, mentor system, special projects.
Goals: To integrate behavior therapy into the medical setting.
Content: Psychopharmacology; neuropsychology; behavior genetics; collection
              and inclusion of medical data in functional behavioral analysis;
              behavior therapy in health care delivery to special groups; behavior

therapy in prevention; behavior therapy in special areas of health care (e.g., specific nursing problems; pediatrics; urology; obstetrics; dentistry; rehabilitation; medicine; medical research).

Evaluation: By behavioral ratings and fulfillment of special requirements such as projects.

Time Arranged
E. Specialized Courses

Procedure: Readings, mentor system, practica, small groups.

Goals: To gain knowledge and skill in areas that are not a part of the basic core or to gain a greater depth of knowledge and skill in areas that were taught in the basic core.

Content: Arranged according to interest and need. Intensive courses in particular treatment techniques (systematic desensitization; sexual dysfunction; etc.) or in application to particular areas of the health field (health care delivery to rural or urban populations; risk factors and prevention; rehabilitation nursing and physical therapy); research in these areas. All are appropriate after the basic core has been fulfilled.

Evaluation: By behavioral ratings, fulfillment of special requirements such as projects, publications.

Model II

The second model relies heavily on the practicing health care provider's feeling a need for techniques for better health care delivery. It uses the traditional consultation service provided by every hospital department. Control is obtained by formalizing the program to offer in-service or continuing education credit to trainees. The offering of credit has been adapted from the work of Canter and Paulson (1974), who used a college credit model of in-school consultation to train grade-school teachers in the use of behavioral intervention techniques. This is an effective way of offering behavioral knowledge and skills to the large group of practitioners who received their training prior to the introduction of behavior therapy.

Procedure: Trainees are expected to present ongoing problems, which they will analyze and for which they will develop treatment plans. Instructors present learning theory as it pertains to behavioral assessment, treatment, and evaluation. Small-group instruction seems ideal for this model. Case presentation can vary, and trainees may wish to work together on projects. Readings and the mentor system also seem suitable.

Goals: The goals of this model are similar to though less ambitious than those of Model I. Learning theory, behavioral assessment and treatment, and the experimental procedure are taught in the context of the consultation case.

Content: Although cases will vary according to the professional specialties
              represented in the training, an effort should be made to cover each
              area of the basic core (learning theory, behavior therapy, research
              procedure) in each presentation.
Evaluation: By case presentations by trainees; behavioral observations of trainees
              in practical situations; critiques of functional behavioral analyses,
              treatment plans, and progress notes.

Below is an example of the *credit consultation model* presented above in which
practitioners from various aspects of rehabilitation medicine are being trained in
behavioral techniques and treatment.

Presenting Problem

The speech pathologist presents the case of a 50-year-old male stroke patient
hospitalized three weeks prior to consultation. The patient has no expressive speech
and limited receptive speech. He and his wife, both of the upper-middle-socioeco-
nomic level, have been demanding on the entire staff. Total treatment has therefore
been difficult, and speech therapy has particularly suffered because the patient's wife
insists that her husband's wishes be anticipated and that he must not be made to
attempt "what he simply cannot do." Prior attempts to solve the problems consisted
of the social worker's explaining the situation and empathizing with the wife; the
physician's threatening to suspend visitation rights or to discharge the patient; the
staff's ignoring as much as possible both husband and wife; and the speech
therapist's attempting to transfer the patient to another therapist.

This case lends itself very well to use as a training example. Ethical considerations, the inadvertant reinforcement of inappropriate behaviors, and the contributions of behavior therapy to medical care all find a place in small-group discussion
of this problem. *Step 1* also sets the stage for the development of a positive attitude
toward the use of behavior therapy in the medical setting in that a frustrating problem
is analyzed and steps are outlined to resolve it.

Step 2 is a description, in learning principles, of the process that has been
occurring between patient and staff.

Step 3 presents the functional behavioral analysis and allows the trainees
experience in collecting data; identifying target behaviors; and observing, measuring,
and recording behavior.

Step 4 entails choosing treatment techniques, implementing them, and measuring outcome. The trainees will also use the literature and set up appropriate designs.

One would expect this training model to produce positive results not only
because of the continuing credits offered for completing the program, but also
because trainees come into the course with problem situations that they themselves
have labled as important to solve. They may be skeptical of the means presented
(i.e., the behavioral approach), but unlike many students still in professional training, they are acutely aware that technology alone cannot produce the best health
care delivery. Many trainees have devised their own methods of coping: the patient
who continues to overeat is reprimanded, the young couple experiencing sexual prob-

lems are advised to "relax and wait," and the dying patient is given misinformation or, often, simply avoided. The general practitioner has not had guidance in handling such problems and has had to rely on his/her own resources. At times, results have been good; at other times, they have hindered treatment. For all these reasons, the already-practicing health care provider is a gratifying trainee.

FUTURE TRENDS

Training will take new forms as we begin to collect data on procedural efficacy and as other disciplines begin to be included in the training process. The specialist in behavioral medicine will act as consultant and educator to the general medical staff and as primary care giver. In turn, the medical staff will share their skills and knowledge with the behavioral medicine specialist. Problem solving and cognitive strategies will probably also see more use both in training and in treatment.

CONCLUDING REMARKS

Specialization has probably seen its limits; the pendulum has begun to swing back to the more fully rounded practitioner. This trend comes at a fortunate time for behavior therapy; techniques are now available that can address problems that have long been of concern in medicine (compliance problems; the effects of emotion on the body; pain; sexual dysfunctions; prevention; etc.). As more professionals become familiar with the theory and techniques of behavior therapy, we expect to find its use expanded.

SUMMARY

Interest in behavioral medicine has become intense over the past year. General hospitals and clinics are seeking behavioral medicine specialists to treat patients, train staff, and consult. The need for models for training in behavioral medicine is immediate. In this chapter, we have begun to address the need by presenting issues pertinent to behavioral competency and models for training practitioners in the use of behavior therapy.

The behaviorally competent practitioner is one who is capable of assessing a problem and applying behavioral treatment in a systematic, quantifiable manner. The setting and problems may be changed somewhat—for example, treatment of a seizure disorder on an inpatient medicine service—but the principles and procedures remain essentially the same.

Bringing behavior therapy into closer union with medical treatment and issues is a means of dealing with problems that have been resistant to solution. Problems such as patient compliance have lately been approached behaviorally and with good results. Indeed, behavioral medicine does seem "an idea whose time has come" (Blanchard, 1977, p. 2).

REFERENCES

Agras, W. S. The role of behavior therapy in teaching medical students. *Journal of Behavior Therapy and Experimental Psychiatry*, 1971, *2*, 219–221.

Agras, W. S. *Behavior modification: Principles and clinical applications*. Boston: Little, Brown, 1972.

Agras, W. S. Foreword. In R. C. Katz & S. Zlutnick (Eds.). *Behavior therapy and health care: Principles and applications*. New York: Pergamon, 1975.

Aiken, L. M. Patient problems are problems in learning. *American Journal of Nursing*, 1970, *70*, 1916–1918.

American Psychological Association. *Ethical standards of psychologists*. Washington, D.C.: Author, 1953.

Andrews, J. M. Neuromuscular re-education of hemiplegia with aid of electromyograph. *Archives of Physical Medicine and Rehabilitation*, 1964, *45*, 530–532.

Armstrong, H. E., & Bakker, C. B. Behavioral self-analysis in the medical curriculum. *Journal of Medical Education*, 1976, *51*, 758–762.

Ayllon, T., & Michael, J. The psychiatric nurse as a behavioral engineer. *Journal of the Experimental Analysis of Behavior*, 1959, *2*, 323–334.

Bandura, A. *Principles of behavior modification*, New York: Holt, Rinehart, & Winston, 1969.

Barnard, K. Teaching the retarded child is a family affair. *American Journal of Nursing*, 1968, *68*, 305–311.

Benassi, V., & Lanson, R. A survey of the teaching of behavior modification in colleges and universities. *American Psychologist*, 1972, *27*, 1063–1969.

Bigelow, G., Strickler, D., Liebson, I., & Griffiths, R. Maintaining disulfiram ingestion among the out-patient alcoholics: A security-deposit contingency contracting procedure. *Behavior Research and Therapy*, 1976, *14*, 378–381.

Birk, L. (Chair). *Behavior therapy in psychiatry. A report of the American Psychiatric Association on behavior therapy*. New York: Aronson, 1974.

Blanchard, E. B. Behavioral medicine: A perspective. In R. B. Williams & W. D. Gentry (Eds.), *Behavioral approaches to medical treatment*. Cambridge, Mass.: Ballinger, 1977.

Bonica, J. J. (Ed.). *The management of pain* (2nd ed.). Philadelphia: Lea & Fehiger, 1975.

Borkovec, T. D. Insomnia. In R. B. Williams & W. D. Gentry (Eds.), *Behavioral approaches to medical treatment*. Cambridge, Mass.: Ballinger, 1977.

Brady, J. P. Behavior therapy: Origins and opportunities. *Career Directions*, 1971, *2*, 125–133.

Brady, J. P. Research and training needs in behavior therapy. *Seminars in Psychiatry*, 1972, *4*(2), 185–190.

Brady, J. P. The place of behavior therapy in medical student and psychiatric resident training. *Journal of Nervous and Mental Diseases*, 1973, *157*, 21–26.

Brown, J. H. U. Behavioral science and the medical school. *Science*, 1969, *163*, 964–967.

Burnet, F. M. The role of the behavioral sciences in medicine: Introduction. *Medical Journal of Australia*, 1969, *2*, 33–35.

Cameron, S. N., & Schmauk, F. J. An undergraduate course in behavior modification. *Psychological Reports*, 1977, *40*, 159–164.

Canter, L., & Paulson, T. A college credit model for inschool consultation: A functional behavioral training program. *Community Mental Health Journal*, 1974, *10*, 268–275.

Clark, F. W., Evans, D. R., & Hamerlynck, L. A. (Eds.). *Implementing behavioral programs for schools and clinics*. Champaign, Ill.: Research, 1972.

Cole, P., & Emmanuel, S. Drug consultation: Its significance to the discharged hospital patient and its relevance as a role for the pharmacist. *American Journal of Hospital Pharmacy,* 1971, *28,* 954–960.

Davidson, P. O., & Costello, C. G. *N = 1: Experimental studies of single cases.* New York: Van Nostrand Reinhold, 1969.

Davidson, G., Goldfried, M., & Krasner, L. A postdoctoral program in behavior modification: Theory and practice. *American Psychologist,* 1970, *25,* 767–772.

Dixon, W. M., Stradling, P., & Wooton, I. Outpatient P.A.S. therapy. *Lancet,* 1957, *2,* 871–872.

Earley, L. W. (Chair). *Teaching psychiatry in medical school.* Washington, D.C.: American Psychiatric Association, 1969.

Epstein, L., & Cincirpini, P. Behavioral medicine III. *Association for the Advancement of Behavior Therapy Newsletter,* 1977, *4*(5), 7–9, 27.

Epstein, L., & Masek, B. J. Behavioral control of medicine compliance. *Journal of Applied Behavioral Analysis,* 1978, *11,* 1–9.

Fink, R., Shapiro, S., & Lewison, J. The reluctant participant in a breast cancer screening program. *Public Health Reports,* 1968, *83,* 479–484.

Fordyce, W. E. *Behavioral methods for chronic pain and illness.* St. Louis: Mosby, 1976.

Franks, C. M. (Ed.). *Behavior therapy: Appraisal and status.* New York: McGraw-Hill, 1969.

Gelfand, S. A behavior modification training program for psychiatric residents. *Journal of Behavior Therapy and Experimental Psychiatry,* 1972, *3,* 147–151.

Goldstein, M. K., Stein, G. H., Smolen, D. M., & Perlini, W. S. Bio-behavioral monitoring: A method for remote health measurement. *Archives of Physical Medicine and Rehabilitation,* 1976, *57,* 253–258.

Grout, R., & Watkins, J. The nurse and health education. *International Nursing Review,* 1971, *18,* 248–257.

Guze, S., Matarazzo, J., & Saslow, G. A formulation of principles of comprehensive medicine with a special preference to learning theory. *Journal of Clinical Psychology,* 1953, *9,* 127–136.

Hahn, A., & Dolan, N. After coronary care—Then what? *American Journal of Nursing,* 1970, *70,* 2350–2352.

Hecht, A. B. Self medication, inaccuracy, and what can be done. *Nursing Outlook,* 1970, *18,* 30–31.

Hersen, M., & Barlow, D. H. *Single case experimental designs.* New York: Pergamon, 1976.

Hooper, D., & Roberts, J. Teaching behavioral science to medical students in some U.S. medical schools—A report. *Social Science and Medicine,* 1968, *2,* 217–219.

Horner, R. D. Establishing use of crutches by a mentally retarded spina bifida child. *Journal of Applied Behavior Analysis,* 1971, *4,* 183–191.

Ince, L. P. *PSRO charting: Behavior modification in rehabilitation medicine.* Springfield, Ill.: Charles C Thomas, 1976.

Kanfer, F. H., & Phillips, J. S. *Learning foundations of behavior therapy.* New York: Wiley, 1970.

Kanfer, F. H., & Saslow, G. Behavioral analysis: An alternative to diagnostic classification. *Archives of General Psychiatry,* 1965, *12,* 529–538.

Kanfer, F. H., & Saslow G. Behavioral diagnosis. In C. M. Franks (Ed.), *Behavior therapy: Appraisal and status.* New York: McGraw-Hill, 1969.

Katz, R., & Zlutnick, S. *Behavior therapy and health care: Principles and applications.* New York: Pergamon, 1975.

LeBow, M. D. Applications of behavior modification in nursing practice. In M. Hersen, R. Eisler, & P. Miller (Eds.), *Progress in behavior modification,* Vol. 2. New York: Academic, 1976.

Levene, H., Breger, L., & Patterson, V. A training and research program in brief psychotherapy. *American Journal of Psychotherapy,* 1972, *26,* 90–100.

Lewis, D. J., Schriver, C. R., & MacDonald, N. R. A behavior, growth, and development course in first-year medicine. *Canadian Medical Association Journal,* 1969, *100,* 641–645.

Lidz, T., & Edelson, M. Towards schools of psychiatry. In T. Lidz & M. Edelson (Eds.), *Training tomorrow's psychiatrists.* New Haven: Yale University Press, 1970.

Linkewich, J. A., Catalano, R. B., & Flack, H. L. The effect of packaging and instructions on outpatient compliance with medication regimens. *Drug Intelligence and Clinical Pharmacy,* 1974, *8,* 10–15.

Mahoney, M. J., & Thoresen, C. E. *Self-control: Power to the person.* Monterey, Calif.: Brooks/Cole, 1974.

Mastria, M. A., & Hosford, R. H. *New and innovative trends in clinical psychology training throughout the United States.* Paper presented at the meeting of the American Psychological Association, Washington, D.C., September 1976.

Mastria, M. A., Robertson, S. J., & Sanders, S. H. *Controlled fluid intake training for end stage renal patients.* Paper presented at the meeting of the Association for the Advancement of Behavior Therapy, Atlanta, December 1977.

Maxmen, J. S. *The post-physician era: Medicine in the twenty-first century.* New York: Wiley, 1976.

Meichenbaum, D. *Cognitive-behavior modification.* New York: Plenum, 1977.

Melzack, R., & Chapman, C. Psychological aspects of pain. *Postgraduate Medicine,* 1973, *53,* 69–75.

Miller, P. M. The use of behavioral contracting in the treatment of alcoholism: A case study. *Behavior Therapy,* 1972, *3,* 593–596.

Miller, P. M., & Mastria, M. A. *Alternatives to alcohol abuse.* Champaign, Ill.: Research, 1977.

Moss, G. R., & Boren, J. J. Specifying criteria for the completion of psychiatric treatment: A behaviorist approach. *Archives of General Psychiatry,* 1974, *24,* 441–447.

Pasternack, S. B. Annual well-child visits. *American Journal of Nursing,* 1974, *74,* 1472–1475.

Patel, C. Reduction of serum cholesterol and blood pressure in hypertension patients by behavior modification. *Journal of the Royal College of General Practioners,* 1976, *26*(164), 211–215.

Putt, A. M. One experiment in nursing adults with peptic ulcers. *Nursing Research,* 1970, *19,* 484–494.

Ratliff, R. G., & Stein, N. H. Treatment of neurodermatitis by behavior therapy: A case study. *Behavior Research and Therapy,* 1968, *6,* 397–399.

Renne, C. M., & Creer, T. L. Training children with asthma to use inhalation therapy equipment. *Journal of Applied Behavior Analysis,* 1976, *9,* 1–12.

Roberts, A. H., Dinsdale, S. M., Matthews, R. E., & Cole, T. M. Modifying persistent undesirable behavior in a medical setting. *Archives of Physical Medicine and Rehabilitation,* 1969, *50,* 147–153.

Rubin, R. D., Brady, J. P., & Henderson, J. D. *Advances in behavior therapy,* Vol. 4. New York: Academic, 1976.

Sackett, D. L., & Haynes, R. B. (Eds.). *Compliance with therapeutic regimens.* Baltimore: Johns Hopkins University Press, 1976.

Scheflen, A. E. An analysis of a thought model which persists in psychiatry. *Psychosomatic Medicine,* 1958, *20,* 235–241.

Schwartz, M. M., & White, M. A. Motivating clinic patients. *Supervisor Nurse,* 1977, *8,* 48–49.

Shumway, S., & Powers, M. The group way to weight loss. *American Journal of Nursing,* 1973, *73,* 269–272.

Stern, R. S. The medical student as behavioral psychotherapist. *British Medical Journal,* 1975, *2,* 78–81.

Stuart, R. B. A three-dimensional program for the treatment of obesity. *Behavior Research and Therapy,* 1971, *9,* 177–186.

Ullman, L. P., & Krasner, L. *Case studies in behavior modification.* New York: Holt, Rinehart, & Winston, 1965.

Usdin, G. (Ed.). *Psychiatry: Education and image.* New York: Brunner/Mazel, 1973.

Wexler, M. Behavioral sciences in medical education. *Study for teaching behavioral sciences in medical schools—First year progress report.* Rockville, Md.: National Center for Health Services Research and Development. Rockville, Md.: Author, 1970.

Wexler, M. The behavioral sciences in medical education: A view from psychology. *American Psychologist,* 1976, *31,* 275–283.

Wiley, L. Coping with chronic complainers. *Nursing,* 1973, *3,* 12–14.

Wittkower, E. D., & Dudek, S. Z. Psychosomatic medicine: The mind–body–society interaction. In B. Wolman (Ed.), *Handbook of general psychology.* Englewood Cliffs, N.J.: Prentice-Hall, 1973.

Wolpe, J. *The practice of behavior therapy.* New York: Pergamon, 1969.

Yates, A. *Behavior therapy.* New York: Wiley, 1970.

Yates, A. Research methods in behavior modification: A comparative evaluation. In M. Hersen, R. Eisler, & P. Miller (Eds.), *Progress in behavior modification,* Vol. 2. New York: Academic, 1976.

Yen, S. *Survey of courses in behavior modification at higher learning institutions.* Paper presented at the meeting of the Association for the Advancement of Behavior Therapy, Washington, D.C., December 1971.

Zifferblatt, S. M. Increasing patient compliance through the applied analyis of behavior. *Preventive Medicine*, 1975, *4*, 173–182.

Zigler, E., & Phillips, L. Psychiatric diagnosis: A critique. *Journal of Abnormal and Social Psychology*, 1961, *63*, 607–618.

Zlutnick, S., Mayville, W. J., & Moffat, S. Modifications of seizure disorders: The interruption of behavioral chains. *Journal of Applied Behavior Analysis*, 1975, *8*, 1–12.

4

A Behavioral Conceptualization of Psychosomatic Illness: Psychosomatic Symptoms as Learned Responses

WILLIAM E. WHITEHEAD, AL. S. FEDORAVICIUS, BARRY BLACKWELL, AND SUSAN WOOLEY

INTRODUCTION

The purpose of this chapter is to review existing theories of etiology of psychosomatic disorders and to describe a theory of psychosomatic etiology based on learning theory. This task carries with it an obligation to define what is meant by *psychosomatic symptoms* or *psychosomatic disorders* because these terms have become controversial. Some writers have proposed that the term *psychosomatic* be applied to all illnesses, since susceptibility to and recovery from most illnesses seem to be influenced by psychological and social variables (Wolf & Goodell, 1976). Others have proposed that the term *psychosomatic* be dropped as useless (Lader, 1972) because it is both misleading and too inclusive. Many contemporary writers lump together under the term *psychosomatic* a variety of symptoms that have traditionally been distinguished, such as conversion reactions, hypochondriacal behaviors, somatopsychic disorders, and psychological disturbances produced directly by insult to or degenerative changes in the nervous system (e.g., Wright, 1977).

In this chapter, we do not take a position on what the boundaries of the term *psychosomatic* ought to be, but we arbitrarily limit our use of the term to symptoms

WILLIAM E. WHITEHEAD • Psychophysiology Laboratory, Departments of Psychiatry and Physical Medicine and Rehabilitation, University of Cincinnati, Cincinnati, Ohio 45267.   AL. S. FEDORAVICIUS • Psychology Service, Veterans Administration Hospital, Albuquerque, New Mexico 87108.   BARRY BLACKWELL • Department of Psychiatry, Wright State University School of Medicine, Dayton, Ohio 45324.   SUSAN WOOLEY • Department of Psychiatry, University of Cincinnati School of Medicine, Cincinnati, Ohio 45267. Preparation of this paper was supported in part by United States Public Health Services Training Grant MH08018.

that (1) are associated with abnormal physical changes in organs innervated by the autonomic nervous system and (2) are influenced by environmental events possessing psychological (i.e., symbolic) significance. Thus, we are maintaining the traditional distinction between psychosomatic symptoms such as peptic ulcer and hypertension, on the one hand, and conversion reactions involving musculoskeletal or sensory anomalies and hypochondriacal complaints such as chronic pain syndromes, on the other hand. We are also excluding the various somatopsychic syndromes in which psychological disturbances occur as a result of physiological changes that have nonpsychological causes (e.g., senility, toxic psychoses). This narrow definition of psychosomatic symptoms may turn out to be indefensible in the light of future research findings, but for the present, it permits us to focus on a set of questions that have been neglected by recent theorists. These questions deal with the extent to which pathological physical changes, as opposed to verbal somatic complaints, can be accounted for by a learning model.

Traditional Theories of Psychosomatic Etiology

The prevailing view of the etiology of psychosomatic disorders is that psychosomatic symptoms are the normal physiological sequelae of chronic emotional states (*Diagnostic and Statistical Manual of Mental Disorders*, 1968). These emotional states are chronic because they are unconscious or suppressed, and they are unconscious or suppressed, according to the most prevalent explanation (Alexander, 1950), because they derive from a conflict. Table 1, derived from Alexander, French, and Pollock (1968), illustrates the psychoanalytic theory of psychosomatic etiology. The importance of these conflicts is that they determine the nature of the emotion that is suppressed or rendered unconscious, and they account for the suppression or denial that results in the emotional state's being chronically present.

The specific emotion hypothesis proposed by Alexander and his colleagues is related to two other theories of psychosomatic etiology: the specific personality hypothesis proposed by Dunbar (1943) and later by Harold Wolff (1968) and the specific attitude hypothesis proposed by Graham (1972). Dunbar (1943) has suggested that there are specific personality traits associated with each psychosomatic symptom. For example, she described the diabetic personality as indecisive, passive, and frequently homosexual. Wolff (1963) later popularized this point of view by referring, for example, to the compulsive migraine personality. However, Wolff's theory of psychosomatic etiology combined the concepts of stress reaction and organ weakness (concepts that are discussed below) with the notion of specific personalities so that the importance of personality traits as causes of psychosomatic symptoms was obscured. The specific personality hypothesis continues to be referred to by many medical practitioners but has disappeared from the scientific literature because of its lack of empirical support.

Graham and his colleagues proposed that specific attitudes are causally related to specific psychosomatic symptoms (Graham, Lundy, Benjamin, Kabler, Lewis, Kunish, & Graham, 1962). *Attitudes* were defined as statements containing two parts: "(a) what the person feels is happening to him, and (b) what he wishes to do

Table 1. Psychoanalytic Concepts of Psychosomatic Specificity[a]

Bronchial asthma: "The central conflict in cases of bronchial asthma stems from internal impulses that threaten a person's attachment to mother or a mother substitute. . . . The most specific feature of these patients . . . is their conflict about crying. Crying, the child's first device for calling mother, is inhibited because of fear of maternal repudiation. . . . Asthmatic attacks can be understood as an inhibition of the expiratory act for communication, either by crying or confession." (p. 12)

Ulcerative colitis: "The central dynamic constellation in ulcerative colitis consists in losing hope that a task involving responsibility, effort, and concentration can be accomplished. These patients are inclined to give up hope easily in the face of obstacles. . . . The typical onset situation is a hopeless struggle for achievement." (p. 13)

Essential hypertension: "In cases of essential hypertension the central findings are the patient's continuous struggle against expressing hostile aggressive feelings and his difficulty in asserting himself. These patients fear losing the affection of others and so control the expression of their hostility. . . . The characteristic onset situation consists in life circumstances that mobilize hostility and the urge for self-assertion and at the same time prohibit their free expression." (pp. 13–14)

Neurodermatitis: "We find a complex configuration between exhibitionism, guilt, and masochism, combined with a deep-seated desire to receive physical expression of love from others. . . . The disease, as a rule, is precipitated after the patient achieves some form of exhibitionistic victory. The victory arouses guilt and creates a need for suffering in the precise part of the body that is involved in the exhibitionistic success." (p. 14)

Thyrotoxicosis: "The central dynamic issue in thyrotoxicosis is a constant struggle against fear concerning the physical integrity of the body and more specifically, fear of biological death. Even more characteristic is the attempt to master fear by denying it and counterphobically seeking dangerous situations and coping with them alone. . . . The precipitating situation is often some kind of threat to survival, in which the counterphobic defense breaks down." (p. 15)

Duodenal peptic ulcer: "The central dynamic feature in duodenal peptic ulcer is the frustration of dependent desires originally oral in character. The craving to be fed appears later as a wish to be loved, to be given support, money, and advice. . . . Onset of illness occurs when the intensity of the patient's unsatisfied dependent cravings increase because of external deprivation or . . . increased responsibilities." (pp. 15–16)

---

[a] From Alexander, F., French, T. M., and Pollock, G. H. *Psychosomatic Specificity*, Vol. 1. Copyright 1968, The University of Chicago Press, Chicago, Illinois. Reprinted with permission of the publisher.

about it" (Graham, 1972, p. 857). Table 2 lists the specific attitudes described by Graham's group and the psychosomatic symptoms to which they refer.

Graham (1972) has reviewed the research literature on the specific attitude hypothesis. Briefly, there have been two studies in which blind judges rated transcripts of interviews for the presence of these attitudes after the interview transcripts had been expurgated of clues as to physical diagnosis. The judges selected the appropriate attitude at better than chance levels, although their accuracy was not high enough to be of clinical usefulness. There followed three studies in which the attitudes presumed to be associated with Raynaud's disease, urticaria, and essential hypertension were suggested to normal subjects during a hypnotic trance. These hypnotic suggestions generally produced differential physiological changes appropriate to these three diseases—a decrease in skin temperature for Raynaud's attitude, an increase in skin temperature for the urticaria attitude, and a rise in blood pressure

Table 2. Specific Attitude Hypothesis of Psychosomatic Etiology[a]

Urticaria: Felt he was taking a beating and was helpless to do anything about it (was being knocked around, hammered on, being mistreated or unfairly treated).

Ulcerative colitis: Felt he was being injured and degraded and wished he could get rid of the responsible agent (was being humiliated, screwed; wanted the situation to be finished, over and done with, disposed of).

Eczema: Felt he was being frustrated and could do nothing about it except take it out on himself (felt interfered with, blocked, prevented from doing something, unable to make self understood).

Acne: Felt he was being picked on or at and wanted to be let alone (being nagged at).

Psoriasis: Felt there was a constant gnawing at him and that he had to put up with it (a steady boring, a constant nagging or irritation or annoyance).

Bronchial asthma: Felt left out in the cold and wanted to shut the person or situation out (felt unloved, rejected, disapproved of, shut out, and wished not to deal with the person or situation, wished to blot it or him out, not have anything to do with it or him).

Hyperthyroidism: Felt might lose somebody or something he loved and took care of and tried to prevent loss of the loved person or object (tried to hold on to somebody loved and taken care of).

Vomiting: Felt something wrong had happened, usually something for which the patient felt responsible, and wished it hadn't happened (was sorry it happened, wished could undo what happened, wished things were the way they were before, wished he hadn't done it).

Duodenal ulcer: Felt deprived of what was due him and wanted to get even (didn't get what he should, what was owed or promised, and wanted to get back at, get revenge, do to him what he did to me).

Constipation: Felt in a situation from which nothing good could come but kept on with it grimly (felt things would never get any better but had to stick with it).

Essential hypertension: Felt threatened with harm and had to be ready for anything (felt in danger, anything could happen at any time from any side; had to be prepared to meet all possible threats, be on guard).

Migraine: Felt something had to be achieved and then relaxed after the effort (had to accomplish something, was driving self, striving, had to get things done, a goal had to be reached; then let down, stopped the driving).

Multiple sclerosis: Felt he was forced to undertake some kind of physical activity, especially hard work, and wanted not to (had to work without help, had to support self and usually others; wanted not to and might or might not express wish for help or support).

Metabolic edema: Felt he was carrying a heavy load and wanted somebody else to carry all or part of it (had too much on his shoulders, too much responsibility; wanted others to take their share of it).

Rheumatoid arthritis: Felt tied down and wanted to get free (felt restrained, restricted, confined, and wanted to be able to move around).

Raynaud's disease: Wanted to take hostile physical action (wanted to hit or strangle, wanted to take action of any kind, had to do something).

Regional enteritis: Felt had received something harmful and wanted to get rid of it (had been given or received something damaged or inferior, felt had been poisoned, wanted the situation to be finished, over and done with, disposed of).

Low backache: Wanted to run away (wanted to walk out of there, get out of there).

---

[a] From Graham, D. T., Lundy, R. M., Benjamin, L. S., Kabler, J. D., Lewis, W. C., Kunish, N. D., and Graham, F. K. Specific attitudes in initial interviews with patients having different "psychosomatic diseases," *Psychosomatic Medicine*, 1962, *24*, 257–266. Reprinted with permission of Dr. Graham and Elsevier North-Holland, Inc.

for the hypertension attitude. These hypnosis experiments provided rather impressive support for the specific attitude hypothesis. However, subsequent studies in which the appropriate attitudes were suggested to nonhypnotized subjects generally failed to produce the expected changes in physiological responses, and the specific attitude hypothesis seems not to have generated much research in the last 10 years. The specific emotion hypothesis proposed by Alexander (1950) and formalized in the *Diagnostic and Statistical Manual of Mental Disorders* of the American Psychiatric Association has clearly dominated practice and research in psychosomatic medicine until recently.

The specific emotion hypothesis, however, has generally not been supported by empirical research. In studies that utilize objective psychological tests in randomly selected groups of people, patients with hypertension are not distinguishable from nonpatients with respect to hostility, neuroticism, or anxiety (Cochrane, 1973; Davies, 1970). Individuals with migraine headaches (Henryk-Gutt & Rees, 1973) and those with asthma (Rees, 1976) are found to be more neurotic and anxious than nonpatients and they lack social skills, but no specific emotional states or personality characteristics are found that are uniquely associated with either disorder.

There are two notable exceptions to the generalization that the specific emotion hypothesis lacks empirical support. In the large study by the Chicago Psychoanalytic Institute (Alexander *et al.*, 1968), analysts were able to predict the physical diagnosis of psychosomatic patients at better than chance levels from transcribed diagnostic interviews that had been expurgated of direct clues as to physical diagnosis. However, methodological problems limit the generality of these findings. Specifically, the interviewers who collected the data were not blind to the diagnosis and may have been biased by their theoretical assumptions in the kinds of material they elicited in unstructured interviews.

A second study (Weiner, Thaler, Reiser, & Mirsky, 1957), which was replicated (Cohen, Silverman, Waddell, & Zuidema, 1961), also tended to support the specific emotion hypothesis. Army recruits in basic training were subdivided into two groups based on their biological predisposition to develop peptic ulcer as reflected in an indirect measure of basal rates of gastric acid and pepsin secretion. They were then tested with projective tests for conflicts relating to dependency versus autonomy. Based on the psychological material alone, raters were able to predict which recruits had preexisting ulcers, or would develop ulcers during basic training. This evidence, too, is of limited generality because it could be argued that recruits with a similar set of psychological characteristics and who had a different biological predisposition would have developed symptoms consistent with their unique biological predisposition. For example, those with a predisposition to develop hypertension would have become hypertensive. It is unfortunate that other psychosomatic disorders were not included in the study.

Basic laboratory experiments on the physiology of emotion have also failed to support the specific emotion hypothesis of psychosomatic etiology. It is rare that different emotions have been found to be associated with qualitative differences in physiological states (Blackwell & Whitehead, 1975). Ax (1953) and later J. Schachter (1957) reported being able to distinguish between epinephrine and norepinephrine responses to anger and fear, respectively, but the systematic studies of Frankenhaeuser (1975) show that these differences could be accounted for on the basis of differences in the level of nonspecific arousal rather than by the type of emotion. Frankenhaeuser showed that both epinephrine and norepinephrine release could be produced by a variety of affects, including that produced by comic films. The physiological indicators that do covary with subjective reports of emotion—forearm blood flow (Kelly & Walter, 1968) and rate of habituation of the electrodermal response (Lader & Wing, 1964) for anxiety; electrodermal response amplitude (Greenfield, Katz, Alexander, & Roessler, 1963; McCarron, 1973) and rate of salivation (Palmai, Blackwell, Maxwell, & Morgenstern, 1967) for depression—typically correlate less than $r = 0.50$ with the subjective report of the emotion, suggesting less specificity than is demanded by the specific emotion hypothesis.

There are also marked individual differences between people in the pattern of physiological response to stress or emotion (Engel & Bickford, 1961; Lacey, Bateman, & Van Lehn, 1953). For example, Figure 1 shows the responses of 26 normal medical students to the Autonomic Perception Questionnaire (Mandler, Mandler, & Uviller, 1958). These subjects were asked to mark how frequently they noticed each of the symptoms indicated on the graph when they felt anxious. Assuming that anxiety is a single emotion, the specific emotion hypothesis would predict

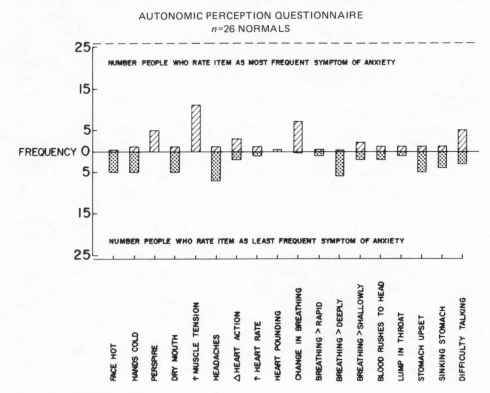

Figure 1. Individual differences in physiological response to anxiety. Shown on the ordinate are the number of people who marked each symptom as their most prominent (top half) and least prominent (bottom half) physical symptom of anxiety.

that all subjects would mark the same symptom as the most common physiological sequel to anxiety and the same symptom as the least common sequel to anxiety. This did not occur; there were marked differences between people in what they perceived as the most frequent symptom of anxiety.

Other basic laboratory studies that tend to disconfirm the specific emotion hypothesis of psychosomatic etiology are those in which epinephrine was injected into human subjects to mimic the physiological arousal characteristic of fear or anxiety. Either the subjects were asked to report what emotions they had subjectively experienced, or the type of emotion was inferred from behavioral observations. S. Schachter and Singer (1962) demonstrated that the type of emotion experienced—either anger or euphoria—was determined by cues in the environment, such as the behavior modeled by a stooge of the experimenter, rather than being determined by the injection of epinephrine. The epinephrine injection did affect the perceived intensity of the emotion, however.

Basic laboratory experiments such as these raise serious problems for the specific emotion hypothesis of psychosomatic etiology.

Perhaps as important as its lack of empirical verification is the fact that the specific emotion hypothesis has not led to effective treatments for psychosomatic disorders. For example, follow-up studies of the treatment of irritable bowel syndrome (Waller & Misiewicz, 1969) and its juvenile equivalent, recurrent abdominal pain (Apley & Hale, 1973; Christensen & Mortensen, 1975), show that insight-oriented psychotherapy has no long-term effects on the course of these disorders. Kellner's (1975) review of the psychotherapeutic treatment of other psychosomatic disorders suggests that insight-oriented psychotherapy is relatively ineffective, and the primary treatment of psychosomatic disorders continues to be pharmacological or surgical management of symptoms.

Recent Developments in Psychosomatic Etiology: The Stress Hypothesis and the Social Learning Hypothesis

In response to growing dissatisfaction with the specific emotion hypothesis, several people have offered new conceptual models that emphasize the role of interactions between the individual patient and the social environment for determining the genesis and course of certain illnesses. In addition, these new models have in common a tendency to lump together several traditional diagnostic categories: hysterical conversion reactions, hypochondriasis, psychosomatic disorders, and somatopsychic disorders.

These new models of psychosomatic etiology are of two types: those emphasizing the biological response to stressful aspects of the environment and those etiological models that emphasize the role of learning and socialization.

Stress models of psychosomatic etiology began with Hans Selye's (1956) description of the general adaptation syndrome to nonspecific stressors such as infection, exposure to cold, and exercise to the point of exhaustion. The general adaptation syndrome, as described by Selye, was a relatively fixed biological response, and for this reason, it had little appeal initially as a model of psychosomatic etiology; it did not seem able to account for symptom choice. Interest in stress models was renewed, however, by two developments. The first was the demonstration by Lacey *et al.* (1953) and by others (e.g., Engel & Bickford, 1961) that many human subjects have stereotyped patterns of physiological response to a variety of stressful stimuli. These responses are stereotyped in the sense that they differ between individuals but are relatively constant from stimulus to stimulus and from time to time for a given individual. These experiments did not explain why individual differences in the physiological response stereotype occur, but they did provide empirical support for a stress model because they showed that individual differences in symptoms might be taken into account without dropping the stress concept. The experiments accomplished this by suggesting that individual differences in stress response might be stable characteristics of organisms rather than being due to differences in the stressful stimuli to which the individual is exposed.

The second development that stimulated interest in a stress model of psychosomatic etiology was the report by Holmes and Rahe (1967) that the incidence of illnesses and injuries of all types could be predicted, within broad limits, from a knowledge of the number of nonspecific stressors the subject had experienced in the recent past. Following these developments, George Engel (1977), Wolf and Goodell (1976), and Rees (1976), among others, published models of psychosomatic etiology that emphasized the role of stress.

The social learning model of psychosomatic etiology began with Parsons (1951), who first described the fact that there is a socially sanctioned sick role that prescribes how an individual is expected to act when he is ill and how the rest of society should respond to him. Mechanic (1962, 1972) subsequently described as illness behavior the different ways in which illness is perceived by different people and their different responses to illness. Mechanic attempted to account for the tendency of some people to deny illness and not seek medical help when it would be appropriate as well as the tendency of other people to overutilize medical care facilities.

Pilowsky (1969) used the term *abnormal illness behavior* and Blackwell, Wooley, and Whitehead (1974) used the term *chronic illness behavior* to describe essentially the same syndrome. This syndrome is characterized by complaints of pain or disability that are disproportionate to physical findings, a lifestyle arranged around the sick role, a constant search for diagnosis and treatment, and interpersonal behaviors that elicit caretaking responses from physicians and relatives. Sternbach (1974) has described a similar syndrome in chronic pain patients, which he labeled *pain behavior*. Evidence in support of these social learning hypotheses of psychosomatic etiology is reviewed below.

This social learning model, which lumps hypochondriacal and hysterical complaints together with psychosomatic symptoms and which emphasizes the role of feedback from the social environment in the course of the illness, has been very useful, but it has several limitations. First, the social learning model emphasizes what people say about their bodies and how they utilize medical facilities; the model does not address the issue of whether actual physiological changes are influenced by the social environment in the same way that verbal behavior and care-seeking behavior are influenced by the environment. Such a distinction may have important consequences for treating disorders such as peptic ulcer in which tissue damage is occurring. Second, the model of chronic illness behavior may be less general than is supposed since it is derived from observations of the relatively few patients who have persistently (and usually insistently) sought medical care for their symptoms. The majority of psychosomatic patients, who get by with infrequent visits to a physician, may be quite different. Large-scale studies of the social learning hypothesis in unselected groups of people have not been reported. Third, this social learning model does not attempt to account for symptom choice—the tendency of one patient to develop ulcers while another develops migraine or muscle contraction headaches. It is the thesis of this chapter that a more detailed analysis of the kinds of learning that may occur in relation to physiological symptoms and the conditions under which such learning may occur may contribute to a better understanding of symptom choice as well as suggesting more specific treatment procedures.

The model of psychosomatic etiology that is presented in this chapter is based on learning theory and on the concept of stress. A major emphasis is placed on the role that perception and awareness of abnormal physiological events play in determining the kinds of learning that may occur. We propose that psychosomatic symptoms characterized by actual physiological changes in autonomically innervated physiological functions may be viewed as (1) simple stress reactions; (2) operantly learned responses; or (3) classically conditioned responses. We also discuss how distinguishing between these three possible causes of symptoms influences the choice of treatment and its outcome.

STRESS AS A CAUSE OF PSYCHOSOMATIC SYMPTOMS

Levi's (1974) stress model is representative of current stress theories of psychosomatic etiology (e.g., Engel, 1977; Rees, 1976; Wolf & Goodell, 1976). Levi proposed that aspects of the person, such as personality, interact with aspects of the psychosocial environment to produce physiological reactions that, if they are prolonged, may lead to psychosomatic disease.

Levi's model is a useful way of organizing the data, but we believe that it obscures some important differences in the etiology of psychosomatic disorders, and that these differences have implications for the treatment of psychosomatic disorders. Specifically, we believe that Levi's reference to interactions between aspects of the environment and aspects of the person should be further divided into (1) physiological responses to aspects of the environment that are aversive to almost all people independent of their learning history (e.g., having to work very rapidly to avoid aversive consequences); and (2) physiological responses to aspects of the environment that are aversive only to people who have a specific past learning experience (e.g., a phobic patient confronting the object he fears). This division corresponds to the difference between unconditioned responses to unconditional stimuli and conditioned responses to conditional stimuli. If pathophysiological changes are the result of a conditioning history, then one can effectively treat them with classical extinction procedures such as flooding or systematic desensitization. If, on the other hand, the pathophysiological changes are evoked by events that are experienced as stressful by essentially everyone, as seems to be the case with occupational stressors like time pressure and responsibility, then classical extinction procedures would be of little value. In this chapter, we restrict the use of the term *stress* to unconditional responses to the environment, and we use the term *classically conditioned response* to describe pathophysiological responses that are the result of a particular learning history. Rules for distinguishing between the two types of responses are discussed in the sections of this chapter on diagnosis.

Several studies have attempted to identify which aspects of environments, especially work environments, make them stressful. The most systematic of these studies are Jay Weiss's (1970, 1971a,b) experiments on the determinants of gastric ulceration in laboratory rats. Weiss used as a paradigm of stress the situation in which rats received electric shock to the tail, and Weiss varied the rat's control over the shock and the amount of information the rat received to guide his performance. Weiss was able to isolate the following factors as being significantly related to the probability that rats would develop gastric ulcers:

1. *Control of aversive events.* Rats that could press a lever to avoid some of the shocks developed fewer ulcers and lost less weight than rats that received exactly the same shocks but were helpless to prevent them. The fact of being helpless to prevent shock made the shock more stressful. The relevance of this control factor to human stress reaction is illustrated by Seligman's (1975) work on learned helplessness and by reports (French & Caplan, 1974) that the incidence of coronary heart disease is positively correlated with the degree of extrinsic motivation in a work environment and negatively correlated with intrinsic motivation. *Extrinsic motivation* refers to the control of work by machines or supervisors, whereas *intrinsic motivation* refers to independent work.

2. *Predictability of aversive events.* Weiss found that rats who received a warning prior to shocks got fewer ulcers than rats who received no warning, even when the shocks were unavoidable for both groups of rats. This finding suggests that human work situations that are characterized by routine and by the absence of unexpected demands should be experienced as less stressful than jobs in which one is frequently required to deal with the unexpected. There is some evidence that this is the case. In a study of NASA personnel, administrators were found to experience their jobs as more stressful than either blue-collar workers or scientists (French & Caplan, 1974).

3. *Feedback about the effectiveness of one's behavior.* Rats who were given a signal to indicate when they had successfully postponed shock developed fewer ulcers than rats who were given no relevant feedback but who could also postpone the shocks. The low feedback condition corresponds to human situations in which feedback about the adequacy of one's performance is very infrequent and situations in which the criteria by which one is judged are vague and subjective.

Weiss also noted that differences between rats influenced their susceptibility to developing gastric ulcers when exposed to stress. Rats who made the most excess responses and who responded fastest in the shock avoidance task developed the most ulcers. This is reminiscent of the reported correlation between Type A personality in humans (hard driving, rushed) and coronary heart disease (Rosenman, Friedman, Straus, Wurm, Jenkins, & Messinger, 1966). Weiss's studies illustrate how aspects of the environment and aspects of the individual may make independent contributions to the development of psychosomatic signs or symptoms.

It has been well documented that stressful environmental circumstances can lead to abnormal physiological responses in some individuals, and that these abnormal responses may develop into psychosomatic symptoms if exposure to the stressful situation is prolonged. To give a few examples, Cobb and Rose (1973) noted that hypertension is four times more prevalent in air traffic controllers as compared to second-class airmen, that the number of new cases per year is six times greater in air traffic controllers, and, furthermore, that the number of new cases per year is correlated with traffic density at the place of work. Cobb and Rose (1973) also reported an excess incidence of peptic ulcer and diabetes in air traffic controllers. Approximately a decade ago, in their review of psychosomatic aspects of hypertension, Gutmann and Benson (1971) noted that hypertension is more common in a variety of environments—in urban as compared to rural areas, in recent migrants to cities as compared to second-generation city dwellers, and so on. Jenkins, Tuthill, Tannenbaum, and Kirby (1977) have recently reported that a variety of socioeconomic conditions, such as income below the poverty level, substandard housing, and crowded living conditions, are significantly correlated with death due to coronary heart disease.

Holmes and his colleagues (Bramwell, Masuda, Wagner, & Holmes, 1975; Holmes & Masuda, 1974; Holmes & Rahe, 1967; Rahe, 1972); have done a series of studies showing that the incidence of illnesses and injuries is correlated with the cumulative number of life events requiring social readjustment that have befallen an individual in the last 6 or 12 months. This literature was reviewed critically by Rabkin and Struening (1976), who concluded that despite methodological limitations, a particular relationship between such life events and illness has been convincingly demonstrated. However, this literature relating acute stressors to acute illness is of limited value in accounting for psychosomatic symptoms that are chronic or recurrent. To account for psychosomatic disorders, one must examine long-term stressors.

As these studies suggest, the nature of the stressor does not determine the type of sign or symptom that develops. An additional assumption is required to account for symptom choice. The simplest assumption is that many people, if not all people, have a predisposition to respond to all stressors in some single characteristic way that differs for different individuals. This concept has been variously termed *somatic compliance* (Wolff, 1968) and *individual response stereotype* (Lacey et al., 1953). This notion has empirical support. Lacey and his colleagues demonstrated 25 years ago that if normal subjects were exposed to a variety of aversive stimuli, about a third would respond to all stimuli with the same pattern of physiological changes, and that these patterns differed for different people. The remaining two-thirds of subjects showed, to varying degrees, different patterns of response to different stimuli. Engel and Bickford (1961) and Malmo and Shagass (1949) have shown that the tendency to respond to all stressors with the same pattern of physiological changes is more common in psychosomatic patients than in normals, and that psychosomatic patients tend to respond to all stressors with the symptomatic response; that is, hypertensives tend to show a rise in blood pressure, ulcer patients tend to show a change in gastric secretion or motility (Walker & Sandman, 1977), and so on.

Importance of Symptom Perception

Although the kinds of symptoms that may result as responses to environmental stressors vary widely, some selection appears to be involved. Symptoms such as migraine headache, functional diarrhea, and asthma are not typically reported to be associated with environmental stressors. They were not reported by Cobb and Rose (1973) to be associated with the job of air traffic controller (Cobb and Rose noted specifically that migraine occurred too infrequently to be studied), and these disorders have generally not been reported to vary as a function of low socioeconomic status or type of employment. Migraine incidence, according to Henryk-Gutt and Rees (1973), is unrelated to social class.

We believe that a subgroup of psychosomatic disorders can be distinguished that are primarily stress responses and that do not appear to be influenced by operant learning or classical conditioning. This group of disorders includes hypertension, coronary heart disease, peptic ulcer, and possibly diabetes. This group of disorders is distinguished by the fact that they are not found in association with characteristics of the person such as anxiety or neuroticism or social inadequacy (e.g., Cochrane, 1973). The association of coronary heart disease with Type A personality is a possible exception, but note that Type A personality (Rosenman et al., 1966) is characterized by excessive drive, aggressiveness, ambition, and a sense of time urgency; it is not characterized by anxiety or deficient social skills.

A second distinguishing characteristic is that there is little or no subjective perception of the physiological changes associated with these diseases. Luborsky, Brady, McClintock, Kron, Bortnichak, and Levitz (1976) studied the ability of subjects to estimate their systolic blood pressure. Although accuracy improved with feedback, improvements could be attributed to the subjects' learning the normal (expectable) range of their blood pressure. Most clinicians report that patients are not able to perceive their blood pressure. There seems to be very little subjective awareness of physiological changes such as coronary blood flow, gastric acid secretion, or blood sugar levels in the early stages of these diseases, although when the pathophysiology is advanced, there are subjective symptoms such as angina, ulcer pain, and the thirst associated with diabetes. For example, in pilot experiments on the discriminability of hydrochloric acid solutions perfused into the stomach of a normal subject, we found that discrimination even of 1.5 pH solutions (highly acidic) was at no better than chance levels. This finding contrasts with the high degree of subjective perception associated with the symptoms of headache, asthma, and irritable bowel syndrome.

These two distinguishing attributes of stress responses we believe to be causally related: stress responses about which people have little subjective perception are unlikely to be influenced by operant learning or classical conditioning. On the other hand, psychosomatic symptoms about which people have good subjective perception may initially be elicited by stressful environmental circumstances, but once learning has occurred, these symptoms are likely to occur in new circumstances that are not aversive to most people, and thus the link between stressor and response is likely to be broken or obscured. There are, of course, instances in which high-perception symptoms such as muscle contraction headache and temporomandibular joint pain continue to occur as simple stress reactions. The point is that low-perception symptoms are not likely to come under the control of operant reinforcers; high-perception symptoms may, but not necessarily will, come under the control of operant reinforcers. Subjective awareness of the physiological changes associated with the symptom is seen as a necessary but not a sufficient condition for the symptom to come under the control of operant reinforcers.

Diagnosis

Psychophysiological disorders should be diagnosed as stress responses only when it can be shown that fluctuations in a physiological response covary with the presence or absence of conditions that are aversive for most people. For example, Figure 2 shows fluctuations in blood pressure in a 50-year-old white male who took his blood pressure three times each day after having been taught how to do so by a medical technician. It may be observed that his blood pressure was extremely variable and was likely to be highest in the middle of the day. This man worked as a bartender in a bar where, according to his report, fights were common, and he experienced his job as very stressful.

It is often difficult to diagnose a stress reaction on the basis of an interview because many psychophysiological reactions that occur as stress reactions are not perceived by the patient. Hypertension provides the best example; the patient cannot report whether his blood pressure goes up when he is at work because he is never aware of what his blood pressure is except when he is at the physician's office. It is possible in an interview to determine whether the patient's lifestyle involves repeated exposure to common stressors and to determine whether an abrupt change in lifestyle was associated with the onset (or discovery) of the disorder. However, this information does not establish a covariation between aversive events and physiological changes.

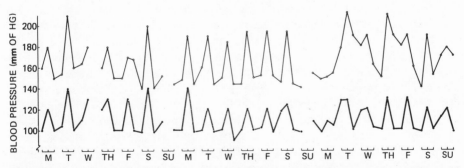

Figure 2. Variations in systolic (top line) and diastolic (bottom line) blood pressure in a 50-year-old white male who took his own blood pressure three times a day at standard times. Blood pressure was consistently higher in the middle of the day when the subject was at work. Days of the week are given on the abscissa.

Somewhat better information may be obtained by the stressful interview technique developed by Harold Wolff (1968). Wolff found that he could identify areas of a patient's life that were stressful and then introduce these topics in the midst of a conversation about more neutral topics. He did this while continuously measuring changes in the physiological response of interest and was able to demonstrate correlations between the topic of conversation and physiological changes in many cases.

In our experience, however, the most reliable method of establishing the diagnosis of a stress reaction is to have subjects self-monitor physiological events over a lengthy period of time while they go about their ordinary daily activities. For example, we (Whitehead, Blackwell, DeSilva, & Robinson, 1977) recently had a group of borderline hypertensive patients measure and record their blood pressure four times each day at predetermined times and had them indicate on analog scales how anxious and how angry they felt at the same time. Since these were not generally anxious people (as measured by the State Trait Anxiety Inventory of Spielberger, Gorsuch, & Lushene, 1970), variations in what they marked on anxiety scales presumably reflected their subjective reaction to different situations. For each subject, we computed the correlation between blood pressure and subjective emotional reactions (anxiety). These correlations varied from $r = .05$ to $r = .79$ with a median of $r = .36$. This finding suggests that blood pressure elevations occurred as stress responses in some subjects (those who showed strong correlations between blood pressure and situational anxiety) but that elevations in blood pressure were unrelated to environmental events in other subjects. Further study would be required to determine whether the events that covaried with blood pressure increases were of the conditional or the unconditional sort.

This approach involving self-monitoring by the patient would not be applicable to all psychophysiological disorders—for example, to coronary blood flow—but is possible in many cases. It should be possible to have diabetics monitor urine sugar levels. It is also possible to have patients self-monitor gastric acid secretion and gastric motility using disposable telemetric transducers.

Not all psychophysiological responses that covary with the presence or absence of specific situations are stress reactions. When the situation that regularly elicits the physiological response is not aversive for most people (such as the agoraphobic leaving his home), or when the triggering situation owes its ability to elicit the physiological response to an occasional association with aversive stimuli (such as the adolescent male approaching a female to arrange a date), then it would not be appropriate to diagnose a stress reaction. An analysis in terms of Pavlovian conditioning would be more appropriate. Also, when the physiological response appears to be instrumental in avoiding or escaping the aversive situation, such as complaining of a migraine headache that results in being exempted from work, an analysis in terms of operant conditioning would be more appropriate. Environmental stressors are aspects of the environment that would be perceived as aversive by all people if they were sufficiently prolonged or intense, although individuals may differ with respect to the threshold for occurrence of a stress response and the type of physiological response that occurs when this threshold is exceeded.

Treatment

When psychosomatic symptoms appear to be primarily or exclusively stress responses, the most appropriate psychological treatments appear to be those that modulate the stressful effects of the environment, treatments that cause the environment to be reinterpreted in ways that lead to its being perceived as less stressful, or treatments that alter the environment. This approach differs from the Pavlovian and operant extinction procedures recommended for the treatment of other kinds of psychosomatic disorders discussed later on.

Progressive muscle relaxation, in which a patient is taught a set of exercises to produce relaxation and is instructed to practice these daily, is an example of a technique designed to counteract the effects of a stressful environment (Benson, Alexander, & Feldman, 1975; Patel, 1977; Stone & DeLeo, 1976). Biofeedback training has been used to lower blood pressure (Shapiro, Schwartz, Ferguson, Redmond, & Weiss, (1977) in hypertensive patients, although its efficacy is not well established. Transcendental meditation (Blackwell, Hanenson, Bloomfield, Magenheim, Gartside, Nidich, Robinson, & Zigler, 1976), which combines a relaxation procedure with a metaphysical belief system, has also been used successfully to lower blood pressure. By contrast, the only controlled study of psychotherapy in hypertension found that psychotherapy was not beneficial (Titchener, Sheldon, & Ross, 1959). It is perhaps also relevant that antianxiety drugs do not significantly lower blood pressure in hypertension (*Medical Letter*, 1974).

Techniques for treating stress reactions that involve a reinterpretation of events leading to their being interpreted as less stressful would include the cognitive restructuring techniques recommended by Meichenbaum and Turk (1976). The only published application of such procedures to a psychosomatic disorder was reported more than 40 years ago (Chappell, Stefano, Rogerson, & Pike, 1936; Chappell & Stevenson, 1936). These investigators studied 52 patients with lengthy histories of ulcer symptoms and with radiological confirmation of peptic ulcer. All were put on a bland diet involving frequent feedings, and 32 were assigned to an experimental treatment group. The experimental treatment involved didactic group sessions seven days each week for six weeks, while the controls were not seen. The experimental treatment involved several elements that would today be called *cognitive restructuring:* patients were taught that worrying caused physiological changes that resulted in ulcer pain and were taught several coping strategies to achieve self-control over worrying. When worrying occurred, patients were to distract themselves by switching to thinking about pleasant periods of their lives. The patients were assured frequently that they could overcome their symptoms and were instructed to repeat aloud to themselves several times each day that they were recovering. The investigators also desensitized their patients to cancer phobia and to various food phobias, which occurred frequently, and they encouraged them to avoid discussing their symptoms with friends and relatives. The results were rather dramatic. Within one month of the termination of treatment 31 of 32 patients in the experimental group had returned to a normal diet and were symptom-free, whereas only 2 of the 20 control subjects were able to return to a normal diet without a return of symptoms. At follow-up 6–10 months after treatment, 26 experimental patients were in excellent health, 1 had had a recurrence of symptoms, and 4 were not examined. At the end of three years' follow-up, 15 experimental subjects were in excellent health, 9 had had numerous occurrences of mild symptoms, 2 had had recurrence of severe symptoms, and 3 could not be located. The authors noted that 15 additional subjects had started the experimental group but dropped out after one or two sessions. Even so, these results provide strong evidence for the efficacy of a treatment program based on cognitive restructuring principles.

The technique of actually altering stressful aspects of the environment as a means of controlling stress reactions may take the form of resolving marital difficulties or providing help with job retraining or housing.

OPERANT CONDITIONING AS A CAUSE OF PSYCHOSOMATIC SYMPTOMS

When any behavior is followed immediately by any desirable consequence, it is more likely to recur in the future. This type of learning is called *operant conditioning* or *trial-and-error learning* or *instrumental learning*. The consequence, which is called a *reinforcer*, need not bear any relationship to the behavior other than temporal contiguity, and it may include escape from aversive events, such as the threat of electric shock, as well as the occurrence of pleasant events, such as food presentation. Thus, any desirable event can be arbitrarily used to increase the frequency of any response. The most common reinforcers of human behavior are the interest and approval of other people and avoidance of social disapproval or embarrassment. More concrete reinforcers, such as monetary incentives and penalties, are also used to control human behavior.

Some kinds of somatic symptoms—those called *hypochondriacal complaints* and *hysterical conversion reactions*—are generally recognized to be influenced by the consequences they produce. These consequences are typically sympathetic attention from other people, financial compensation, or escape from situations that produce anxiety. For example, Sternbach (1974) and Timmermans and Sternbach (1974) described how chronic pain patients tend to exaggerate their reports of pain in ways that establish dependent, caregiving relationships with physicians; and Farbman (1973) reported that the length of physical disability following neck sprain is positively correlated with litigation to secure financial compensation, with a history of prior similar injuries, with pressure at work prior to injury, and with symptoms of nervousness or other psychiatric symptoms. Pain complaints such as these would probably be classified as hypochondriacal reactions. Hysterical conversion reactions are also commonly observed to produce desirable consequences for the patient (*Diagnostic and Statistical Manual of Mental Disorders*, 1968).

The desirable social consequences that occur contingent on somatic complaints are regarded as important by most theorists, but they are assigned different labels depending on the theoretical orientation. Dynamic theorists believe that these consequences help to maintain conversion symptoms and hypochondriacal complaints but that they play no role in the etiology of these symptoms. They refer to such consequences as secondary gain. Behavioral theorists, on the other hand, believe that these symptoms are learned as well as maintained by the effects they produce on the environment, and they refer to such consequences as *operant reinforcers*.

Although the hypothesis that social consequences play a role in the etiology of hypochondriacal and hysterical symptoms has been accepted without much protest, it is only within the last few years that Miller (1972, 1975, 1976; Miller & Dworkin, 1977) and others have begun to suggest that psychosomatic symptoms involving abnormal responses of the autonomic nervous system may be caused by reinforcing social consequences. The biofeedback experiments reported in the literature provide a model of such learning. They show that most autonomically mediated responses can be altered if subjects are provided with mechanical or electronic feedback on small changes in the response (Miller, 1969).

Figure 3 provides an illustration of such learning. It shows the motility in the colon of a patient with irritable bowel syndrome (spastic colon). This woman experienced severe abdominal pain, diarrhea, gas distension of the abdomen, and loud bowel sounds on a daily basis. The pressure recording showed her bowel to be quite active although normal subjects rarely show any activity. She was given biofeedback on the occurrence of the largest pressure waves and instructed to increase or decrease the frequency of these events. The figure is a recording of the fifth training session, which shows that she was able to increase and decrease colonic motility on command, although she required about five minutes to effectively decrease motility. In the first session, she could not decrease motility at all. This gradual acquisition of control over bowel motility was associated with some relief of symptoms between training sessions, but these improvements were not well maintained when she discontinued treatment.

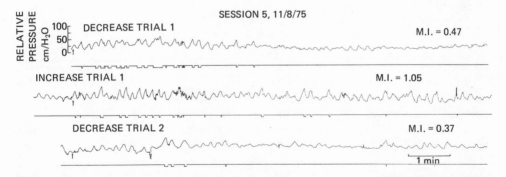

Figure 3. Pressure recordings from the sigmoid colon of a patient with irritable bowel syndrome. Consecutive 10-minute segments of the fifth biofeedback training session are shown. In the first segment (at the arrow), the subject was instructed to decrease the frequency with which the feedback light came on; in the second segment, she was instructed to increase it; and in the third segment, she was instructed to decrease it again. Downward deflections of the straight line below each pressure recording show where the feedback light came on. This light was activated by pressure waves above a fixed amplitude.

Since contractions of the bowel are relatively easy to perceive for some patients, it is possible that this same type of learning could occur in response to social reinforcement and without biofeedback training. Miller (1972) has speculated, by analogy from such experiments, that children may inadvertently learn to produce gastrointestinal symptoms if their mothers respond to stomach complaints by letting them stay home from school, or they may learn to produce other abnormal physiological responses in a similar way.

Importance of Symptom Perception

Naturally occurring contingencies of reinforcement, such as that suggested by Miller, differ, however, in several respects from biofeedback experiments. In Miller's example, the reinforcing consequence of avoiding school is not directly contingent on a change in a physiological response; it is contingent on a verbal report of a physiological response, whereas in the biofeedback experiment, reinforcement is contingent on mechanical detection of the physiological change itself. What are the conditions under which reinforcement of a verbal complaint will result in a change in the frequency of a physiological response rather than simply a change in verbal behavior (that is, in hypochondriasis)? The conditions are (1) that the subject be able to accurately and sensitively detect changes in the physiological response and (2) that he report on them accurately.

It is reasonable to suppose that Miller's child tells the truth, although some children have been known to exaggerate or misrepresent their symptoms. However, the other condition, that subjects be able to accurately and sensitively detect the pathophysiological response, is obviously not true for all physiological responses. Subjects seem unaware, for example, of fluctuation in blood pressure and of the physiological changes associated with the early stages of peptic ulcer, coronary artery disease, or diabetes.

Two deductions follow from this analysis. First, psychosomatic symptoms that are associated with a high degree of subjective perception of the pathophysiological response, such as migraine headaches and diarrhea, are more apt to come under the control of reinforcing environmental consequences than are psychosomatic symptoms that are associated with poor subjective perception of the pathophysiological response, such as hypertension, peptic ulcer development, coronary artery disease, and diabetes. This deduction is consistent with the research literature. It is consistent, for example, with the observation that the incidence of high-perception psychosomatic symptoms, such as migraine, asthma, and irritable bowel syndrome, tend not to be associated with stressful environmental circumstances, whereas hypertension, peptic ulcer, and diabetes do tend to be associated with environmental stressors. Moreover, the high-perception symptoms tend to be associated with a higher incidence of anxiety and neuroticism and with inadequate social skills (Rees, 1976), whereas this is not the case with hypertension, at least (Cochrane, 1973). One might expect inadequate social skills, anxiety, and neuroticism to covary with the adoption of illness as a way of relating to other people, although there is no logical necessity in this association.

Additional evidence comes from the second volume published on the Midtown Manhattan Project (Langner & Michael, 1963). This study showed that children of parents with psychosomatic symptoms are more likely themselves to have psychosomatic symptoms than children of parents without psychosomatic symptoms. Moreover, occurrence of psychosomatic symptoms in the mother (who typically spends more time with the children than the father) was associated with a greater risk of psychosomatic symptom development in offspring than occurrence of symptoms in the father. These data are consistent with the hypothesis that modeling or differential reinforcement of somatic complaints by a similarly affected parent plays an etiological role in psychosomatic disorders, although heritability cannot be ruled out as an explanation of these data. Of more direct relevance to the hypothesized role of perception in the etiology of psychosomatic disorders is the finding reported by Langner and Michael (1963) that people tend to develop the same psychosomatic symptoms their parents had, and that this tendency is generally greater for high-perception symptoms, such as asthma, colitis, hay fever, and skin trouble (diagnostic categories used by Langner and Michael), than for low-perception symptoms, such as stomach ulcer and high blood pressure. If we assume that heritability played no role in these correlations, the data are consistent with, and tend indirectly to support, the hypothesis that high-perception symptoms are more likely to come under the control of social reinforcement contingencies than low-perception symptoms.

Consistent with the findings of Langner and Michael (1963), several investigators (Christensen & Mortensen, 1975; Hill & Blendis, 1967; Oster, 1972; Stone & Barbaro, 1970) have reported that recurrent abdominal pain in children—which appears to be a juvenile equivalent of irritable bowel syndrome, since the underlying physiological mechanisms appear to be the same (Kopel, Kim, & Barbero, 1967)—occurs most frequently in families where one or both parents have *current* gastrointestinal symptoms. This finding suggests that modeling and reinforcement play a role in the etiology of this childhood disorder. The alternative explanation that there exists an inherited predisposition for the disorder is inconsistent with the observation that a *history* of gastrointestinal symptoms as opposed to current symptoms is no more common in parents of children with recurrent abdominal pain than in parents of children without this syndrome (Christensen & Mortensen, 1975). Recurrent abdominal pain is also more common in large families than in small families (Hill & Blendis, 1967). Hill and Blendis suggested that this relationship to family size occurs because illness is the only way to get attention in a large family.

The clearest support for the distinctions we are attempting to make between high-perception and low-perception symptoms comes from a telephone survey that we recently conducted. A random sample of people from metropolitan Cincinnati were asked a series of questions about what symptoms they currently had and about their early experiences in relation to illness. Of the 832 respondents, 67 were classified as having probable irritable bowel syndrome on the basis of their answering "yes" to the question, "Are you often troubled with intestinal gas distension or abdominal pain?" and answering "yes" to the question, "Are you often troubled with constipation or diarrhea?" Two hundred and twenty were classified as having hypertension on the basis of their answering "yes" to the question, "Have you ever been told by a doctor or nurse that you have high blood pressure?" There was some overlap between these groups. All these people were asked what was the occupation of the highest paid member of the household, and the response was classified as either low SES (blue-collar or public assistance) or high SES (white-collar or professional). All subjects were also asked, "Did your parents show special consideration for you when you had a cold or flu (as a child) by giving you special foods, toys, or other gifts?"

People with irritable bowel syndrome had been rewarded for illness more frequently as children than had people without irritable bowel syndrome, whereas people with hypertension had not been rewarded for illness significantly more than people without hypertension. The results were most striking for female subjects. Women with irritable bowel syndrome had been rewarded by parents for illness twice as often as women without irritable bowel syndrome (65% versus 33%). Socioeconomic status, which was inferred from occupation, was assumed to reflect differences in the amount of chronic stress to which people were exposed. Chi-square analysis indicated that persons who reported having hypertension were significantly more likely to come from the lower SES grades than were people without hypertension, whereas there were no significant differences in SES associated with irritable bowel syndrome.

These data support the hypothesis that high-perception psychosomatic symptoms, such as irritable bowel syndrome, are more likely to be associated with a history of reinforcement for illness than are low-perception symptoms, such as hypertension, whereas low-perception symptoms (e.g., hypertension) are more likely to be associated with chronic stressors (as reflected in occupation) than are high-perception symptoms.

The second logical deduction that one could draw from the analysis of how psychosomatic symptoms might come to be operantly conditioned is that patients with symptoms ought to have a greater subjective awareness of sensations associated with the pathophysiological response than people without these symptoms. Where there are research data available, this seems to be the case. Ritchie (1973) has shown that patients with irritable bowel syndrome have a lower threshold for pain produced by inflating a balloon in the colon than do nonpatients, and Schuster (1977) indicated that these patients also report subjective sensations other than pain at lower thresholds of distension than nonpatients. These data showing greater perceptual sensitivity for the symptomatic response in irritable bowel patients are not conclusive because it could be argued that greater sensitivity is the result rather than the cause of bowel symptoms. However, there is no inflammation in the bowel of these patients that would make this a likely explanation for the data, since occurrence of inflammation would lead to a diagnosis other than irritable bowel syndrome.

In contrast to these data suggesting that irritable bowel patients are more aware than nonpatients of sensations originating in the bowel, we have not observed a relationship between autonomic perception and voluntary control of an autonomic response in nonpatients. We (Whitehead, Drescher, Heiman, & Blackwell, 1977) studied the relationship between individual differences in awareness of heartbeat and individual differences in ability to voluntarily increase and decrease heart rate in 54 normal subjects and found the correlation to be near zero. Also, awareness of heartbeat did not correlate with learned increases or decreases in heart rate during biofeedback training. This finding contrasts with the modest positive correlations (rho approximately equal to 0.50) between heart rate perception and learned increases in heart rate that were reported by McFarland (1975) and by Clemens and MacDonald (1976).

We believe that our data showing a lack of relationship between heartbeat awareness and heart rate control in normal subjects do not disconfirm the hypothesized relationship between awareness and occurrence of symptoms in psychosomatic patients for the following reasons. As previously stated, awareness is a necessary but not a sufficient condition for the acquisition of voluntary control over an autonomic response in the absence of mechanical feedback. The other requisite conditions include motivation to control the response and an opportunity to engage in extended practice. The normal subjects whom we studied were motivated by the offer of money for a successful performance, but they had never been motivated to control their heart rate before and had never practiced prior to the test session. Had they practiced for several sessions prior to the test session (without mechanical feedback), we would predict that awareness of heartbeat would have correlated with voluntary control of heart rate.

One of the implications of the hypothesis that psychosomatic symptoms may be learned because of the reinforcing consequences that follow them is that operant psychosomatic symptoms and hysterical conversion symptoms are functionally equivalent. They develop in the same way and may be treated in the same way. Miller (1975) has also discussed this point.

Diagnosis

It is usually possible to determine when operant reinforcers are maintaining psychosomatic symptoms by a careful interview directed at discovering what the patient does when he is ill and how other people respond to him when he is ill. The patient with operantly conditioned symptoms is more likely to exempt himself from his regular duties, to consult a physician, and to go to bed than is another patient with physiological changes that a physician would expect to result in comparable subjective distress. Family members and friends of a patient with operantly reinforced symptoms are more likely to take over the patient's duties when he is ill and to show him special consideration. Such patients are also likely to have poor social skills and to appear mildly depressed. In social interactions, they frequently focus on their somatic symptoms in ways that elicit caretaking responses from others, and they reward caretaking responses by expressions of gratitude (Wooley & Blackwell, 1975). They often have a long history of frequent visits to doctors and multiple hospital admissions, and they are frequently taking excessive amounts of medication, especially analgesics and tranquilizers.

An example of a patient with a psychosomatic symptom that appeared to be maintained by operant reinforcers is the following. A 20-year-old married woman was referred by her internist with complaints of frequent diarrhea and tension headaches. She had had extensive diagnostic workups for both symptoms, but with the exception of multiple allergies, nothing had been found. Treatment of the allergies had not reduced her symptoms. She appeared to be depressed and reported that she avoided social activities. Prior to marriage, she had had few female friends but mostly male friends whom she dated. After her marriage, these male friends related only to her husband, so that her limited social skills were no longer appropriate. She was unable to assert herself at work when other employees took advantage of her and was unable to assert herself in family gatherings other than by means of her symptoms. Her headaches did not interfere with her work. Diarrhea had interfered with a previous factory job that she did not like but did not interfere with her current job as a storeroom clerk. Diarrhea also interfered with her social life; she would not have guests to dinner and would avoid other social activities because of it. Symptoms of irritable bowel syndrome were most likely to occur when she was with her husband or her mother-in-law, whom she liked. A typical instance of diarrhea was as follows. She was visiting her husband's parents, and her father-in-law was talking endlessly about hunting or about auto accidents. She wanted to leave but did not want to offend people. She got nervous, and her stomach began to hurt. She did not say anything, but eventually her husband and her mother-in-law noticed that she was squirming and grimacing, and they decided to end the evening.

It is important to note that even though psychosomatic symptoms may appear to be under the control of operant reinforcers, the patient is not intentionally acting ill—vomiting or whatever—in order to get attention. Rather, it appears that these symptoms are usually inadvertently learned responses over which the patient feels he has no control. Confrontations with the patient about the cause of his symptoms is perceived as threatening. The therapist must be sensitive in how he deals with these issues with the patient and his family. Techniques that we have found helpful are (1) simply suggesting that paying attention to symptoms by thinking about them and talking about them can make them worse and (2) suggesting that, just as with biofeedback, in which people can be taught to lower their heart rate or change autonomic responses in desired directions, people may accidently be exposed to biofeedback contingencies that cause their bodies to learn inappropriate physiological responses. A third technique for reducing the threat is (3) to use a patient group in which most of the information is transmitted by peers who have had similar problems rather than by therapists.

Treatment

When psychosomatic symptoms are under the control of operant reinforcers, two strategies are used to treat them. The first is extinction, in which the aim of treatment is to stop the reinforcement of illness behavior, and the second technique is to teach the patient alternative social skills for getting attention from others or for controlling the occurrence of aversive events.

In our inpatient psychosomatic service, extinction of somatic complaints is accomplished by having the staff systematically ignore somatic complaints, and the patient is instructed to discuss his symptoms only at scheduled times with his primary physician. Other staff members do not listen to complaints, and the patient group is encouraged to behave in the same way toward new patients. Physical signs are also ignored insofar as this is possible while maintaining adequate medical coverage, and the patient is given responsibility for managing his own symptom. Thus, for example, a patient who vomits is ignored and is expected to clean up after himself. He is also given daily feedback on his electrolyte balance and is expected to regulate this himself. Failure to maintain his electrolytes within acceptable limits will result in a transfer to medicine.

It is possible to extinguish somatic complaints in outpatients as well. For example, one patient who made multiple somatic complaints was told that her therapist would talk with her about somatic complaints only during the last 10 minutes of the hour; at other times, he wanted to discuss her accomplishments since the last meeting. This tactic successfully reduced the amount of somatic complaining to the point that she sometimes forgot to engage in it, and alternative, more healthy behaviors increased in frequency.

In the inpatient treatment program we (Wooley, Blackwell, & Winget, 1978) find it especially important to counsel families around the issue of ignoring somatic complaints. Family counseling is, of course, not restricted to a discussion of how to ignore symptoms. Typically, it involves a discussion of what kinds of behaviors family members want from each other and how they can get these behaviors and manage to reinforce them without using the illness of one family member to accomplish these goals.

The importance of social reinforcers in maintaining somatic complaints and the effectiveness of extinction procedures are illustrated by an analog study carried out on the inpatient psychosomatic service at Cincinnati General Hospital (Wooley, Epps, & Blackwell, 1975). Inpatients were asked to hold their hands in ice water for as long as possible and were tested under two conditions. In one condition, the experimenter dressed in a white coat and provided encouraging comments at 15-second intervals (e.g., "You are doing fine"). In the other condition, subjects were told that it was up to them to figure out how to tolerate the cold water because the staff had no idea, and we would be interested in what they came up with (i.e., self-responsibility was emphasized). Also, the experimenter dressed in street clothes and made no comment during the test. Figure 4 shows the dramatic differences between these two test conditions. When the medical care establishment was present in the form of a white-coated and solicitous experimenter, pain tolerances were uniformly below one minute. However, when the patient was put on his own and the experimenter's social role and behavior were neutral with respect to the patient's history of reinforcement, pain tolerances were unusually high—11 of 12 patients reached the maximum of six minutes.

This analog study does not address the issue of whether abnormal physiological events change in response to reinforcement and extinction, since the study dealt only with overt behaviors and verbal behaviors. It is our contention that for high-perception symptoms, at least, physiological events may respond in the same way to reinforcement and extinction.

The second treatment strategy for dealing with operantly reinforced symptoms—namely, training patients in alternative behaviors to get what they want from others—is achieved primarily through social skills training. Through the use of

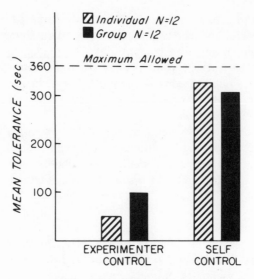

MEAN ICE WATER TOLERANCE

Figure 4.   Effects of experimenter control versus self-control on the behavior of psychosomatic patients undergoing a cold pressor test. When discriminative stimuli previously associated with reinforcement of illness behaviors were presented (a solicitous experimenter dressed in a white coat), pain tolerance was lower than when no such discriminative stimuli were present (self-control condition).

didactic instruction, modeling, and practice with feedback, patients are taught how to stick up for their rights, how to express affection as well as anger or other feelings, how to carry on conversations in ways that convey interest, shaping as a means of modifying the behavior of others, and problem solving. The rationale for social skills training is the assumption that people need to obtain certain kinds of attention from other people and that if they do not learn new ways of getting it, they will fall back on their symptoms as a means of obtaining this attention. Sometimes remedial education or job training are also used to establish behaviors incompatible with illness.

An example of the application of social skills training to the treatment of psychosomatic symptoms is contained in a study by Mitchell and Mitchell (1971). They compared relaxation alone, systematic desensitization, and social skills training plus desensitization in the treatment of migraine headaches. Social skills training consisted of modeling appropriate behaviors by the therapist, rehearsal by the patient with feedback from the therapist, and behavioral assignments to carry out outside of treatment sessions. The training emphasized "frank verbalization and spontaneous expression of basic feelings and emotions such as love, affection, and hostility," in a social context such as asking for a date where the patient reported having difficulty. Patients treated with social skills training showed a significant reduction in frequency of migraine headaches compared to the other groups.

CLASSICAL CONDITIONING AS A CAUSE OF PSYCHOSOMATIC SYMPTOMS

When some neutral stimulus such as a bell sound is repeatedly paired with a stimulus that elicits a reflex (such as electric shock eliciting increases in blood pressure), eventually the neutral stimulus (bell) alone will elicit the reflex (DeLeon, 1972). This form of learning is called *classical conditioning*, *Pavlovian conditioning*, or *respondent conditioning*. The stimulus eliciting the reflex need not be aversive. For example, we have classically conditioned decreases in blood pressure by pairing a bell with tilting the subject 15° head down from the horizontal, which is a mild stimulus (Whitehead, Lurie, & Blackwell, 1976a).

Some psychosomatic symptoms seem more likely than others to become classically conditioned. The best evidence for classical conditioning exists for asthma, in which the occurrence of conditioned responses to artificial flowers and oxygen masks, for example, is well documented in papers reviewed by Moore (1965). There is also evidence for classical conditioning in the etiology of irritable bowel syndrome. Chudhary and Truelove (1962) found that 25% of their patients dated the onset of symptoms from an attack of dysentery but continued to have periodic symptoms following the elimination of amoebas from the bowel. Other studies reviewed by Thompson (1974) found that altered bowel habits persisted well after adequate organic causes ceased to be present. Vomiting may also occur as a classically conditioned response.

Importance of Symptom Perception

Laboratory experiments and clinical observations suggest that awareness of the physiological response is not necessary for the occurrence of classical conditioning. As a matter of fact, it is not even necessary that the response occur (Crisler, 1930; Solomon & Turner, 1962), provided the conditional stimulus and an adequate unconditional stimulus are appropriately paired. It is thus possible that many poorly perceived physiological responses, such as blood pressure elevation may become classically conditioned to aspects of the environment that are intermittently paired with stressors without the subject's knowledge or his physician's knowledge that this has occurred.

It is our impression, however, that the symptoms that are most susceptible to classical conditioning (e.g., asthma, irritable bowel syndrome, and vomiting) are those that have an abrupt onset rather than a gradual onset, such as occurs in migraine. This observation, if it is accurate, may simply reflect the fact that the required temporal relationship between the conditional stimulus and the unconditional stimulus is more likely to occur when the unconditional stimulus and its associated response are discrete and follow the conditional stimulus immediately. Naturally occurring conditional stimuli are likely to be time-limited.

Diagnosis

A psychosomatic symptom is designated a classically conditioned response if the symptom occurs reliably in one or more specific situations that are not considered aversive by most people and if there is no evidence that the symptom is differentially affected by the response of other people to it. This information can be obtained by interview, but it is more reliable to have the patient keep records of the antecedents and consequences of the symptomatic response.

Classical conditioning is sometimes confused with the effects of situational stressors because both may be associated with the occurrence of abnormal physiological responses only in specific situations. The difference is that in simple stress reactions, the physiological responses are appropriate to the situation, whereas in classically conditioned responses, the physiological responses are not appropriate to or are not adequately accounted for by the situations that appear to elicit them. For example, elevations in blood pressure that occur when the air traffic controller is at work would be regarded as stress reactions because the situation remains stressful, whereas the asthmatic attack that occurs when an asthmatic sniffs a paper flower (cf. Moore, 1965) would be regarded as a classically conditioned response because the paper flower is in fact harmless.

It is often difficult in practice to decide whether a response is classically conditioned or not on the basis of whether the situation appears stressful, especially if the triggering situation is an interpersonal one, such as dinnertime in a family. Social interactions between family members at dinnertime may occasionally be highly stressful for the patient but may usually be relatively innocuous. In such a case, we would infer that classical conditioning had occurred if the patient's symptoms occurred every time he sat down to dinner and that a simple stress reaction was occurring if the patient's symptoms occurred only on the days when his environment was stressful.

Psychosomatic symptoms that appear to be classically conditioned are often associated with or mediated by anxiety. All situations that make the patient anxious cause the psychosomatic symptom to be elicited even though in many of these situations, there may never have been a sequence of events that could account for the classical conditioning of the symptom. For example, it is easy to understand how an asthmatic reaction to a plastic flower could have developed by classical conditioning but not an asthmatic reaction to having to talk to one's boss. In such individuals, one cannot arouse significant amounts of anxiety without eliciting the psychosomatic symptom, although the converse is not true; one can trigger the symptom when the patient is not anxious. This finding suggests that some aspect of the anxiety state itself comes to act as a conditional stimulus that elicits the psychosomatic symptom because of its frequent association with unconditional stimuli that do produce the symptom. It is possible to eliminate such classically conditioned responses by the usual classical extinction procedures described below as long as the anxiety and the psychosomatic symptoms are elicited by only a limited number of identifiable situations.

Treatment

Classically conditioned symptoms are treated by classical extinction procedures, namely, systematic desensitization and flooding. In both cases, treatment consists of exposing the patient to the harmless situation until it no longer elicits the conditioned response.

In systematic desensitization, the therapist teaches the patient to relax so that muscular relaxation can be used to counteract or suppress the anxiety or the psychosomatic symptoms during exposure to the situations that evoke symptoms. The therapist arranges the situations that produce symptoms into a hierarchy, beginning with those situations that produce the most intense symptoms. Desensitization is accomplished by having the patient visualize the hierarchy items for periods of about six seconds while relaxed. When visualization of items at the bottom of the hierarchy no longer leads to symptoms (or arousal), the therapist moves up to the next hierarchy item. In this way, the conditioned symptomatic response is eliminated from each item in the hierarchy. Toward the end of the hierarchy, the patient may be instructed to put himself into the actual situation.

Moore (1965) reported a study that illustrates the use of systematic desensitization in the treatment of bronchial asthma. She compared systematic desensitization as described above with a treatment that involved relaxation only and to another treatment that involved relaxation training plus suggestions that improvement would occur. Asthmatic patients in all three groups showed a decrease in the number of attacks that they reported having outside the hospital, but only the desensitization treatment produced a significant improvement in objective pulmonary function tests (i.e., an increase in maximum peak flow).

Cohen and Reed (1968) reported on the use of systematic desensitization to treat six patients with psychosomatic symptoms (two with nausea and vomiting when eating in public, two with frequency of defecation when traveling, one with frequency of micturation when traveling, and one with excessive sweating when traveling). These patients were selected for treatment because their symptoms appeared to be restricted to specific situations that were not objectively stressful; that is, their symptoms appeared to be classically conditioned. Two hierarchies were used—one involving the situations eliciting symptoms and one involving occurrence of the symptoms themselves. The five patients who completed the treatment showed marked improvement, which was maintained at follow-up six months later. The number of sessions ranged from 6 to 19.

Another classical extinction procedure that is frequently used to treat conditioned anxiety responses is flooding. Flooding usually involves exposure of the patient to the actual situation that elicits his symptoms, and exposure begins at the top of the hierarchy rather than being gradual. Also, muscle relaxation is not used to inhibit anxiety or symptoms during exposure. Another critical element is that the patient cannot escape from or rapidly terminate exposure to the situation because the occurrence of an escape response followed by an abrupt reduction in symptoms prevents extinction from occurring. Flooding seems to lead to more rapid reduction in phobic symptoms than does systematic desensitization (e.g., Marks, 1975). Flooding has not been reported as a treatment for psychosomatic symptoms. There are some symptoms, such as asthma, that one would not want to elicit in a maximal form, but other symptoms, such as vomiting, could be extinguished using a flooding procedure.

INTERACTIONS BETWEEN CLASSICAL AND OPERANT CONDITIONING AND STRESS RESPONSES

We have emphasized the distinctions between classical and operant conditioning and stress responses in order to underscore the fact that they make independent contributions to the etiology of psychosomatic disorders and to point out that different treatment strategies are appropriate, depending on how the abnormal physiological response is currently maintained. Many psychosomatic disorders, however, are the result of interactions between stress reactions and classical and operant conditioning.

It is probable that many, if not most, psychosomatic symptoms first arise as reactions to environmental stressors because most of these symptoms tend to occur in situations that are perceived by the patient as stressful or anxiety-arousing at least some of the time. When these stress responses are easily perceived by the patient and others in his environment, they may quickly come under the control of operant conditioning contingencies. This may occur in the same way that pain complaints in chronic pain patients come under the control of social consequences even though the pain may originally have had a quite adequate physical cause (Timmermans & Sternbach, 1974). When this happens (i.e., when a stress response comes under the control of an operant conditioning contingency), the relationship between the stressful aspects of the environment and occurrences of the symptom is obscured; the symptom begins to occur in new situations in which the stressor is not present. It is then more appropriate to disregard the stressor and to treat the problem as an operantly conditioned response, since these contingencies will ordinarily account for more occurrences of the response than the stressor.

Hypertension provides a revealing example of this kind of interaction. It was originally supposed that hypertension was caused by suppressed hostility (Alexander, 1950; Hokanson & Burgess, 1962; Hokanson, Burgess, & Cohen, 1963), and some early studies of clinic populations of hypertensives supported this view by showing that hypertensive clinic-attenders were more neurotic, anxious, or hostile than nonpatients. When studies came to be focused on random samples of people with hypertension, including those who were unaware of having elevated blood pressure, the correlations between personality traits and blood pressure no longer obtained;

hypertensives were no more neurotic, anxious, or hostile than people in general (Cochrane, 1973; Davies, 1970). Cochrane (1969) has directly compared hypertensives attending medical clinics with those who do not and finds that the clinic attenders score high on tests on neuroticism, whereas the clinic nonattenders are indistinguishable from the general population. These differences between hypertensive patients who attend clinics and those who do not suggest that when people become aware of a physical disorder, they may then secondarily use somatic complaints in ways that produce favorable consequences for them but that also lead them to be described as neurotic. This interpretation is underscored by the results of a recent Canadian study (Sackett, 1977) in which a group of factory workers who were newly discovered to have hypertension were educated about their disease and encouraged to seek treatment; not many workers sought treatment by a physician, but absenteeism from work increased substantially.

In hypertension, social consequences that are contingent on somatic complaints appear to increase somatic complaints and sick-role behaviors, but such social consequences probably do not account for blood pressure elevations because blood pressure elevations are not perceived by the patient. However, if the physiological response (such as spasm of the colon) is distinctly perceived by the patient or is observable to others, we would expect social consequences contingent on somatic complaints to increase the frequency of the physical event as well as the verbal complaint.

Interactions between classical and operant conditioning also appear to be common. Thus, symptoms such as asthma and irritable bowel syndrome that may have occurred as classically conditioned responses at some earlier stage may come to be influenced by social consequences. For example, the young woman with headaches and irritable bowel syndrome referred to earlier had begun to have diarrhea in connection with eating in the presence of strangers. This was probably a simple classically conditioned response. Gradually, however, the symptoms of spastic colon came to be reinforced by her husband and mother-in-law and began to occur in situations having nothing to do with eating. As one might expect, once the symptoms of irritable bowel syndrome were under the control of operant reinforcement, then systematic desensitization, which is based on classical extinction, was ineffectual for this symptom, even though it did reduce the frequency of her tension headaches.

Interactions such as these between classical and operant conditioning contingencies are exactly what one would expect based on the laboratory study of learning. Mellgren and Ost (1969); Whitehead, Lurie, and Blackwell, (1976b); and others (Grant, Kroll, Kantowitz, Zajano, & Solberg, 1969) have shown that learning achieved with a classical conditioning paradigm transfers readily to an operant conditioning task, and these studies suggest that such transfer results in more rapid acquisition of operant control over the response than is possible with an operant conditioning contingency alone.

Interactions such as these are particularly appealing in attempts to account for the learning of abnormal physiological responses because classical and operant conditioning procedures have complementary advantages and limitations. In accounting for the acquisition of abnormal physiological responses, classical conditioning provides a more plausible model than operant conditioning because classical conditioning of large-magnitude physiological responses may occur after only a few pairings of the neutral (conditional) stimulus and the unconditional stimulus (e.g., Whitehead *et al.*, 1976a). By contrast, the operant conditioning of some physiological responses is slow and difficult if one is restricted to reinforcing naturally occurring (unelicited) physiological changes. In laboratory studies or biofeedback training situations, the experimenter must usually begin by rewarding small deviations from baseline and gradually shaping the desired response by a process of reinforcing successively better approximations to the desired response (Miller, 1969; Fields, 1970). However, if one can apply the reinforcement to a physiological response that is already large and easily distinguished from baseline activity by eliciting a classically conditioned response, acquisition of large-magnitude physiological responses appears to be more rapid (Whitehead *et al.*, 1976b).

In attempting to account for the maintenance of learned physiological responses, on the other hand, operant conditioning has advantages over classical conditioning procedures. Classically conditioned responses typically extinguish quite rapidly. For example, Ottenberg, Stein, Lewis, and Hamilton (1958) established classically conditioned respiratory abnormalities in guinea pigs that mimicked asthmatic symptoms, but these symptoms extinguished after relatively few (up to 12) unreinforced trials. This extinction is uncharacteristic of naturally occurring psychosomatic symptoms, which may persist for many years. Classically conditioned responses are also difficult to establish and maintain on intermittent schedules of reinforcement (e.g., where the unconditioned stimulus is presented only occasionally following the conditioned stimulus; Ross, 1959), although under natural conditions, the unconditional stimuli that elicit psychosomatic symptoms reflexively usually occur only infrequently.

By contrast, operant conditioning procedures have two advantages: (1) operant responses are easily maintained on intermittant schedules of reinforcement and are very resistant to extinction when reinforcement is unpredictable (e.g., Reynolds, 1968; and (2) the class of events that may serve as operant reinforcers is much more inclusive than the class of events that may serve as unconditional stimuli for eliciting a given physiological response. Operant reinforcers may include avoidance of or escape from any aversive situation and may include attention from other people. Thus, the possibilities of maintaining an abnormal physiological response once it has been learned are greater with operant conditioning than with classical conditioning.

As the preceding analysis suggests, most of the high-perception psychosomatic symptoms have an etiology that reflects an interaction between stress reactions, classical conditioning, and operant conditioning. (This is not the case with psychosomatic disorders that are not perceived, such as high blood pressure, because they cannot be exposed to operant conditioning contingencies.) When psychosomatic symptoms are multiply determined in this way, diagnosis should be directed at determining the relative contribution of these different factors to the way the symptoms are *currently* maintained. The most appropriate treatment strategy will usually follow from such an analysis.

SUMMARY

The theoretical formulation presented here may be summarized as follows:

1. There are three determinants of psychosomatic symptoms: environmental stressors, operant reinforcement, and classical conditioning.

2. Psychosomatic symptoms that are difficult for people to perceive (e.g., hypertension, coronary heart disease) are more likely to occur as stress reactions, whereas symptoms that are easily perceived (e.g., migraine headaches, diarrhea) are more likely to occur as operantly conditioned symptoms. Either high-perception or low-perception symptoms may become classically conditioned, but symptoms that involve abrupt onset of pain or discomfort are more likely to become classically conditioned that symptoms having a gradual onset.

3. The etiological distinction has treatment implications. Stress reactions are treated by techniques that modulate the effects of stress (such as relaxation exercises or meditation) by techniques that cause the environment to be perceived differently (such as cognitive restructuring), or by modifying the stressful environment. Operantly conditioned symptoms are treated by discontinuing the reinforcement of symptoms and by teaching alternative behaviors. Classically conditioned responses are treated by classical extinction procedures, such as systematic desensitization or flooding.

4. It is not useful to distinguish between psychosomatic symptoms and hysterical conversion symptoms because the symptoms so labeled have similar etiologies and can be treated by similar techniques. The functional analysis described above is more useful for planning treatment.

ACKNOWLEDGMENTS

Francisco Barrios, Ph.D., contributed greatly to the review of previously published work. Bernard T. Engel, Ph.D., Chief of the Laboratory for Behavioral Sciences, Gerontology Research Center, National Institute on Aging, reviewed and made helpful suggestions for revising this paper. An abstract of this paper was presented at the Fourth International Congress of Psychosomatic Medicine in Kyoto, Japan, 1977.

REFERENCES

Alexander, F. *Psychosomatic medicine: Its principles and applications.* New York: W. W. Norton, 1950.

Alexander, F., French, T. M., & Pollock, G. *Psychosomatic specificity: Experimental study and results,* Vol. 1. Chicago: University of Chicago Press, 1968.

Apley, J., & Hale, B. Children with recurrent abdominal pain: How do they grow up? *British Medical Journal,* 1973, *3*, 7–9.

Ax, A. F. The physiological differentiation between fear and anger in humans. *Psychosomatic Medicine,* 1953, *14*, 433–442.

Benson, H., Alexander, S., & Feldman, C. L. Decreased premature ventricular contractions through use of the relaxation response in patients with stable ischaemic heart-disease. *Lancet*, 1975, *2*(7931), 380–382.

Blackwell, B., & Whitehead, W. E. Behavioral evaluation of antianxiety drugs. In A. Sudilovsky, S. Gershon, & B. Beer (Eds.), *Predictability in psychopharmacology—Preclinical and clinical correlations*. New York: Raven, 1975.

Blackwell, B., Wooley, S., & Whitehead, W. E. Psychosomatic illness: A new treatment approach. *Journal of Cincinnati Academy of Medicine*, 1974, *55*, 95–98.

Blackwell, B., Hanenson, I., Bloomfield, S., Magenheim, H., Gartside, P., Nidich, S., Robinson, A., & Zigler, R. Transcendental meditation in hypertension: Individual response patterns. *Lancet*, 1976, *1*(7953), 223–226.

Bramwell, S., Masuda, M., Wagner, N., & Holmes, T. Psychosocial factors in athletic injuries. *Journal of Human Stress*, 1975, *1*, 6.

Chappell, M. N., & Stevenson, T. I. Group psychological training in some organic conditions. *Mental Hygiene*, 1936, *20*, 588–597.

Chappell, M. N., Stefano, J. J., Rogerson, J. S., & Pike, F. H. The value of group psychological procedures in the treatment of peptic ulcer. *American Journal of Digestive Diseases*, 1936, *3*, 813–817.

Christensen, M. F., & Mortensen, O. Long-term prognosis in children with recurrent abdominal pain. *Archives of Diseases of Children*, 1975, *50*, 110–114.

Chudhary, N. A., & Truelove, S. C. The irritable colon syndrome. *Quarterly Journal of Medicine*, 1962, *31*, 307–322.

Clemens, W. J., & MacDonald, D. F. Relationship between heart beat discrimination and heart rate control. *Psychophysiology*, 1976, *13*, 176.

Cobb, S., & Rose, R. M. Hypertension, peptic ulcer, and diabetes in air traffic controllers. *Journal of the American Medical Association*, 1973, *224*, 489–492.

Cochrane, R. Neuroticism and the discovery of high blood pressure. *Journal of Psychosomatic Research*, 1969, *13*, 21–25.

Cochrane, R. Hostility and neuroticism among unselected essential hypertensives. *Journal of Psychosomatic Research*, 1973, *17*, 215–218.

Cohen, S. I., & Reed, J. L. The treatment of "nervous diarrhea" and other conditioned autonomic disorders by desensitization. *British Journal of Psychiatry*, 1968, *114*, 1275–1280.

Cohen, S. I., Silverman, A. J., Waddell, W., & Zuidema, G. D. Urinary catecholamine levels, gastric secretion and specific psychological factors in ulcer and non-ulcer patients. *Journal of Psychosomatic Research*, 1961, *5*, 90–115.

Crisler, G. Salivation is unnecessary for the establishment of the salivary conditioned reflex induced by morphine. *American Journal of Physiology*, 1930, *44*, 553–556.

Davies, M. Blood pressure and personality. *Journal of Psychosomatic Research*, 1970, *14*, 89–104.

DeLeon, G. Classical conditioning and extinction of human systolic blood pressure. *Conditioned Reflex*, 1972, *7*, 193–209.

Diagnostic and Statistical Manual of Mental Disorders (2nd ed.). Washington, D.C.: American Psychiatric Association, 1968.

Dunbar, F. *Psychosomatic diagnosis*. New York: Paul B. Hoeber, 1943.

Engel, B. T., & Bickford, A. F. Response specificity: Stimulus–response and individual-response specificity in essential hypertensives. *Archives of General Psychiatry*, 1961, *5*, 478–489.

Engel, G. L. The need for a new medical model: A challenge for biomedicine. *Science*, 1977, *196*, 129–136.

Farbman, A. A. Neck sprain: Associated factors. *Journal of the American Medical Association*, 1973, *223*, 1010–1015.

Fields, C. Instrumental conditioning of the rat cardiac control system. *Proceedings of the National Academy of Sciences*, 1970, *65*, 293–299.

Frankenhaeuser, M. Experimental approaches to the study of catecholamines and emotion. In L. Levi (Ed.), *Emotions: Their parameters and measurement*. New York: Raven Press, 1975.

French, J. R. P., Jr., & Caplan, R. D. Psychosocial factors in coronary heart disease. In P. M. Insel & R. H. Moos (Eds.), *Health and the social environment*. Lexington, Mass.: Lexington, 1974.

Graham, D. T. Psychosomatic medicine. In N. S. Greenfield & R. A. Sternbach (Eds.), *Handbook of psychophysiology*. New York: Holt, Rinehart & Winston, 1972.

Graham, D. T., Lundy, R. M., Benjamin, L. S., Kabler, J. D., Lewis, W. C., Kunish, N. O., & Graham, F. K. Specific attitudes in initial interviews with patients having different "psychosomatic diseases." *Psychosomatic Medicine*, 1962, *24*, 257–266.

Grant, D. A., Kroll, N. E., Kantowitz, B., Zajano, M. J., & Solberg, K. G. Transfer of eyelid conditioning from instrumental to classical reinforcement and vice versa. *Journal of Experimental Psychology*, 1969, *82*, 503–510.

Greenfield, D., Katz, D., Alexander, A., & Roessler, R. The relationship between physiology and psychological responsivity: Depression and galvanic skin response. *Journal of Nervous and Mental Disease*, 1963, *136*, 535–539.

Gutman, M. C., & Benson, H. Interaction of environmental factors and systemic arterial blood pressure: A review. *Medicine*, 1971, *54*, 543–553.

Henryk-Gutt, R., & Rees, W. L. Psychological aspects of migraine. *Journal of Psychosomatic Research*, 1973, *17*, 141–153.

Hill, O. W., & Blendis, L. Physical and psychological evaluation of "non-organic" abdominal pain. *Gut*, 1967, *8*, 221–229.

Hokanson, J. E., & Burgess, M. The effects of three types of aggression on vascular processes. *Journal of Abnormal and Social Psychology*, 1962, *64*, 446–449.

Hokanson, J. E., Burgess, M., & Cohen, M. F. Effects of displaced aggression on systolic blood pressure. *Journal of Abnormal and Social Psychology*, 1963, *67*, 214–218.

Holmes, T., & Masuda, M. Life changes and illness susceptibility. In B. S. Dohrenwend & B. P. Dohrenwend (Eds.), *Stressful life events*. New York: Wiley, 1974.

Holmes, T. H., & Rahe, R. H. The social readjustment rating scale. *Journal of Psychosomatic Research*, 1967, *11*, 213–218.

Jenkins, C. D., Tuthill, R., Tannenbaum, S. I., & Kirby, C. Community stressors predicting death from hypertensive heart disease. Paper presented at the annual meeting of the American Psychosomatic Society, March 1977.

Kellner, R. Psychotherapy in psychosomatic disorders: A survey of controlled studies. *Archives of General Psychiatry*, 1975, *32*, 1021–1028.

Kelly, D. H. W., & Walter, C. J. S. The relationship between clinical diagnosis and anxiety assessed by forearm blood flow and other measurements. *British Journal of Psychiatry*, 1968, *114*, 611–626.

Kopel, F. B., Kim, I. C., & Barbero, G. J. Comparison of rectosigmoid motility in normal children, children with recurrent abdominal pain, and children with ulcerative colitis. *Pediatrics*, 1967, *39*, 539–545.

Lacey, J. I., Bateman, D. E., & Van Lehn, R. Autonomic response specificity: An experimental study. *Psychosomatic Medicine*, 1953, *15*, 8–21.

Lader, M. Psychophysiological research and psychosomatic medicine. In R. Porter & J. Knight (Eds.), *Physiology, emotion, and psychosomatic illness*. New York: Elsevier, 1972.

Lader, M. H., & Wing, L. Habituation of the psycho-galvanic reflex in patients with anxiety states and in normal subjects. *Journal of Neurology and Neurosurgical Psychiatry*, 1964, *27*, 210–218.

Langner, T. S., & Michael, S. T. *Life stress and mental health: The Midtown Manhattan study*, Vol. 2. London: Free Press of Glencoe, 1963.

Levi, L. Stress, distress and psychosocial stimuli. In A. McLean (Ed.), *Occupational stress*. Springfield, Ill.: Charles C Thomas, 1974.

Luborsky, L., Brady, J. P., McClintock, M., Kron, R. E., Bortnichak, E., & Levitz, L. Estimating one's own systolic blood pressure: Effects of feedback training. *Psychosomatic Medicine*, 1976, *38*, 426–438.

Malmo, R. B., & Shagass, C. Physiologic study of symptom mechanisms in psychiatric patients under stress. *Psychosomatic Medicine*, 1949, *11*, 25–29.

Mandler, G., Mandler, J., & Uviller, E. Autonomic feedback: The perception of autonomic activity. *Journal of Abnormal and Social Psychology*, 1958, *56*, 367–373.

Marks, I. Behavioral treatments of phobic and obsessive-compulsive disorders: A critical appraisal. In M. Hersen, R. M. Eisler, & P. M. Miller (Eds.), *Progress in behavior modification*, Vol. 1. New York: Academic, 1975.

McCarron, L. T. Psychophysiological discriminants of reactive depression. *Psychophysiology*, 1973, *10*, 223–230.

McFarland, R. A. Heart rate perception and heart rate control. *Psychophysiology*, 1975, *12*, 402–405.

Mechanic, D. The concept of illness behavior. *Journal of Chronic Disease*, 1962, *15*, 189–194.

Mechanic, D. Social psychologic factors affecting the presentation of bodily complaints. *New England Journal of Medicine*, 1972, *286*, 1132–1139.

Medical Letter, Diazepam (Valium) in hypertension. *Medical Letter Drug Therapy*, 1974, *16*(23), 96.

Meichenbaum, D., & Turk, D. The cognitive-behavioral management of anxiety, anger, and pain. In P. O. Davidson (Ed.), *The behavioral management of anxiety, depression and pain*. New York: Brunner/Mazel, 1976.

Mellgren, R. L., & Ost, J. W. P. Transfer of Pavlovian differential conditioning to an operant discrimination. *Journal of Comparative and Physiological Psychology*, 1969, *67*, 390–394.

Miller, N. E. Learning of visceral and glandular responses. *Science*, 1969, *163*, 434–445.

Miller, N. E. Interactions between learned and physical factors in mental illness. *Seminars in Psychiatry*, 1972, *4*, 239–254.

Miller, N. E. Applications of learning and biofeedback to psychiatry and medicine. In A. N. Freedman, H. I. Kaplan, & B. J. Sadock (Eds.), *Comprehensive textbook of psychiatry* (2nd ed.). Baltimore: Williams & Wilkins, 1975.

Miller, N. E. Learning, stress, and psychosomatic symptoms. *Acta Neurobiologica Experimentia*, 1976, *36*, 141–156.

Miller, N. E., & Dworkin, B. R. Effects of learning on visceral functions—Biofeedback. *New England Journal of Medicine*, 1977, *296*, 1274–1278.

Mitchell, K. R., & Mitchell, D. M. Migraine: An exploratory treatment application of programmed behavior therapy techniques. *Journal of Psychosomatic Research*, 1971, *15*, 137–157.

Moore, N. Behavior therapy in bronchial asthma: A controlled study. *Journal of Psychosomatic Research*, 1965, *9*, 257–276.

Oster, J. Recurrent abdominal pain, headache, and limb pains in children and adolescents. *Pediatrics*, 1972, *50*, 429–435.

Ottenberg, P., Stein, M., Lewis, J., & Hamilton, C. Learned asthma in the guinea pig. *Psychosomatic Medicine*, 1958, *20*, 395–400.

Palmai, G., Blackwell, B., Maxwell, A. E., & Morgenstern, F. Patterns of salivary flow in depressive illness and during treatment. *British Journal of Psychiatry*, 1967, *113*, 1297–1308.

Parsons, T. *The social system*. New York: Free Press, 1951.

Patel, C. H. Biofeedback-aided relaxation and meditation in the management of hypertension. *Biofeedback and Self-Regulation*, 1977, *2*, 1–41.

Pilowsky, I. Abnormal illness behavior. *British Journal of Medical Psychology*, 1969, *42*, 347–351.

Rabkin, J. G., & Struening, E. L. Life events, stress, and illness. *Science*, 1976, *194*, 1013–1020.

Rahe, R. H. Subjects' recent life changes and their near-future illness reports. *Annals of Clinical Research*, 1972, *4*, 250–265.

Rees, W. L. Stress, distress and disease. *British Journal of Psychiatry*, 1976, *128*, 3–18.

Reynolds, G. S. *A primer of operant conditioning*. San Diego: Scott, Foresman, 1968.

Ritchie, J. Pain from distension of the pelvic colon by inflating a balloon in the irritable colon syndrome. *Gut*, 1973, *14*, 125–132.

Rosenman, R. H., Friedman, M., Straus, R. Wurm, M., Jenkins, C. D., & Messinger, H. B. Coronary heart disease in the Western collaborative group study. *Journal of the American Medical Association*, 1966, *195*, 130–136.

Ross, L. E. The decremental effects of partial reinforcement during acquisition of the conditioned eyelid response. *Journal of Experimental Psychology*, 1959, *57*, 74–82.

Sackett, D. Personal communication, 1977.

Schachter, J. Pain, fear, and anger in hypertensives and normotensives: A psychophysiological study. *Psychosomatic Medicine*, 1957, *19*, 17–29.

Schacter, S., & Singer, J. E. Cognitive, social, and psychological determinants of emotional state. *Psychological Review*, 1962, *69*, 379–399.

Schuster, M. M. Personal communication, 1977.

Seligman, M. E. P. *Helplessness: On depression, development, and death.*San Francisco: W. H. Freeman, 1975.

Selye, H. *The stress of life.* New York: McGraw-Hill, 1956.

Shapiro, A. P., Schwartz, G. E., Ferguson, D. C. E., Redmond, D. P., & Weiss, S. M. Behavioral methods in the treatment of hypertension: A review of their clinical status. *Annals of Internal Medicine,* 1977, *86,* 626–636.

Solomon, R. L., & Turner, L. H. Discriminative classical conditioning in dogs paralyzed by curare can later control discriminative avoidance responses in the normal state. *Psychological Review,* 1962, *69,* 202–219.

Spielberger, C. D., Gorsuch, R. L., & Lushene, R. E. *Manual for the state-trait anxiety inventory.* Palo Alto: Consulting Psychology Press, 1970.

Sternbach, R. A. *Pain patients: Traits and treatment.* New York: Academic, 1974.

Stone, R. A., & DeLeo, J. Psychotherapeutic control of hypertension. *The New England Journal of Medicine,* 1976, *294,* 80–84.

Stone, R. T., & Barbero, G. J. Recurrent abdominal pain in childhood. *Pediatrics,* 1970, *45,* 723–738.

Thompson, W. G. The irritable colon. *Canadian Medical Association Journal,* 1974, *111,* 1236–1244.

Timmermans, G., & Sternbach, R. A. Factors of human chronic pain: An analysis of personality and pain reaction variables. *Science,* 1974, *184,* 806–808.

Titchener, J. L., Sheldon, M. B., & Ross, W. D. Changes in blood pressure of hypertensive patients with and without group psychotherapy. *Journal of Psychosomatic Research,* 1959, *4,* 10–12.

Walker, B. B., & Sandman, C. A. Physiological response patterns in ulcer patients: Phasic and tonic components of the electrogastrogram. *Psychophysiology,* 1977, *14,* 393–400.

Waller, S. L., & Misiewicz, J. J. Prognosis in the irritable-bowel syndrome. *Lancet,* 1969, 753–756.

Weiner, H., Thaler, M., Reiser, M. F., & Mirsky, I. A. Etiology of duodenal ulcer. *Psychosomatic Medicine,* 1957, *19,* 1–10.

Weiss, J. M. Somatic effects of predictable and unpredictable shock. *Psychosomatic Medicine,* 1970, *32,* 397–408.

Weiss, J. M. Effects of coping behavior in different warning signal conditions on stress pathology in rats. *Journal of Comparative and Physiological Psychology,* 1971, *77,* 1–13. (a)

Weiss, J. M. Effects of coping behavior with and without a feedback signal on stress pathology in rats. *Journal of Comparative and Physiological Psychology,* 1971, *77,* 22–30. (b)

Whitehead, W. E., Lurie, E., & Blackwell, B. Classical conditioning of decreases in human systolic blood pressure. *Journal of Applied Behavior Analysis,* 1976, *9,* 153–157. (a)

Whitehead, W. E., Lurie, E., & Blackwell, B. Classical conditioning procedures facilitate biofeedback training to lower blood pressure in essential hypertension. *Psychophysiology,* 1976, *13,* 176–177. (b)

Whitehead, W. E., Blackwell, B., DeSilva, H., & Robinson, A. Anxiety and anger in hypertension. *Journal of Psychosomatic Research,* 1977, *21,* 383–389.

Whitehead, W. E., Drescher, V. M., Heiman, P., & Blackwell, B. Relation of heart rate control to heart beat perception. *Biofeedback and Self-Regulation,* 1977, *2,* 371–392.

Wolf, S., & Goodell, H. *Behavioral science in clinical medicine.* Springfield, Ill.: Charles C Thomas, 1976.

Wolff, H. G. *Headache and other head pain.* New York: Oxford University Press, 1963.

Wolff, H. G. *Stress and disease* (2nd ed.). Revised and edited by S. Wolf and H. Goodell. Springfield, Ill.; Charles C Thomas, 1968.

Wooley, S. C., & Blackwell, B. A behavioral probe into social contingencies on a psychosomatic ward. *Journal of Applied Behavioral Analysis,* 1975, *8,* 337–339.

Wooley, S. C., Epps, B., & Blackwell, B. Pain tolerance in chronic illness behavior. *Psychosomatic Medicine,* 1975, *37,* 98.

Wooley, S. C., Blackwell, B., & Winget, C. The learning theory model of chronic illness behavior: Theory, treatment, and research. *Psychosomatic Medicine,* 1978, *40,* 379–401.

Wright, L. Conceptualizing and defining psychosomatic disorders. *American Psychologist,* 1977, *32,* 625–628.

5

Assessment Strategies in Behavioral Medicine

FRANCIS J. KEEFE

Recently, there has been a great deal of interest in the application of behavioral treatment techniques to the modification of physiological function and disease. A wide array of techniques have been employed including autogenic training (Surwit, Fenton, & Pilon, 1978), progressive relaxation training (Freedman & Papsdorf, 1976), biofeedback training (Blanchard & Young, 1974; Keefe & Surwit, 1978; Shapiro & Surwit, 1976), and positive reinforcement procedures (Fordyce, Fowler, Lehmann, & DeLateur, 1968). While the importance of *treatment techniques* in the emerging field of behavioral medicine has been clearly recognized, little has been written regarding *assessment* in behavioral medicine. The relevance of behavioral assessment to the acquisition and maintenance of clinically significant changes in physiological function and disease, however, is becoming increasingly apparent (Epstein, 1976; Feuerstein & Schwartz, 1977; Schwartz, 1973, 1977; Shapiro & Surwit, 1976).

The present chapter reviews the role that assessment strategies play in behavioral medicine. The major focus is on practical aspects of the behavioral assessment process. The chapter is divided into two sections. In the first section, the theoretical foundations and basic principles underlying behavioral assessment strategies are considered. In the second section, the major methods of assessment that are currently used in the field of behavioral medicine are reviewed.

THEORETICAL FOUNDATIONS AND BASIC PRINCIPLES

The focus in behavioral assessment is on behavior. Behavior is broadly defined. The term *behavior* can refer to how a patient acts, to how he responds physiologi-

FRANCIS J. KEEFE • Department of Psychiatry, Behavioral Physiology Laboratory, Duke University Medical Center, Durham, North Carolina 27710.

cally, or to his subjective view of his own behavior. From a theoretical standpoint, the major interest is identifying the factors that account for observed behaviors and understanding how these factors function over time.

The theoretical foundation for behavioral assessment strategies comes from the work of experimental psychologists interested in conditioning and learning. These investigators emphasize the interrelationship between behavior and the environment. The two models of learning that have had the most influence on behavioral assessment methodology are (1) classical conditioning and (2) operant conditioning.

Classical Conditioning

Classical conditioning emphasizes the importance of *antecedents*—the stimuli that precede behavior. Through classical conditioning, environmental antecedents acquire the ability to elicit particular responses. Pavlov (1927) studied this phenomenon in a series of laboratory experiments. Pavlov knew that the delivery of an *unconditioned stimulus* (dry powdered food) into a dog's mouth invariably produced an *unconditioned response* (salivation). He also observed that a salivary response often occurred in response to other stimuli associated temporally with delivery of the food, such as the sight of the experimenter. This observation was an important discovery that was systematically investigated by use of the paradigm illustrated in Figure 1. A neutral stimulus (a bell) that initially elicited no salivary response was paired with the unconditioned stimulus. Early in conditioning, a salivary response was noted only after delivery of the food. However, after a number of pairings of the bell and the food, a conditioned salivary response occurred prior to

Procedural Steps	ANTECEDENTS	BEHAVIOR
1	Neutral stimulus (bell)	No response
2	Unconditioned stimulus (food)	Unconditioned response (salivation)
	After few pairings	
3	Neutral stimulus and Unconditioned stimulus	Unconditioned response
	After many pairings	
4	Neutral or *conditioned* stimulus and Unconditioned stimulus	Conditioned response (salivation prior to delivery of food) and Unconditioned response

Figure 1

the actual delivery of the food. Thus, through temporal pairing, previously neutral environmental stimuli acquired the ability to elicit a physiological response. Pavlov called these neutral stimuli *conditioned stimuli*. The process of learning he discovered has been called *Pavlovian* or *classical conditioning*.

Research has demonstrated that classical conditioning is a basic form of learning evident in species ranging from the simple planarian (flatworm) (Thompson & McConnell, 1955) to newborn infants (Marquis, 1931). Recent studies have suggested that classically conditioned physiological reactions can play a major role in the disease process. Animals who develop classically conditioned emotional responses show a lower threshold of vulnerability to ventricular fibrillation (Lown, Verrier, & Rabinowitz, 1977). While similar classical conditioning experiments have not been conducted in man, evidence strongly suggests that environmental stimuli associated with stressful events can induce ventricular arrhythmia, which may play a role in the phenomenon of sudden death (Lown *et al.*, 1977).

Behavior therapists (Wolpe, 1969) have used the classical conditioning model to explain the acquisition of behavioral disorders, such as phobias. Through a process of classical conditioning, previously neutral stimuli, such as elevators, cars, or crowds, can acquire the ability to elicit conditioned physiological responses such as increases in heart rate, in respiration, and in blood pressure. These classically conditioned physiological responses, perceived by the patient as increasing anxiety, may trigger inappropriate behavior patterns, such as avoidance or escape.

Behavioral assessment attempts to identify the conditioned environmental stimuli that elicit inappropriate behaviors on the part of the patient. The conditioned stimuli may be physical or social. For example, the sight of falling snow may be a powerful conditioned stimulus for a patient suffering from Raynaud's disease, whereas watching a spouse munch junk food may be a potent conditioned stimulus for an obese patient. The maladaptive response patterns that can be elicited by such stimuli include physiological, cognitive, and motor components.

In summary, classical conditioning provides a theoretical formulation that helps us understand how certain environmental stimuli come to exert control over responding. This model directs our attention in behavioral assessment to the environmental stimuli that precede target behavior.

Operant Conditioning

A second model of learning that has had a profound impact on assessment strategies in behavioral medicine is that of operant or instrumental conditioning. B. F. Skinner (1953) and his colleagues (Ferster & Skinner, 1957) were among the first to systematically investigate this type of conditioning. Operant conditioning emphasizes the relationship between behavioral responses and their *consequences*.

The basic paradigm used to demonstrate operant conditioning is a simple one. An animal emits a particular motor response, such as a key peck. As a result of this response, some consequence is delivered. The likelihood that the response will recur depends on the type of consequence that is delivered. Delivery of a positive reinforcer (a reward) increases the likelihood of responding. Delivery of an aversive stimulus (a punisher) decreases the likelihood of reponding. Another major element in this paradigm is the contingency relationship or the schedule under which the consequences are deliverd. This variable influences the rate of acquisition and the rate of extinction of responses. For example, a response that is reinforced on a partial reinforcement schedule shows a greater resistance to extinction than a response reinforced under a continuous reinforcement schedule (Ferster & Skinner, 1957).

The field of behavior modification developed mainly from attempts to apply the operant conditioning model to the analysis and treatment of clinical problems. Through the systematic manipulation of environmental consequences, a wide variety of behavior disorders have been treated. The focus in these applications of operant conditioning has primarily been the modification of overt motor responses.

It is only relatively recently that operant conditioning techniques have been extended to the modification of physiological responses. The major reason is that autonomic physiological responses were once thought to be involuntary and therefore not subject to the principles of operant conditioning. However, laboratory studies have convincingly demonstrated that through a process of operant conditioning, normal human subjects can exert some degree of voluntary control over such "involuntary functions" as heart rate (Engel & Chism, 1967), blood pressure (Shapiro, Tursky, & Schwartz, 1970), and vasomotor responses (Christie & Kotses, 1973; Keefe, 1975; Surwit, Shapiro, & Feld, 1976).

The operant conditioning model directs our attention in behavioral assessment to the effects that environmental consequences can have on behavior. Environmental consequences can be used to modify a wide variety of behavior, including the behavior of complex physiological systems (Schwartz, 1972, 1977).

The S-O-R-K-C Model

Kanfer and Phillips (1970) combined the basic elements of the classical and operant conditioning models to form the S-O-R-K-C model. The synthesis of these two models provides for a more comprehensive description of behavior. The S-O-R-K-C model is used to analyze complex sequences of behavior occurring in the natural environment. The basic components are shown in Figure 2.

S—*stimulus conditions* are those that immediately precede the occurrence of the target response. Physical or social stimuli may serve to set the occasion for responding. Stimulus factors may also include the behaviors of others or one's own behavior.

ANTECEDENTS	S—*Stimulus conditions:* relevant physical, social, and internal stimuli
	O—*Organismic variables:* biologic state of the organism
BEHAVIOR	R—*Response repertoire:* motor, subjective, and physiological components
CONSEQUENCES	K—*Contingency relationships:* schedule of reinforcement
	C—*Consequences:* positive and aversive stimuli

Figure 2.   The S-O-R-K-C model.

O—*organismic variables* include the biological state of the individual. The effects of physical handicaps, medication, genetic background, and biological cycles are included in this class of variables. Organismic variables are particularly important in the behavioral medicine area. Organismic variables often impose certain biologically determined limits on the modification of a target response.

R—the *response repertoire*, or the description and specification of responses, is fundamental to behavioral assessment. Responses are considered to occur in the motor, the physiological, or the subjective (self-report) response systems. Specification of the patient's repertoire of responses is critical for behavioral assessment.

K—the term *contingency relationships* refers to the correlation that occurs between the target response and its consequences. The likelihood that an obese patient may receive social reinforcement for certain health-related activities, such as jogging, is quite variable. The contingency relationship describes the likelihood that such a response will be reinforced, that is, the schedule of reinforcement.

C—*consequences* are those stimuli, both positive and aversive, that follow the response.

The S-O-R-K-C model integrates what is known about conditioning and learning into a behavioral equation. This equation provides a conceptual framework for the *functional analysis* (Ferster, 1965) of behavior.

Basic Principles

As we have seen, the major goal of assessment in behavioral medicine is to discover the relationships that exist between a target behavior and its environment. There are several basic principles that guide the clinician in his attempts to conduct this analysis. These include the following: (1) problems are defined in observable terms; (2) measurements are repeated over time; (3) assessment information is used to plan treatment; (4) interventions are introduced systematically; and (5) generalization and maintenance of behavior change are planned, not expected.

Presenting Problems Defined in Observable Terms

Behavioral assessment focuses upon target responses that are potentially observable and measurable. Vague, general patient complaints, such as "I always have a headache," are defined in more specific terms, for example, as excessive muscle tension in the trapezius or frontalis muscle group. Problems are defined in terms that are relevant and meaningful to both the patient and the therapist. The key feature of these definitions is that they refer to observable and measurable behaviors. In many medical problems, symptoms are readily observable. For example, in Raynaud's disease, vasospastic attacks cause actual changes in the color of the patient's hands. With other medical problems, such as hypertension, clearly observable referents are more difficult to identify. In the latter case, the patient may need to use a measurement device (e.g., a portable blood pressure cuff) in order to observe the behavior of interest (Epstein & Blanchard, 1977).

Presenting problems are typically defined as occurring in one or more of the following response systems: motor, physiological, or subjective (self-report). In behavioral medicine, the physiological response system typically constitutes the major target. However, this does not mean that assessment of motor or subjective responses is contraindicated. For example, Fordyce (Fordyce, Fowler, Lehmann, & DeLateur, 1968) has worked extensively with patients whose chronic complaints of pain have a physiological basis. He routinely assesses self-report of pain (the subjective response system) and the patient's activity level (the motor response system).

Measurements Repeated over Time

Once problems have been defined clearly, in terms of one or more of the three response systems, an attempt is made to measure the target response at several points in time. Measurements may be taken during different experimental sessions, over several weeks, or on several different days in a naturalistic setting. For example, migraine headache patients might be asked to monitor hand temperature repeatedly over several weeks. Initial measurements provide a *baseline* indicating the pretreatment level of a target response. This baseline permits later comparisons of treatment effectiveness. A second advantage of repeated measurements is that they demonstrate the variability in responding that may occur. Examination of this variability provides important clues for the behavioral treatment of medical disorders.

Assessment Information Used to Plan Treatment

Behavioral assessment strategies provide case formulations and clues that serve to specifically guide the progress of therapy. Adherence to this basic principle means that in behavioral assessment, the focus is narrowed. Only those factors that are deemed relevant to treatment are included in the scope of assessment. Specific, current, and maintaining or controlling factors are given more attention than remote historical events.

In behavioral medicine, assessment procedures are a continuing and integral part of the treatment itself. Methods that are used to evaluate a patient's pretreatment are often employed as a means of inducing therapeutic change. For example, recording equipment used initially to monitor target physiological response may later be used to provide biofeedback to enhance control of these responses. In behavioral medicine, assessment is not limited to a pretreatment workup. Rather, assessment information is gathered each step of the way from the initial contact with the patient through to termination. Keefe, Kopel, and Gordon (1978) have presented a five-stage procedural framework outlining this process. Table 1 is a summary of this framework.

Systematic Introduction of Interventions

A fourth guiding principle of behavioral assessment is that interventions, once selected, are introduced systematically, thus permitting ongoing evaluation of the

Table 1. A Procedural Framework for Behavioral Assessment[a]

Assessment stage	Tasks	Methods
Problem identification	Pinpoint presenting problems Determine response characteristics Obtain problem history Identify probable controlling variances Select tentative behavioral targets	Interviews with patient and significant others Questionnaires
Measurement and functional analysis	Measure problem Determine relationship between behavior, antecedents, and consequences	Self-observation Direct observation Laboratory observation
Matching treatment to client	Assess client's motivation Assess client's skills and resources Select treatment procedures Conduct sharing conference	Review all data Interview for sharing conference
Assessment of ongoing therapy	Check application of treatment techniques Monitor efficacy of treatment techniques Modify treatment program as needed	Interviews Questionnaires Self-, direct, and laboratory observations
Evaluation of therapy	Evaluate treatment outcome Assess maintenance and generality of behavior changes	Interviews Questionnaires Self-, direct, and laboratory observations

[a] Based on Ch. 2, A Procedural Framework for Behavioral Assessment. In F. J. Keefe, S. A. Kopel, and S. B. Gordon, *A Practical Guide to Behavioral Assessment*. New York: Springer Pub. Co., 1978.

effectiveness of intervention procedures. A number of strategies have been developed to evaluate the effectiveness of interventions with individual patients.

The A-B Design. Probably the single most popular method of evaluating the effectiveness of an intervention is to compare measurements of behavior taken during therapy intervention with those taken prior to that intervention. Such comparisons allow one to make tentative conclusions about therapy effectiveness. However, they do not rule out the possibility that extraneous influences may have produced the clinical changes and the improvement noted. Nevertheless, in clinical settings, a comparison of baseline versus intervention data is often the only realistic alternative (Liberman, King, & DeRisi, 1976).

The A-B-A-B Design. This design, also called the reversal design, allows the clinician to make a much more precise evaluation of behavioral treatment procedures. Following baseline (A phase), a given intervention is systematically instituted (B phase), withdrawn and returned to baseline (A phase), and finally reinstated (B phase).

The reversal design rules out rival hypotheses, such as maturation or coinciding extraneous events, that could have accounted for therapeutic effects. Only by systematically withdrawing and reinstituting treatment can these explanations be ruled out.

While the A-B-A-B design does permit a more precise evaluation of treatment effectiveness, it does have certain drawbacks. First, if treatment procedures have been in effect for long periods of time, withdrawal of those treatments may not produce the desired return to baseline. In such instances, other environmental contingencies acquire control over behavior and maintain those behaviors (Leitenberg, 1973). A second problem is that ethical considerations or the need to respond to a crisis in treatment may make it impossible to exercise the degree of control needed. In such cases, the use of other experimental designs is indicated.

The Multiple-Baseline Design. The multiple-baseline design involves the systematic application of a single treatment procedure across several target behaviors, several patients, or several environmental settings. The multiple-baseline design has several advantages for applied clinical research in behavioral medicine. First, large groups of patients are not required. This can be a real asset when presenting medical complaints are fairly rare or the population of the patients is too heterogeneous to allow for large-group designs. A second advantage is that the multiple-baseline design does not require the reversability of behavior change.

Planned Generalization and Maintenance

This is one of the most important principles that underpin assessment strategies in behavioral medicine. Numerous research reports have demonstrated that physiological function can be controlled under controlled laboratory conditions. One assumption that is not made in behavioral medicine is that the degree of physiological self-control demonstrated under laboratory conditions will *automatically* transfer to the patient's natural environment. Assessment strategies, thus, typically must involve measurement of the target responses across several different settings. This kind of measurement permits evaluation of the generality of treatment effects. Procedures are implemented to enhance generalization when the data indicate that they are necessary.

The maintenance of behavior change is likewise not expected. In order to evaluate the maintenance of behavior change, measurements are taken over long time periods, for example, months to several years, thus permitting long-term feedback to both the clinician and the patient. Long-term follow-up is particularly important in disorders in which seasonal variations may influence the targeted behavior. For example, in the behavioral treatment of Raynaud's disease, measurements must be taken over several winter seasons before therapy can be considered a "success."

METHODS OF ASSESSMENT

In behavioral medicine, a wide variety of techniques are used in assessment. In this section, we focus on five methods that are commonly used. These include (1) the interview; (2) questionnaires; (3) self-observation; (4) direct observation in a naturalistic setting; and (5) laboratory observation. The purpose of this section is to illustrate how these strategies are applied in the practice of behavioral medicine.

The Behavioral Interview

The interview is probably the most widely used of all behavioral assessment methods (Keefe *et al.*, 1978). Most contact with patients occurs in an interview setting. Behavioral interviews may take a variety of forms. They may have little formal structure, with the main focus being on letting the patient "tell his own story," as in an initial intake interview. Interviews may be structured around a specific task, such as identifying probable controlling variables in the patient's environment through a review of his "typical day." Highly structured interviews in which a predetermined set of questions are asked by either a live or an "automated" (Keefe & Webb, 1974) interviewer are also sometimes used in behavioral assessment.

While the format for a behavioral interview may vary, the basic rationale for its use as a tool for behavioral assessment is a simple one: the interview provides one of the most expedient means of gathering data about the patient.

The Interview to Gather History Information

Prior to seeking behavioral treatment, the patient has undoubtedly sought help from a number of medical specialists. These specialists have used the interview to obtain a detailed *medical history*. In behavioral medicine, the interview is used to develop a *behavioral learning* history. The major task is to discover the learned habit patterns that constitute or contribute to the presenting problem. In terms of history, the behavioral interviewer is interested in how these patterns initially developed, how they have been modified over time, and what are the factors that currently maintain them. Particular attention is paid to the social history of the patient. There is a great deal of evidence that social factors play an important part in the success or failure of treatment programs in behavioral medicine. For example, a spasmodic torticollis patient whose spouse and friends are enthusiastic and supportive about her biofeedback program is much more likely to practice developing skills in physiological self-control in the home setting than a patient who does not have these social resources.

The learning history gathered by means of the behavioral interview is viewed as a supplement to, but not a replacement for, a good medical history. The major strength of the medical history is that it provides detailed information about the pathophysiological processes responsible for physical illness and disease. The major strength of the learning history is that it identifies and clarifies sociopsychological processes that may affect the course of a physical disease or illness. Thus, the medical history and the learning history each provide a unique perspective on medical disorders. Each of these perspectives can complement the other. It is becoming increasingly clear that both the medical and the behavioral models of physical illness can and should be used to examine similar phenomena (Begelman, 1976; Schwartz & Weiss, 1978).

The Interview as a Method of Specifying and Defining Problems

"I always have a headache," "I'm never able to get an erection," "The muscle spasms come and go on their own." General complaints such as these are very common. Patients tend to define their problems in global terms. One of the major uses of the behavioral interview is to help define such complaints in more specific terms. For example, in the case of headache pain, it is important to determine where the pain occurs (for example, in the occipital region or in the cephalic vasomotor region). It is also important to determine how the patient experiences the pain—whether it is a pounding sensation or a feeling of tightness like a band around the head (Lance, 1975). The interview can be employed to reduce vague physical complaints to specific observable referents that can be monitored by the patient.

The Interview to Identify Current Environmental Controlling Factors

The behavioral learning history provides a great deal of information. Typically, the most relevant information for treatment purposes comes from a close examination of the patient's current environment. The presenting target behavior needs to be placed in its situational context. Relevant environmental antecedents and their consequences can thereby be evaluated. One approach that is very helpful in identifying probably controlling variables is to ask a patient to describe a typical day in his life from the time he wakes up in the morning until the time he retires. This single question often yields enough detailed information to require a full interview session. The following transcript taken from an interview with a patient suffering from spasmodic torticollis illustrates the process employed:

THERAPIST: Up to this point, we've talked about your problem with the torticollis in general terms.

I'd like to try to obtain some more specific, detailed information from you today. I am particularly interested in exploring with you how the torticollis affects you on a day-to-day basis. I'd like to review a typical day in your life. Could you describe for me a typical day, starting from the time you get up to the time you go to bed? I'd like you to be as specific as you can.

PATIENT: Well, I usually get up before anyone else at about 6:45. The alarm on the clock radio usually wakes me. When I awake, I am aware of the pain in my neck and also a feeling of tenderness and soreness.

THERAPIST: Could you rate the pain that you feel at that point using a 10-point scale, with 10 being the most pain you've ever experienced and 1 being the least pain?

PATIENT: Well, I guess I'd have to rate it at about 3. It's not really that high, but it sure is noticeable.

THERAPIST: What happens next?

PATIENT: Well, I usually go into the bathroom and take my shower. I turn the hot water on and can stand under it or feel that I can stand under it for hours.

THERAPIST: How long do you stay there?

PATIENT: Well, probably only for 3 to 5 minutes, but it feels good. This is one of the most relaxing times of my day. In fact, it's one of the few times that I can bring my head back toward the midline.

THERAPIST: How would you rate your pain at this point?

PATIENT: Oh, it's much better. I'd rate it about a 1. It's really very relaxing for me to take a warm shower. After I finish my shower, I usually go down to eat breakfast; then my husband comes down and we sit for a few minutes having breakfast together.

THERAPIST: Can you tell me what typically happens during this time?

PATIENT: Well, we talk about a lot of things, work, what I have planned for the day. You know, just a lot of different things. My husband usually asks me about how I'm dealing with the pain. He tends to be very supportive and sympathetic about this whole thing.

THERAPIST: What do you do at this point?

PATIENT: Well, I start to think about how I'm going to get to work and the endless details that I have to attend to. I'm very conscious of time. I feel as if I have to rush in order to get anything done. That's when I really start to have trouble. When I begin thinking about the day and work. I really have trouble keeping my head straight.

THERAPIST: What does your husband do at this point?

PATIENT: Usually, he notices that I'm having trouble and tells me to try to relax. Sometimes, if things are too bad, he drives me to work so I don't have to take the bus.

THERAPIST: What happens next?

PATIENT: Well, if my husband doesn't drive me, he leaves for work and then I walk to the bus. At this point, I'm usually really worried about getting to work late, even though I usually leave very early. I have a lot of trouble with the pain. I guess I'd give it a very high rating, maybe a 7 or 8 on that scale. The walking, the traffic really seem to bother me a lot. I usually get to work around 9:00.

THERAPIST: What happens then?

PATIENT: Well, if I walk in and no one is there, I really feel much more relaxed. I feel as if I can take my time and just unwind. The pain seems a lot better and I'm able to move to keep my head more centered. The problems really begin when my boss comes in. He's very tense and tries to run the business in a high-powered way. I find it really hard to relax around him.

The interview continues in this manner until the entire day is covered. This type of interview highlights many of the problem situations as well as the nonproblematic periods of the day. As the therapist proceeds through a review of the typical day, he begins to develop hypotheses about what factors control the problem behavior.

The Interview as a Sample of Behavior

The interview provides an opportunity to observe the patient's behavior. This sample of behavior is an important one. The patient's mannerisms, use of gestures, and physical appearance may suggest the need to focus on problems that were not initially reported. For example, the patient who suffers from bruxism may show signs of high levels of general muscular tension in an interview setting. He may, for example, sit on the edge of his chair, repeatedly clench and unclench his fists, and tap his feet. Such overt signs of general muscle tension suggest the need for a general relaxation strategy rather than a strategy that focuses only on lowering levels of masseter (jaw) muscle activity.

The Interview as a Setting for Sharing Information

One of the major purposes of the interview in behavioral medicine is to educate the patient about the behavioral approach to medical problems. A great deal of care is taken to explain concepts and methods of behavioral medicine to patients. One format for doing this is the "sharing conference" usually conducted at the end of preliminary assessment and prior to the introduction of intervention procedures. The importance of the patient's understanding of the behavioral approach in medical treatment cannot be overstressed. Most intervention strategies need to be applied by the patient on a long-term basis. Without a full understanding of the rationale for this approach, patients may find it difficult, if not impossible, to meet this goal.

Concepts are presented to the patient in terms that are clear and understandable. Simple diagrams and illustrations may be used to make basic principles clear. Table 2 presents a topical outline for a sharing conference.

Social Reinforcement in the Interview

In behavioral medicine, the interviewer plays a major role in behavior change efforts. A common misconception about behavior therapy is that the relationship with the patient is unimportant. Evidence from controlled research studies clearly demonstrates that the quality of the therapeutic relationship can influence the success of behavioral treatment procedures (Morris & Suckerman, 1974). By developing a therapeutic relationship with the patient, the interviewer acquires value as a social reinforcer (Birk, 1968). Through the judicious application of reinforcement procedures, the behavior therapist can help the patient move toward the attainment of treatment goals, such as compliance with medication regimens, weight reduction, and increased exercise.

Early in assessment, the therapist may restrict the use of his value as a social reinforcer to minimize bias in the assessment process (Thomas, 1973). However, as assessment proceeds, the therapist typically drops his stance as a neutral figure in order to facilitate the assessment process. Thus, the therapist is aware of and

Table 2. The Sharing Conference in Behavioral Medicine: A Topical Outline

I. Presenting problems: Definition and brief review.

II. Problem history: An historical review of behavioral learning history, highlighting any significant events important in the development of maladaptive behavior patterns. Identify behavior patterns other than presenting ones that contribute to dysfunction.

III. Functional analysis: Summary of data gathered during measurement. Problematic behaviors are related to current antecedents and consequences. Simple diagrams used to illustrate concepts such as classical conditioning, reinforcement, and stimulus generalization.

IV. Basic tenets of behavioral medicine: Research demonstrates that behavioral factors can influence development and course of physical illness and disease. Principles of learning may well be important in understanding patient's present physical disorder. Changes in patterns of behavior depend on learning new patterns of physiological, cognitive, and motor behavior.

V. Proposed treatment program: Need for setting specific goals. Importance of practice. Rationale for specific treatment strategy (e.g., biofeedback, autogenic training, or progressive relaxation training). Use of reinforcement principles in structuring treatment. Final goal of treatment is self-control of physiological function in the natural environment.

systematically uses his value as a source of social reinforcement. Verbal praise, smiles, nods, and encouragement are used to reward progress in the therapeutic direction.

Selective social reinforcement occurs in almost every interview situation, even if the therapist is "nondirective" (Truax & Mitchell, 1971). In behavioral assessment, there is an attempt to make the use of social reinforcement much more explicit. Over the course of behavioral treatment, the targets for social reinforcement in interview sessions are changed. Initially, the patient may be reinforced for his efforts to develop a heightened awareness of his own behavior and how it relates to current environmental stimuli. Later, the patient may be reinforced for systematic collection of data. Still later in treatment, reinforcement may be made contingent on correct and consistent application of an intervention procedure such as relaxation training.

Most treatment procedures in behavioral medicine are based on a self-control model (Epstein & Blanchard, 1977). Self-control techniques require extensive practice on the part of the patient and therefore his active involvement in the therapy. The therapist's use of his own value as a social reinforcer is one of the most important factors influencing and guiding the client toward this goal. Social reinforcement in the interview process, therefore, has a pivotal position in the practice of behavioral medicine.

Questionnaires in Behavioral Assessment

Historically, behaviorally oriented therapists have scorned the use of questionnaires as an assessment tool (Azrin, Holz, & Goldiamond, 1961). However, as behavioral approaches are becoming more widely used to modify physiological function and disease, the utility of questionnaires for a comprehensive assessment of the patient is becoming clear. A broad spectrum of questionnaires is currently being used in behavioral medicine. These include (1) traditional psychological tests; (2) general history questionnaires; (3) problem-oriented questionnaires; and (4) questionnaires that identify controlling factors.

Traditional Psychological Tests

One of the major contributions that clinical psychologists have made to the field of mental health has been in the area of psychological testing. Standards for such tests have been refined, strengthened, and codified. Psychological test instruments have been developed for intellectual and neuropsychological evaluation and for personality assessment.

Traditional psychological tests are widely used in behavioral assessment for purposes of intellectual and neuropsychological evaluation. Examples include the Wechsler series of intelligence tests (WAIS, WISC-R, WPPSI) and the Halstead–Reitan battery for evaluating central nervous system dysfunction. Tests such as these provide valuable information for treatment planning. For example, the patient who has very low verbal IQ or whose intellectual efficiency is impaired because of a cerebral vascular accident or disease may not be able to understand the concept of biofeedback. These patients may fail to find a feedback signal "reinforcing." Such a patient may respond more readily to concrete extrinsic rewards that are made contingent upon control of the physiological response being monitored (see, for example, Finley, Niman, Standley, & Wansley, 1977). Information from intellectual and neuropsychological tests may thus help specify the realistic limits of behavioral performance that can be expected from a patient.

Behaviorally oriented clinicians have strongly objected to the methods of traditional personality assessment (Mischel, 1968). They have been particularly critical of *projective* testing. In projective testing, ambiguous stimuli such as inkblots (the Rorschach test) or pictures (the Thematic Apperception Test) are presented to a patient and the patient is requested to make some type of response to them. The projective hypothesis that forms the basis for these tests states that responses to ambiguous stimuli can reveal the structure of personality. The evidence for the validity of the projective hypothesis is meager, however (Mischel, 1968).

Objective tests have also been employed for personality assessment. Examples of objective tests are the Minnesota Multiphasic Personality Inventory (MMPI), the Psychological Screening Inventory (PSI), and the California Psychological Inventory (CPI). These tests are considered objective in that scoring procedures are standardized and the patient's responses are compared to those of a normative reference group. The results of objective tests are typically a "personality profile" indicating the extent to which the patient's responses correspond to those of a normative reference group on a variety of scaled dimensions.

Behavioral clinicians have criticized personality assessment because they disagree with the theoretical model upon which these assessment methods are based. This model essentially states that it is personality structure or dynamics that determine behavior. One unfortunate result of the criticism leveled against personality tests is that behaviorally oriented clinicians are often in the embarrassing position of rejecting tests whose reliability and validity are superior to the ones commonly used in behavioral assessment. Recently, there has been an increasing openness to the use of certain personality tests in behavioral assessment. While projective testing is rarely used, behavior therapists now administer certain objective personality scales such as the D scale in the MMPI (Lewinsohn & Libet, 1972). When the emphasis in assessment is on speed and efficiency, objective personality tests may provide a pragmatic tool. It should be pointed out, however, that results gleaned from such tests are viewed as one limited piece of information that needs to be validated against data gathered through other methods of behavioral assessment.

General History Questionnaires

General history questionnaires are widely used by behavior therapists to quickly gather demographic background data. These questionnaires are comprehensive and are essentially seen as an extension of the interview. They are administered during the early stages of assessment. A variety of general history questionnaires have been developed. Most follow the general format of Lazarus's (1971) Life History Questionnaire, in which information is gathered on a range of topics, including problem history, occupational data, marital history, sexual history, developmental history, and other life problems. In behavioral medicine applications, the major advantages of the Life History Questionnaire are (1) they sample a wide range of potential problem areas; (2) they aid in formulating a behavioral learning history; and (3) they survey the resources of the patient and his environment.

Problem-Oriented Questionnaires

Problem-oriented questionnaires are employed to gather detailed data on a single target behavior. Most of these questionnaires have been developed by practicing clinicians who deal with patients with similar presenting complaints. There are two major advantages in using such questionnaires: (1) they are time saving, and (2) they provide a standard format for collecting a data base (Cautela & Upper, 1975). A number of questionnaires have been described, including the Stuttering History Questionnaire (Martyn & Sheehan, 1968), the Smoking History Questionnaire (Keutzer, 1968), the Alcohol Questionnaire (Cautela, 1977) and the Sexual Interaction Inventory (LoPiccolo & Steger, 1974).

Questionnaires That Identify Probable Controlling Factors

Questionnaires are also used in behavioral assessment to evaluate the patient's view of relevant environmental antecedents and consequences that may influence the target response. One example is the Fear Survey Schedule (FSS) (Wolpe & Lang, 1964). This schedule lists a variety of antecedent stimuli that can elicit physiological arousal or anxiety in a patient. The patient rates the severity of his reaction to each of these stimuli, and this rating is used to plan treatment strategies. Another example is the Reinforcement Survey Schedule (RSS) (Cautela & Kastenbaum, 1967). The RSS is composed of 54 potentially rewarding items, activities, and events. The patient rates each item, indicating its reinforcing value to him on a five-point scale. A list of reinforcers can thereby be generated for use in treatment.

Self-Observation

Self-observation is one of the most basic assessment strategies in behavioral medicine. When behavioral medicine interventions are used with outpatients, the major treatment goal is to enhance self-control of physiological responses. Self-observation is fundamental to the attainment of this goal. The rationale for self-observation is relatively straightforward. Before a client can take steps to alter a physiological response, he must be aware of the occurrence or nonoccurrence of this response.

Self-observation involves three steps. First, the patient learns to discriminate the target behavior. This learning might entail becoming more attentive to the physiological changes occurring during a migraine headache, a muscle spasm, or a Raynaud's attack. Second, the patient makes a record of the behavior he has observed. A variety of characteristics of the behavior may be recorded, such as the intensity of headache pain (Budzynski, Stoyva, & Adler, 1970), the frequency of epileptic seizures (Johnson & Meyer, 1974), or the duration of compulsive-binge eating episodes (Keefe, Birk, & Schoonover, 1977). Finally, the patient analyzes the data gathered by summarizing them and examining patterns of change occurring over time.

The ease of self-observation depends on the discriminability of the physiological response chosen as a target. Some patterns of physiological responding are clearly observable to the patient and thus can be easily monitored through rather simple self-observation procedures. The self-observation of other responses, such as electromyograph (EMG) activity or blood pressure, which are not so readily apparent to the patient, may require the use of portable automatic recording devices.

Simple Self-Observation Procedures

Many of the problematic behaviors in behavioral medicine are highly visible. These include tics, asthmatic attacks, stuttering, spasmodic torticollis, chronic vomiting, enuresis, smoking, eating behaviors, and epileptic attacks. Self-observation techniques generally employed by behavior therapists (Thoreson & Mahoney, 1974) can easily be adapted to the recording of such highly visible behaviors. These techniques are relatively simple and easy to use. They require neither extended training of the patient as an observer nor expensive equipment. Typical recording devices include the daily notebook, counting devices, and charts.

The Daily Notebook. The daily notebook is a comprehensive self-observation strategy. Because of this, the daily notebook is commonly employed in the initial stages of assessment. The patient keeping a daily notebook is asked to make an entry in the notebook each time the target behavior occurs. Each entry includes a description of the problematic sequence of behavior. Essentially, the patient is asked to describe what happened before, during, and after each instance of the target

Table 3. The Daily Notebook

Date: December 12, 1977	Theresa H.
Time: 8:00 A.M.	

What happened before? I was on my way out the door. Everyone else in the house had already left for work. I had listened to the weather forecast and knew it was cold—16°. I went to the closet by the front door to put on my coat. I was really thinking about how cold the steering wheel of my car was going to be.

What happened during? Before getting out the door. I had an *attack*. Bad pain in my hands. They turned whitish, then purple. My feet were OK. I decided not to go to work, took off my coat, and sat down for a half hour. Felt very discouraged and frustrated. Very pessimistic about prospects for changing this.

What happened after? After half hour, hands did warm up. Felt a little more relaxed. Decided to stay home for the day.

Comments: This is the third attack that I've had like this, this week.

behavior. Table 3 is a sample taken from a daily notebook kept by a patient suffering from idiopathic Raynaud's disease. As can be seen, the patient attends to many aspects of the Raynaud's attack, including the time and date of the episode and the physical and social stimuli present before and after the attack. In terms of the actual attack, recording focuses on all three components of the target behavior: physiological, motor, and subjective.

The daily notebook is particularly appropriate for target responses that occur with relatively low frequency, perhaps one to five times per day. The observations generated using the daily notebook are very detailed. Gross changes in the environment that occur in association with the problem behavior can thus be easily identified. These environmental changes may have a functional relationship to the behavior itself. In keeping a daily notebook, the patient is asked to discriminate not only the occurrence of the target behavior but also its environmental antecedents and consequences. The result is a heightened awareness of all three elements in the behavioral equation. This awareness is likely to enhance the patient's ability to take the appropriate steps to change his behavior.

The immediacy and detail of daily notebook records provides the clinician with tentative clues for formulating treatment strategies. The validity of these clues can be established through the use of applied behavior-analysis research strategies such as the A-B-A-B and multiple-baseline designs, in which contingencies are systematically manipulated and the resultant effects carefully observed (Baer, Wolf, & Risley, 1968). For example, daily notebook records may indicate that a 10-year-old epileptic child engages in a great deal of inappropriate behavior that appears to be reinforced by his parents' attention. One hypothesis is that if the parents' attention were made contingent on more appropriate behavior, the frequency of the epileptic attacks would decrease significantly (Mostofsky & Balaschak, 1977). To test this possibility, an A-B-A-B design can be used. First the parents can be asked to record the frequency of epileptic attacks under existing conditions (A phase—or baseline). Next, they can be trained to systematically reward appropriate behavior and to extinguish inappropriate behavior by ignoring it. During this treatment, or B phase, the frequency of epileptic attacks may well decrease. A return to baseline conditions (A phase) can help validate the importance of parental attention in controlling epileptic seizure activity. If epileptic seizure frequency increases during this return to baseline, parental attention is very likely to be an important controlling influence. During the final phase of this design, parents are asked to reinstitute treatment (B phase), and the effects are observed. An abrupt reduction in epileptic attacks provides further confirmation of the initial hypothesis. Thus, by systematically manipulating treatment strategies developed from information supplied by observation devices such as the daily notebook, we can establish the validity of behavioral conceptualizations.

Counting Devices. Behavior therapists have developed a wide variety of ingenious counting devices that can be used for self-observation. Most of these devices are unobtrusive and easy to use. Examples include knitting tallies (Thoreson & Mahoney, 1974), golf counters (Lindsley, 1968), jewelry with moveable abacus counters (Epstein & Hersen, 1974; Mahoney, 1974), and grocery counters. Counting devices may be particularly helpful when there is a need to monitor high-frequency responses such as tics (Azrin & Nunn, 1973) or to monitor several behaviors simultaneously (Epstein & Hersen, 1974).

Charts. Simple data charts can be constructed to facilitate self-observation. These charts are often developed for use with common referral problems. In our laboratory, we use charts in clinical research projects. For example, in the assessment of Raynaud's attacks, patients are asked to make an entry on a chart on a daily basis. They are instructed to record the frequency of attacks, the severity of the worst attack, the side of the body affected, and the external temperature. Once behavioral training has begun, patients also record on the chart their performance in voluntarily warming their hands. The major advantage of charts is that they provide the patient with something concrete on which the behaviors to be monitored are clearly defined and indicated.

It should be noted in closing that these simple self-recording procedures need not be restricted to monitoring inappropriate, maladaptive responses. Self-observation strategies can easily be used to monitor the physiological correlates of appropriate behaviors. For example, patients may be instructed in methods of recording their own pulse before, during, and after periods of exercising, or they may be asked to record the number of aerobic points earned by engaging in various types of exercise (Cooper, 1970; Kau & Fischer, 1974).

Portable Recording Devices

Recently, there has been a great deal of interest in the development and application of portable devices for monitoring physiological responses. These devices extend the range of responses that can be easily discriminated by a patient.

Portable recording devices have been developed for nearly every physiological response that can be noninvasively recorded. Of course, some of these devices are in the early stages of development and field testing and are therefore not widely available. Many portable recording devices, commonly used in behavioral medicine application, can be purchased easily from commercial suppliers (Rugh & Schwitz-gebel, 1975a,b). These include units for recording blood pressure, heart rate, skin resistance, electroencephalogram (EEG), skin temperature, and EMG.

When portable recording devices are used in self-observation, the general procedure is similar to that used in other self-observation strategies. There are, however, several additional details that demand attention. First, there is a need to train the patient in the use of the instrument. Methods for attaching transducers, bringing in the signal, and reading output displays need to be demonstrated to the patient in terms that are easy to understand. The patient's competence in these tasks needs to be evaluated before assessment begins.

A second consideration is specifying the time period for observation. If the portable device is very unobtrusive, recording may take place over long time periods. For example, Rugh and Solberg (1974) described an interesting portable EMG device used in the assessment of bruxism—excessive clenching and grinding of the teeth. In their study, patients were outfitted with a small EMG feedback unit that presented a tone when the level of masseter muscle activity exceeded a criterion level. Patients were instructed to wear the device for several days during activities of daily living. The patients reported that the portable EMG unit helped them to become more aware of their bruxing and also helped them learn to relax the muscles of the jaw.

If the recording is more obtrusive, for example, in monitoring blood pressure, a time-sampling procedure may be used. For time sampling, a hypertensive patient's day would be divided into equal intervals. At the end of each interval, the patient would place the blood pressure cuff on and take a measurement.

A third consideration is the cost involved in the use of portable physiological recording devices. The cost of many of these devices is high, particularly when they are being used only for self-observation. Over time, technological advances may provide less expensive alternatives for the self-recording of physiological responses. For example, we recently have begun using a device called the "physiological trend indicator" (Medical Device Corp., P.O. Box 217, Clayton, Indiana 46118) for the self-monitoring of hand temperature. This is a small ($2\frac{1}{4}$" $\times$ $\frac{1}{4}$") adhesive strip with a temperature-sensitive chemical backing similar to that used in "mood rings." The strip is placed on the finger, and changes in temperature are noted as changes in the number and color of the strip. This strip can be used to monitor temperature in the natural environment or to provide biofeedback as to the success of various hand-warming strategies. The cost of the strip is two dollars.

Direct Observation in a Naturalistic Setting

Direct observation is considered to be the most fundamental and objective method of behavioral assessment (Azrin, Holz, & Goldiamond, 1961; Lipinski & Nelson, 1974). In direct observation, trained observers monitor and record the behavior(s) of interest. An attempt is usually made to observe behavior in "real-world" or naturalistic settings. Direct observations have many advantages. First, the reliability of recording tends to be higher because observers are specially trained.

Second, direct observations often yield information that the patient has failed to report. Third, they provide an opportunity to view directly the controlling effects of situational factors. Fourth, they enable the clinician to check the validity of data gathered through other assessment procedures. Because of these advantages, direct observation procedures are used in behavioral assessment whenever they are practically feasible.

In behavioral medicine, a number of direct observation strategies have been developed. We shall consider three of these: (1) ward observations; (2) home observations; and (3) telemetric recording.

Ward Observations

Patients who are hospitalized for treatment can be easily observed. Frequent observations can be made by staff members throughout the patient's day. Recording procedures may be individually tailored for the particular patient or may be standardized for applications on behavioral medicine wards.

The development and maintenance of recording strategies for ward observation requires considerable time and attention. Observers must be trained and their reliability checked periodically. Procedural details, such as the time of observation, the setting, and special behavior to be recorded, need to be clear to all observers. Particular attention needs to be given to reinforcing data collection on the part of staff members who may view this task as an additional "chore."

Sand, Trieschmann, Fordyce, and Fowler (1970) have described the use of ward observation procedures in the behavioral assessment of a paraplegic patient whose compliance with medical regimens was inconsistent. Self-care behaviors (e.g., catheter irrigation, taking medication, washing) expected to be completed by the patient were targeted for observation on the ward. Observations were carried out during baseline and token reinforcement procedures. Token reinforcement produced a dramatic increase in the number of self-care activities consistently completed.

Ward observations have also been used in the behavioral assessment of patients suffering from anorexia nervosa (Garfinkel, Kline, & Stancer, 1973), asthma (Neisworth & Moore, 1972), Gilles de la Tourette's syndrome (Thomas, Abrams, & Johnson, 1971), chronic vomiting (Wolf, Birnbrauer, Williams, & Lawler, 1965), and a variety of other medical complaints.

Home Observations

Direct observations of behavior in the patient's home setting are a common measurement procedure in behavioral assessment (Eyberg & Johnson, 1974; Lewinsohn, 1975). The basic observation procedures are similar. An observer or a team of observers visits the patient's home for one or two hours. All family members are requested to be present during this time, and the family is additionally instructed to restrict themselves to one area of the home. The family members are encouraged to refrain from interacting with the observers. Behaviors of both the patient and others are recorded. The particular responses measured and the categories used to code the behavior vary according to the target complaint.

Home observations are very often employed in the behavioral assessment of children. For example, Nordquist (1971) employed home observations in his assessment of a 5-year-old enuretic boy. The initial home visit revealed that the child frequently failed to comply with parental requests and engaged in oppositional behaviors, including hitting and yelling. Excessive attention in the form of threats and arguments was given by the parents to disruptive behavior, while very little attention was paid to appropriate behavior. Enuretic episodes decreased significantly once the parents had been trained in behavioral child management techniques of positive reinforcement and time out.

While home observations are less frequently used in the assessment of adult patients, I find that they yield interesting and valuable data. Recently, I conducted a home observation of 28-year-old anorexic patient. The observation was carried out during a typical mealtime hour. Surprisingly, the patient was very active in the kitchen around mealtime. She prepared a gourmet meal for her family. She received a great deal of attention for her efforts and praise for her obvious cooking abilities. In addition, her own unwillingness to eat any food brought forth many protests from other family members and was the major topic of discussion. It was evident from this observation and other data sources that the attention given by family members for this patient's refusal to eat was a major factor in the maintenance of her anorexic behavior.

Telemetric Recording

Telemetric recording devices offer a number of interesting possibilities for the direct observation of physiological responses in natural settings. Telemetric devices eliminate the need for outside observers. As a result, they may be somewhat less intrusive. Telemetric devices consist of monitors worn by the patient that can send information back to a central data location.

Lown *et al.* (1977) have reported using telemetric devices to track cardiac responses of patients suffering from heart disease. Records from these units have helped to pinpoint environmental stresses that can trigger cardiac arrhythmia.

Laboratory Observation

The field of behavioral medicine has drawn heavily upon basic and applied research in human psychophysiology. It is not surprising, therefore, that the psychophysiology laboratory is one of the most common settings for behavioral assessment. The major advantage of the laboratory as an assessment setting is that it allows for precise control over extraneous influences that may confound the data gathered. In the laboratory, multiple physiological responses can be monitored under controlled environmental conditions. The *patterns* of change under different stimulus conditions can thereby be evaluated. It is by examining these patterns that the most valid statements about the relationship between physiological responses and the environment can be made. Practitioners in the field of behavioral medicine have adapted many of the concepts and methods used in human psychophysiology to develop strategies for the applied analysis of physiological behavior.

The Laboratory Setting

The psychophysiology laboratory contains two adjacent rooms consisting of a subject room and a control room. The subject room is equipped with a comfortable chair and a variety of transducers for measuring physiological responses. This room also has a number of display devices, such as lights, meters, and loudspeakers. The subject room is usually soundproof and is maintained at a constant temperature and humidity level. The adjacent control room houses a polygraph and electromechanical programming equipment. The polygraph enables one to simultaneously monitor several physiological responses, such as blood pressure, heart rate, and respiration. Electromechanical programming equipment provides for precise control of all environmental stimuli in the subject room. The laboratory is very flexible. The investigator can easily vary the response monitored and the nature of the stimuli delivered to the subject.

Laboratory Assessment Strategies

A variety of laboratory assessment strategies are used in behavioral medicine. Commonly employed strategies include baseline sessions, biofeedback training, ongoing evaluation of treatment effectiveness, and pre- and posttherapy comparisons.

Baseline Sessions. Baseline sessions are used to establish pretreatment levels of physiological responding and to rationally select target responses for behavioral treatment. During baseline sessions, several relevant responses are monitored under different stimulus conditions.

Van Boxtel and Van der Ven (1978) described the use of baseline sessions to evaluate EMG activity in patients complaining of muscle contraction headache. Electromyographic recordings were taken from four muscle sites: (1) the frontalis; (2) the trapezius; (3) the temporalis; and (4) the forearm flexors. The activity of each muscle group was assessed while the subject rested and during a reading task. The only muscle group that reliably differentiated between headache patients and normals was the frontalis. These results suggested the need for a training procedure such as EMG biofeedback (Keefe & Surwit, 1978) or progressive relaxation training, designed to lower frontalis EMG activity levels.

Another example of the use of baseline sessions in behavioral medicine has been in the assessment of impotence (Rosen & Keefe, 1978). In the normal male, penile erection occurs in association with the beginning and end of rapid eye movement (REM) sleep. Four or five periods typically occur during the average night. This fact has been confirmed by all night baseline sleep recordings of penile erection made using a mercury strain gauge. Recently, similar recording methods have been used in laboratory baseline sessions to differentially diagnose psychogenic versus organic impotence. In men suffering from psychogenic impotence, normal cycles of nocturnal penile erection occur during REM periods. In contrast, patients whose impotence is caused by an underlying disease process show very low levels of penile tumescence during REM periods. Those patients suffering from organically caused impotence require appropriate medical treatment, whereas those with normal REM-associated cycles of sleep erections are likely to respond to sex therapy.

Biofeedback Training. Biofeedback training had its origins in research studies conducted in the laboratory setting. With the growing popularity of biofeedback as a clinical enterprise, training has been shifted from the laboratory to office and home settings. Technological advances in the area of self-contained portable feedback units have made this shift in training settings feasible. Nevertheless, the laboratory remains a very important setting for biofeedback training. There are several reasons for this. First, the psychophysiology lab is very easily adapted to specialized problems. With appropriate modifications of existing equipment, a polygraph can be used to trigger feedback devices for an extraordinary range of physiological responses. This wideness of range may be particularly helpful when working with unique or unusual presenting complaints for which no portable equipment is available. Second, laboratory equipment tends to be more sophisticated than most home biofeedback units. Thus, information can be fed back to the patient at a more refined level. For example, an integrated average of EMG activity rather than the raw signal can be presented to a patient. In the lab, feedback can be made contingent on *patterns* of physiological change such as heart rate up–blood pressure down, rather than on isolated changes in single response systems. Third, the control that the laboratory provides over extraneous stimuli, such as noise, cold, and humidity, can be a real asset in biofeedback training. Eliminating these stimuli can facilitate the development of physiological self-control, particularly when the goal of training is a low arousal state.

Ongoing Evaluation. The laboratory may also be used to monitor the effects of behavioral treatment procedures other than biofeedback training that the patient employs on a self-control basis outside the laboratory. Daily or weekly laboratory sessions may be scheduled to evaluate the patient's ability to control a particular physiological response.

For example, in our laboratory, we recently saw a patient who suffered from a variety of psychogenic facial tics affecting muscle groups throughout the face. Baseline measurement indicated very high levels of resting frontalis EMG activity. The patient was trained in progressive relaxation and instructed to practice at home twice a day. Additional lab measurements were taken on a weekly basis throughout training. Gradual improvement was obtained in the ability to suppress excessive EMG activity during rest and during various activities. In this instance, laboratory measurements provided important feedback to the clinician and the patient that the treatment strategy was working.

Pre- and Posttherapy Comparisons. A very efficient lab assessment strategy is to evaluate patterns of physiological responding before and after behavioral training. We use such strategy to assess the effectiveness of behavioral treatments for Raynaud's disease and Raynaud's phenomenon. The first laboratory test is given one month prior to behavioral training. During the test, the patient wears a terry-cloth robe. Thermistors are placed on the index finger of each hand, and EKG electrodes are attached to each arm. Measures are taken during a 20-minute stabilization period in which the temperature is held constant at 75°F and then during a gradual temperature drop to 60°F. Patients are instructed to keep their hands as warm as possible throughout the laboratory test. A second laboratory test is conducted one month after behavioral training has begun. Our results indicate that after behavioral training, patients can keep their hands 2–5° warmer in this laboratory test. Such lab tests provide a more objective evaluation of the effectiveness of training than is available from the patient's self-report of the frequency and intensity of Raynaud's attacks. Similar pre- versus posttherapy comparisons can be easily made for a variety of conditions treated through behavioral medicine by varying the stimulus or condition used as a stressor.

Methodological Issues in Behavioral Assessment

As behavioral assessment strategies are more broadly applied to the field of behavioral medicine, important methodological issues are raised. Attention to these issues is one of the most important factors responsible for the success or failure of assessment efforts. Two of the most fundamental issues are reliability and validity.

Reliability

Reliability refers to the *consistency* of a measurement procedure. For example, the reliability of a direct observation procedure depends on the extent to which two observers who simultaneously observe a subject can agree that a particular behavior has occurred. Reliability is critical to any attempt to assess human behavior. If measurement procedures have low reliability, it is impossible to evaluate the significance of any behavioral changes that are recorded. With low reliability, the clinician is left with the question "Are these changes 'real' or are they due to a measurement error?"

Recently, there has been a great deal of interest in the reliability of behavioral assessment strategies (Johnson & Bolstad, 1973; Lipinski & Nelson, 1974). Particular attention has been paid to identifying and eliminating those factors that tend to lower reliability. One such factor is *observer bias*. Bias may be caused by the expectations held by the observer about the subject (Rosenthal, 1963). The result is a systematic error in a direction consistent with the observer's expectations. Observer bias may be lessened by restricting the flow of information to observers.

A second factor that tends to lower reliability is *reactivity*. Reactivity is the tendency of the assessment procedure to influence and change the behavior being studied. The effects of reactivity can be minimized by using recording procedures that are less obtrusive than direct observations (such as automatic recording devices).

Assessment methods differ in their inherent reliability. Those methods, such as laboratory observation, that rely on automatic recording devices eliminate many sources of error and tend to be more reliable and precise. Assessment methods that rely on human observers, such as self- or direct observation, are more likely to be subject to observer bias and reactivity. Reactivity is particularly likely to affect self-observation. Because human observers often provide the only feasible method of behavioral assessment, it is important to attempt to minimize factors that tend to lower reliability. When using human observers, the selection of easily observed target behaviors and clear, concise definitions is especially important.

Validity

The *validity* of an assessment strategy refers to the agreement that occurs between two attempts to measure the same behavior. As we have seen, there are five common measurement procedures used in behavioral medicine: (1) interviews; (2) questionnaires; (3) self-observation; (4) direct observation; and (5) laboratory observation. In behavioral assessment, two or more of these methods are typically used to gather data. For example, in the assessment of migraine headache, relevant data may come from interviews with the patient and significant others, self-observation, and laboratory observation. Simultaneous measurement permits one to determine how generalizable are the findings obtained. The higher the agreement among the various sources of data, the greater the validity.

A major advantage of assessment strategies in behavioral medicine is that they are multimodal. It is extremely rare that assessment relies solely upon one source of data gathered in one isolated situation. This reliance on multiple sources of data enhances the validity of behavioral assessment.

CONCLUSIONS

Behavioral medicine represents an innovative approach to the problems of disease and illness. Behavioral assessment strategies have only recently been developed and applied to the field of medicine. The methods we have reviewed are promising and have already yielded interesting and valuable results for certain problems. The reliability, validity, and utility of these methods need to be evaluated on an even broader basis, however. This effort may well yield significant advances in our understanding of physical health and illness.

Behavioral medicine is a promising field that has attracted a great deal of attention and interest. Much of the appeal of behavioral medicine lies in its attempt to integrate knowledge from the behavioral and the biomedical sciences to reach solutions to practical problems of physical health and illness. While a great deal has been written about treatment techniques such as biofeedback, relaxation training, and autogenic training, relatively little has been written regarding the role of assessment in behavioral medicine. In this chapter, assessment methods currently employed in behavioral medicine were reviewed. Many of these methods have only recently been developed and applied. The methods reviewed are promising and have already yielded interesting and valuable data. Most of the assessment strategies discussed in the present chapter have come from the fields of behavior therapy and behavior modification. It should be noted that behavioral medicine has been conceived of as being broad in scope and is not limited to any one discipline or theoretical orientation. In the future, it is likely that the more behavioral methods of assessment discussed in the present chapter will be combined with a wide variety of assessment devices from numerous disciplines, including sociology, internal medicine, epidemiology, physiology, and cardiology. Through this interdisciplinary effort may well come some of the most significant advances in our understanding of physical health and illness.

SUMMARY

Assessment strategies in behavioral medicine are based upon social learning theory. Two models of learning have been influential: classical and operant conditioning. The S-O-R-K-C (Kanfer & Phillips, 1970) model represents an attempt to integrate these two models of learning. This synthesis is particularly important because it directs assessment efforts to a broader range of variables influencing performance. The variables that are considered include S (stimulus conditions), O (organismic variables), R (response repertoire) K (contingency relationship) and C (consequences). Behavioral assessment is guided by five basic principles. These are (1) problems are defined in observable terms; (2) measurements are repeated over time; (3) assessment information is used to plan treatment; (4) interventions are introduced systematically; and (5) generalization and maintenance of behavior change is planned, not expected.

A number of assessment methods are commonly employed in behavioral medicine. Interviews are widely used because of their flexibility. Questionnaires, once shunned by behavioral clinicians, are becoming increasingly popular as a means of assessment in behavioral medicine. Psychological tests are viewed as particularly helpful for purposes of intellectual evaluation and neuropsychological assessment, whereas questionnaires aid in gathering specific historical and current data on presenting problems. Because of the emphasis on self-control strategies in behavioral medicine, self-observation is widely used as an assessment tool. Direct observation of the patient in a naturalistic setting (such as in the patient's home or on a hospital ward) is one of the most objective methods of assessment. Of all the assessment methods reviewed, observations of the patient in a psychophysiology laboratory probably provide the most reliable data on physiological responding. The scientific adequacy of assessment strategies in behavioral medicine depends on their demonstrated reliability and validity.

REFERENCES

Azrin, N. H., Holz, W., & Goldiamond, I. Response bias in questionnaire reports. *Journal of Consulting Psychology*, 1961, *25*, 324–326.

Azrin, N. H., & Nunn, R. G. Habit-reversal: A method of eliminating nervous habits and tics. *Behaviour Research and Therapy*, 1973, *11*, 619–628.

Baer, D., Wolf, M., & Risley, T. Some current dimensions of applied behavior analysis. *Journal of Applied Behavior Analysis*, 1968, *5*, 525–528.

Begelman, D. A. Behavioral classification. In M. Hersen & A. Bellack (Eds.), *Behavioral assessment: A practical handbook*. New York: Pergamon, 1976.

Birk, C. L. Social reinforcement in psychotherapy. *Conditioned Reflex*, 1968, *3*, 116–123.

Blanchard, E. B., & Young, L. D. Clinical applications of biofeedback training: A review of evidence. *Archives of General Psychiatry*, 1974, *30*, 573–589.

Budzynski, T. H., Stoyva, J. M., & Adler, C. Feedback-induced muscle relaxation: Application to tension headache. *Journal of Behavior Therapy and Experimental Psychiatry*, 1970, *1*, 205–211.

Cautela, J. R. *Behavioral analysis forms for clinical intervention*. Champaign, Ill.: Research, 1977.

Cautela, J. R., & Kastenbaum, R. A. A reinforcement survey schedule for use in therapy, training and research. *Psychological Reports*, 1967, *20*, 1115–1130.

Cautela, J. R., & Upper, D. The process of individual behavior therapy. In M. Hersen, R. M. Eisler, & P. M. Miller (Eds.), *Progress in behavior modification*, Vol. 1. New York: Academic, 1975.

Christie, D. J., & Kotses, H. Bidirectional operant conditioning of the cephalic vasomotor response. *Journal of Psychosomatic Research*, 1973, *17*, 167–170.

Cooper, K. H. *The new aerobics*. New York: Bantam, 1970.

Engel, B. T., & Chism, R. A. Operant conditioning of heart rate speeding. *Psychophysiology*, 1967, *3*, 418–426.

Epstein, L. H. Psychophysiological measurement in assessment. In M. Hersen & A. S. Bellack (Eds.), *Behavioral assessment: A practical handbook*. New York: Pergamon, 1976.

Epstein, L. H., & Blanchard, E. B. Biofeedback, self-control, and self-management. *Biofeedback and Self-Regulation*, 1977, *2*, 201–212.

Epstein, L. H., & Hersen, M. A multiple baseline analysis of coverant control. *Journal of Behavior Therapy and Experimental Psychiatry*, 1974, *5*, 7–12.

Epstein, L. E., & Peterson, G. L. Differential conditioning using covert stimuli. *Behavior Therapy*, 1973, *44*, 96–99.

Eyberg, S. M., & Johnson, S. M. Multiple assessment of behavior modification with families: Effects of contingency contracting and order of treated problems. *Journal of Consulting and Clinical Psychology*, 1974, *42*, 594–606.

Ferster, C. B. Classification of behavioral pathology. In L. Krasner & L. P. Ullmann (Eds.), *Research in behavior modification*. New York: Holt, Rinehart, & Winston, 1965.

Ferster, C., & Skinner, B. F. *Schedules of reinforcement*. New York: Appleton-Century-Crofts, 1957.

Feuerstein, M., & Schwartz, G. E. Training in clinical psychophysiology: Present trends and future goals. *American Psychologist*, 1977, *32*, 560–567.

Finley, W., Niman, C., Standley, J., & Wansley, R. Electrophysiologic behavior modification of frontal EMG in cerebral-palsied children. *Biofeedback and Self-Regulation*, 1977, *2*, 59–80.

Fordyce, W. E., Fowler, R. S., Lehmann, J. F., & DeLateur, B. J. Some implications of learning in problems of chronic pain. *Journal of Chronic Diseases*, 1968, *21*, 179–190.

Freedman, R., & Papsdorf, J. D. Biofeedback and progressive relaxation treatment of sleep onset insomnia. *Biofeedback and Self-Regulation*, 1976, *1*, 253–271.

Garfinkel, P., Kline, S., & Stancer, H. Treatment of anorexia nervosa using operant conditioning techniques. *Journal of Nervous and Mental Disease*, 1973, *6*, 428–433.

Johnson, R. K., & Meyer, R. G. Phased biofeedback approach for epileptic seizure control. *Journal of Behavior Therapy and Experimental Psychiatry*, 1974, *5*, 185–188.

Johnson, S. M., & Bolstad, O. D. Methodological issues in naturalistic observation: Some problems and solutions for field research. In L. A. Hamerlynck, L. C. Handy, & E. G. Mash (Eds.), *Behavior change: Methodology, concepts, and practice*. Champaign, Ill.: Research, 1973.

Kanfer, F. H., & Phillips, J. S. *Learning foundations of behavior therapy*. New York: Wiley, 1970.

Kau, M. L., & Fischer, J. Self-modification of exercise behavior. *Journal of Behavior Therapy and Experimental Psychiatry*, 1974, *5*, 213–214.

Keefe, F. J. Conditioning changes in differential skin temperature. *Perceptual and Motor Skills*, 1975, *40*, 283–288.

Keefe, F. J., & Surwit, R. S. Electromyographic biofeedback—Behavioral treatment of neuromuscular disorders. *Journal of Behavioral Medicine*, 1978, *1*, 13–24.

Keefe, F. J., & Webb, J. T. Sex and the automated interview: Interviewer and interviewee sex difference effects. Paper presented at the Southeastern Psychological Association, Jan. 1974, Hollywood Beach, Fla.

Keefe, F. J., Birk, C. L., & Schoonover, S. Behavioral treatment of compulsive eating disorders: A multiple baseline study. Unpublished manuscript, Harvard Medical School, 1977.

Keefe, F. J., Kopel, S. A., & Gordon, S. B. *A practical guide to behavioral assessment.* New York: Springer, 1978.

Keutzer, C. S. Behavior modification of smoking: The experimental investigation of diverse techniques. *Behavior Research and Therapy,* 1968, *6,* 137–158.

Lance, J. W. *Headache: Understanding, alleviation.* New York: Scribner's, 1975.

Lazarus, A. A. *Behavior therapy and beyond.* New York: McGraw-Hill, 1971.

Leitenberg, H. The use of single-case methodology in psychotherapy research. *Journal of Abnormal Psychology,* 1973, *82,* 87–101.

Lewinsohn, P. M. The behavioral study and treatment of depression. In M. Hersen, R. Eisler, & P. M. Miller (Eds.). *Progress in behavior modification.* New York: Academic, 1975.

Lewinsohn, P. M., & Libet, J. Pleasant events, activity schedules, and depression. *Journal of Abnormal Psychology,* 1972, *79,* 291–295.

Liberman, R. P., King, L. W., & DeRisi, W. J. Behavior analysis and therapy in community mental health. In H. Leitenberg (Ed.), *Handbook of behavior modification and behavior therapy.* Englewood Cliffs, N.J.: Prentice-Hall, 1976.

Lindsley, O. R. A reliable wrist counter for recording behavior rates. *Journal of Applied Behavior Analysis,* 1968, *1,* 77–78.

Lipinski, D., & Nelson, R. Problems in the use of naturalistic observation as a means of behavioral assessment. *Behavior Therapy,* 1974, *5,* 341–351.

LoPiccolo, J., & Steger, J. C. The sexual interaction inventory: A new instrument for assessment of sexual dysfunction. *Archives of Sexual Behavior,* 1974, *3,* 585–595.

Lown, B., Verrier, L. R. L., & Rabinowitz, S. H. Neural and psychological mechanisms and the problem of sudden cardiac death. *The American Journal of Cardiology,* 1977, *39,* 890–902.

Mahoney, M. J. *Cognition and behavior modification.* Cambridge: Ballinger, 1974.

Marquis, D. P. Can conditioned responses be established in the newborn infant? *Journal of Genetic Psychology,* 1931, *39,* 479–492.

Martyn, M. M., & Sheehan, J. Onset of stuttering and recovery. *Behaviour Research and Therapy,* 1968, *6,* 295–308.

Mischel, W. *Personality and assessment.* New York: Wiley, 1968.

Morris, R. J., & Suckerman, K. R. Therapist warmth as a factor in automated systematic desensitization. *Journal of Consulting and Clinical Psychology,* 1974, *42,* 244–250.

Mostofsky, D. I., & Balaschak, B. A. Psychological control of seizures. *Psychological Bulletin,* 1977, *84,* 723–750.

Neisworth, J., & Moore, F. Operant treatment of asthmatic responding with the parent as therapist. *Behavior Therapy,* 1972, *3,* 95–99.

Nordquist, V. M. The modification of a child's enuresis: Some response–response relationships. *Journal of Applied Behavior Analysis,* 1971, *4,* 241–247.

Pavlov, I. *Conditioned reflexes.* London: Oxford University Press, 1927.

Rosen, R. C., & Keefe, F. J. The measurement of human penile tumescence. *Psychophysiology,* 1978, *25,* 366–376.

Rosenthal, R. On the social psychiatry of the psychological experiment. The experimenter's hypothesis as unintended determinent of experimental results. *American Scientist,* 1963, *51,* 268–282.

Rugh, J. D., & Schwitzgebel, R. L. Biofeedback apparatus: List of suppliers. *Behavior Therapy,* 1975, *6,* 238–240. (a)

Rugh, J. D., & Schwitzgebel, R. L. Biofeedback apparatus: List of suppliers. *Behavior Therapy,* 1975, *6,* 423. (b)

Rugh, J. D., & Solberg, W. K. The identification of stressful stimuli in natural environments. Paper presented at the Biofeedback Research Society Annual Meeting, Colorado Springs, February 1974.

Sand, P. L., Trieschmann, R. B., Fordyce, W. E., & Fowler, R. S. Behavior modification in the medical rehabilitation setting: Rationale and some implications. *Rehabilitation and Practice Review,* 1970, *1,* 11–24.

Schwartz, G. E. Voluntary control of human cardiovascular integration and differentiation through feedback and reward. *Science,* 1972, *175,* 90–93.

Schwartz, G. E. Biofeedback as therapy: Some theoretical and practical issues. *American Psychologist*, 1973, *28*, 666–673.

Schwartz, G. E. Psychosomatic disorders in biofeedback: A psychobiological model of disregulation. In J. D. Mazer & M. E. P. Seligman (Eds.), *Psychopathology: Experimental models*. San Francisco: W. H. Freeman, 1977.

Schwartz, G. E., & Weiss, S. N. Yale Conference on Behavioral Medicine; a proposed definition and statement of goals. *Journal of Behavioral Medicine*, 1978, *1*, 3–12.

Shapiro, D., & Surwit, R. S. Learned control of physiological function and disease. In H. Leitenberg (Ed.), *Handbook of behavior modification and behavior therapy*. New York: Prentice-Hall, 1976.

Shapiro, D., Tursky, B., & Schwartz, G. E. Control of blood pressure in man by operant conditioning. *Circulation Research*, 1970, *27*, I-27–I-32.

Skinner, B. F. *Behavioral organisms*. New York: Appleton-Century-Crofts, 1938.

Skinner, B. F. *Science in human behavior*. New York: Macmillan, 1953.

Surwit, R. S., Shapiro, D., & Feld, J. L. Digital temperature autoregulation and associated cardiovascular changes. *Psychophysiology*, 1976, *13*, 242–248.

Surwit, R. S., Fenton, C., & Pilon, R. Behavioral treatment of Raynaud's disease. *Journal of Behavioral Medicine*, 1978, *1*, 323–335.

Thomas, E. G. Bias and therapist influence in behavioral assessment. *Journal of Behavior Therapy and Experimental Psychiatry*, 1973, *4*, 107–111.

Thomas, E. J., Abrams, K., & Johnson, J. Self-monitoring and reciprocal inhibition in the modification of multiple ties of Gilles de la Tourette's Syndrome. *Journal of Behavior Therapy and Experimental Psychiatry*, 1971, *2*, 159–171.

Thompson, R., & McConnell, J. Classical conditioning in the planarian: Dugesia Dorotocephala. *Journal of Comparative and Physiological Psychology*, 1955, *48*, 65–68.

Thoreson, C. E., & Mahoney, M. J. *Behavioral self-control*. New York: Holt, Rinehart, & Winston: 1974.

Truax, C. B., & Mitchell, K. M. Research on certain therapist interpersonal skills in relation to process and outcome. In A. E. Bergin & S. L. Garfield (Eds.), *Handbook of psychotherapy & behavior change*. New York: Wiley, 1971.

Van Boxtel, A., & Van der Ven, J. Differential EMG activities in subjects with muscle contraction headaches related to mental effort. *Headache*, 1978, *17*, 233–237.

Wolf, M. M., Birnbrauer, J., Williams, T., & Lawler, J. A note on apparent extinction of the vomiting behavior of a retarded child. In L. Ullmann & L. Krasner (Eds.), *Case studies in behavior modification*. New York: Holt, Rinehart, & Winston, 1965.

Wolpe, J. *The practice of behavior therapy*. New York: Pergamon Press, 1969.

Wolpe, J., & Lang, P. J. A fear survey schedule for use in behavior therapy. *Behaviour Research and Therapy*, 1964, *2*, 27–30.

6
Biofeedback: A Selective Review of Clinical Applications in Behavioral Medicine

EDWARD B. BLANCHARD

THE PLACE OF BIOFEEDBACK WITHIN BEHAVIORAL MEDICINE

At one time, *biofeedback* and *behavioral medicine* were considered synonymous, as evidence by Birk's 1973 book, *Biofeedback: Behavioral Medicine*. As is obvious from the contents of this present book, behavioral medicine encompasses much, much more than biofeedback. However, as pointed out by Blanchard (1977), biofeedback is one important aspect of behavioral medicine. Much of behavioral medicine is concerned with changing gross, observable behavior. This can be accomplished either as direct treatment of a disorder with demonstrable pathophysiology, such as the treatment of obesity through modifying eating behavior and exercise patterns, or as an adjunct to standard medical treatment, such as improving medication-taking compliance in the drug treatment of hypertension. Biofeedback is somewhat different in that it represents psychological intervention delivered directly at the physiological level rather than at the level of gross motor behavior. Thus, in a sense, biofeedback could be seen as applied, or clinical, psychophysiology.

Before going further, let me formally define *biofeedback*: "A process in which a person learns to reliably influence physiological responses of two kinds: either responses which are not ordinarily under voluntary control or responses which ordinarily are easily regulated but for which regulation has broken down due to trauma or disease." (Blanchard & Epstein, 1978, p. 2). Biofeedback is most easily conceptualized as a three-step procedure: (1) the detection and amplification of various

---

EDWARD B. BLANCHARD • Department of Psychology, State University of New York, Albany, New York 12222.

physiological responses; (2) the conversion of the response to some easy-to-process form of information, usually an auditory or visual signal; and (3) the feeding of this information back to the patient on a relatively immediate basis. All three steps are most conveniently accomplished with electronic instruments.

The early work in biofeedback was marked by much speculation as to the potential for the field and the potential for patients to play an active role "in healing themselves." One leader described biofeedback as a "new panacea" (Brown, 1974). This early promise has not yet been fulfilled and may never be. However, the research in biofeedback has sparked a major effort at treating psychophysiological disorders and other medical problems through psychological means. Thus, biofeedback was one of the main forces responsible for the growth of the field of behavioral medicine.

BASES FOR REVIEW AND EVALUATION

As indicated by the title of this chapter, this is a selective review of the clinical applications of biofeedback. Since there are well over 2,000 citations in the biofeedback literature in a recently published bibliography (Butler, 1978), any review must of necessity be selective. Thus, this review, except on rare occasions, omits the whole field of basic research in biofeedback. Moreover, it is my intention primarily to examine a few areas of clinical biofeedback application in which some sizable body of literature exists, with only a brief mention of other areas. Thus, this review is obviously neither exhaustive nor comprehensive; rather, it is intended to summarize the state of the art in certain areas.

For the interested reader, in addition to the recent bibliography by Butler (1978), several more comprehensive reviews of the clinical (and basic) literature are in existence: Blanchard and Young (1974), Blanchard and Epstein (1977, 1978), and Miller (1978).

In evaluating biofeedback, or any other therapeutic endeavor, there are certain factors one should consider. First and foremost is *efficacy*, or whether the treatment works. To a certain extent, the determination of efficacy depends upon the experimental design used to evaluate the therapy. In a previous review (Blanchard & Young, 1974), we listed five classes of designs arranged hierarchically in terms of the strength of the conclusions one could draw from results. These five classes were (1) anecdotal case report; (2) systematic case study; (3) single-subject experiment; (4) single-group outcome study; and (5) controlled-group outcome study. Relatively firm conclusions about efficacy can be drawn from a series of single-subject experiments on the same problem and from single-group outcome studies with adequate baselines. Ultimately, conclusions about efficacy must rely upon controlled-group outcome studies, in which there is an attention–placebo control group. In this review, anecdotal case reports and individual systematic case studies are omitted for the most part. Instances of multiple systematic case studies of the same disorder are included.

After establishing efficacy, the next concern is for *relative efficacy*, or whether the treatment works better than other established treatments. This determination requires controlled-group outcome studies. There are, to my knowledge, no studies comparing biofeedback to conventional pharmacological therapy. There are, however, studies comparing biofeedback with other forms of psychological treatment and studies in which biofeedback is used as an adjunct to standard medical treatment.

Beyond efficacy, there are at least three other issues that should be considered: (1) *efficiency*, or whether biofeedback brings about more rapid removal of symptoms; (2) *generality*, or what proportion of a patient population is helped appreciably by the biofeedback treatment; and (3) *durability*, or what happens to successfully treated patients over long-term follow-up. In most instances, unfortunately, data on these three factors are relatively unavailable. However, they are discussed where possible.

A final issue to which this review attends is the supposed mode of action of the biofeedback treatment. In evaluating biofeedback therapies, it is important to have data on the changes in the physiological response for which feedback was given. The reason is that there are numerous applications of biofeedback for which feedback training is given for one response but the main indication of improvement is either self-report or the measurement of a second response. For example, in the treatment of migraine headaches, feedback is usually given of hand or fingertip temperature, while the primary measure of improvement is self-report of headache activity. In the treatment of hypertension, feedback is usually given on the response of interest, blood pressure. To be convincing, both the physiological response on which feedback is given and the clinical response of interest could change, more or less synchronously.

In an instance in which there is an improvement by self-report in the absence of measurable physiological change, one must suspect a placebo response. Stroebel and Glueck (1973) have aptly described biofeedback as the "ultimate placebo." In this age of space flight and electronic gadgets, a treatment that involves equipment, flashing lights, or moving dials, clicks and changing tones, all housed in impressive wooden or metal cabinets, has much possiblity of evoking a placebo response. While there is nothing inherently evil or wrong about a placebo response, and all good clinicians probably tend to capitalize on it, the effect tends to be transient. If biofeedback is to take its place in the behavioral medicine armamentarium, it should be able to demonstrate that its effects are more than just placebo (Orne, 1978).

MUSCLE–CONTRACTION HEADACHES

Muscle–contraction, or tension, headache is one of the five areas for which the Biofeedback Society of America claims there is demonstrated efficacy of biofeedback therapy. Muscle–contraction headache is believed to arise from "the long sustained contraction of the skeletal muscles of the scalp, shoulders, neck and face in patients suffering from anxiety, environmental and situational tension and depressed states" (Friedman, 1975). Although there are some data (cited by Bakal, 1975) to support the association of increased levels of muscle tension, recent reports by Epstein & Abel (1977) and Phillips (1977) call this relation into question.

Muscle–contraction headaches are usually described as a generalized pain over the entire head, usually starting in the occipital or neck region. The pain is characterized by a dull ache and is frequently described as a band or caplike pressure or tightness. It is not unusual for sufferers of this disorder to experience headache almost every day.

Biofeedback Treatment

In the biofeedback treatment of muscle–contraction headache, the electromyogram (EMG) is measured from electrodes placed on the forehead, approximately one inch above each eyebrow. This placement measures the EMG from the frontalis and other facial muscles. Treatment is thus aimed at reducing the EMG of these muscle groups.

In the first report of this form of treatment, Budzynski, Stoyva, and Adler (1970) treated five patients with chronic muscle contraction headaches in a single-group outcome study. Patients were seen for two or three sessions per week for 4–12 weeks. They also were given instruction in muscle relaxation training and told to practice this at home on a daily basis. All five patients reported marked decreases in headache activity by the end of treatment and for follow-ups of up to three months. On a group basis, EMG levels showed a gradual decrease during treatment. Interestingly, failure to continue regular practice of home relaxation was associated with a return of headaches in two of five cases.

Wickramasekera (1972) provided independent confirmation of the efficacy of EMG feedback training for muscle contraction headaches in a single-group outcome study of five patients. After a baseline phase of three weeks, three weeks of false feedback training were given as a control procedure. Neither headache activity nor EMG decreased. Next, 12 weeks of true feedback training were given, which led to marked decreases in headache reports and EMG.

Very much to their credit, Budzynski and his associates (Budzynski, Stoyva, Alder, & Mullaney, 1973) next completed a small-scale controlled-group outcome study of EMG biofeedback combined with regular home practice of relaxation. After two weeks of baseline headache recording, six patients received 16 sessions of veridical EMG biofeedback training over nine weeks; as a control for attention–placebo effects, six other patients received 16 sessions of nonveridical feedback with instructions to attend to the sound; a final group of six continued to monitor headache activity but received no other treatment. The first two groups were instructed to practice relaxation at home on a daily basis.

Results showed a significant decrease in headache activity only for the group receiving veridical feedback. Four of six patients had marked decreases in headache activity at the end of treatment. The two failures had not practiced relaxation regularly. There was no overall decrease in headache activity in the two control groups. However, one patient in the false feedback group did improve significantly; she had practiced relaxation regularly. Three-month follow-up data showed the same results. At 18 months, four of the patients in the true feedback condition were contacted; the three who had shown initial improvement were still doing well.

At this point, the combination of EMG biofeedback and regular practice of relaxation seemed to have demonstrable efficacy for muscle contraction headaches.

Phillips (1977), in a small-scale refinement of the Budzynski *et al.* (1973) study, compared true and false EMG feedback, *without regular relaxation practice*, in two groups of three patients each. While the patients receiving true feedback showed a significant decrease in EMG at the end of treatment and those receiving false feedback did not, there was no difference in headache report at the end of treatment. However, at a follow-up six to eight weeks after treatment, the true feedback group had shown improvement.

Epstein & Abel (1977) performed six systematic case studies of EMG feedback *alone* for the treatment of muscle–contraction headaches. All patients received 16 sessions of feedback training. Three of the six showed marked reduction in headache activity as measured by a daily headache diary. An analysis of individual data revealed essentially no relationship between self-report of degree of headache pain and EMG level.

Finally, in an uncontrolled clinical trial, Diamond and Franklin (1974) reported a good response in 13 of 31 patients with pure muscle-contraction headaches treated entirely with EMG biofeedback.

Comment

At this point, the efficacy of the combination of frontal EMG feedback and regular practice of relaxation seems adequately demonstrated. The relationship between forehead EMG levels and headache, the physiological basis for the biofeedback treatment, is anything but clear, however.

Comparisons of Biofeedback and Relaxation

Given the success of the combination of frontal EMG biofeedback and relaxation training in treating muscle contraction headaches, it is not surprising that researchers would seek to determine the relative importance of these two components. To date, at least four controlled-group comparisons of frontal EMG biofeedback and relaxation training have been published.

The first, and in many ways the best, study was a comparison by Cox, Freundlich, and Meyer (1975) of (1) frontal EMG biofeedback and instructions to practice cue-controlled relaxation regularly at home; (2) instruction in progressive relaxation and instructions to practice cue-controlled relaxation regularly at home; and (3) a glucose placebo capsule that was given with a strong expectancy that it would relieve headaches. After a two-week baseline of headache recording, nine patients were assigned to each condition and given eight individual treatments over a four-week period. They were then followed up for four and a half months.

Results showed a significant reduction in headache activity for *both* the biofeedback group and the relaxation group, as well as significant reduction in frontal EMG in both groups. Both groups improved more than the placebo group. At follow-up, seven out of eight available patients in each group were still much improved.

Haynes, Griffin, Mooney, and Parise (1975) compared frontal EMG biofeedback alone, relaxation training, and instructions "to try to relax" in college students with chronic tension headaches. Both the patients in the biofeedback condition and the relaxation training condition were significantly improved after the three weeks of treatment (six sessions) and more improved than the "self-relaxed" group. A one-week follow-up showed maintenance of the effects. Loss of subjects prevented any analysis of longer-term follow-up.

Chesney and Shelton (1976), in another study of college volunteers with tension headaches, compared frontal EMG biofeedback training, training in progressive relaxation and regular home practice, and a combination of the two with a no-treatment control condition. Treatment consisted of eight sessions over a two-week interval. Results showed significant improvement for the relaxation training and the combined treatment; moreover, both groups improved more than the biofeedback treatment or the no-treatment group, which did not differ. No follow-up data were available.

In the final report of this series, Hutchings & Reinking (1976) compared frontal EMG biofeedback, instruction in relaxation that the investigators made up, and a combination of the two treatments. All patients were instructed to practice the relaxation at home regularly. After the 10 treatment sessions, approximately twice per week, patients were followed up for one month. Results showed significant reductions (about 66%) in headache activity for the EMG biofeedback group and the combined treatment but little change (about 20%) for the relaxation-only group.

At a follow-up of three months, this same result obtained. However, at follow-ups at six months and one year, all differential treatment effects had vanished, and continued improvement seemed related only to continual regular practice of relaxation (Reinking, 1976).

Comment

In three of four comparisons, relaxation training alone with regular practice leads to results equivalent to those obtained with a combination of frontal EMG and regular practice of relaxation. In the one study that found an advantage for EMG biofeedback training over relaxation training, follow-up revealed that it was more an advantage in efficiency than in long-term efficacy. Certinly, the efficacy of the combined treatment is well documented. The role of the EMG biofeedback and the relationship of EMG levels to headache pain reports remain unanswered.

MYOFACIAL PAIN

Another clinical problem that is rather similar to muscle contraction headaches and that has been successfully treated with EMG biofeedback is myofacial pain. In particular, the pain associated with temperomandibular joint (TMJ) syndrome has been treated by teaching patients to relax the facial muscles, particularly the masseter and the temporalis. Although the standard dental treatment of this disorder is to adjust the occlusion between the upper and the lower teeth, there are some patients for which there is clearly muscle involvement. In advanced cases, the masseter is so hypertrophied that the lower face appears swollen.

In an initial report of the use of biofeedback with this disorder, Gessel and Alderman (1971) gave 11 patients a combination of EMG feedback from the masseter and extensive training in progressive relaxation. Of the 11, 6 were much improved in this single-group outcome study.

In a second study of similar design, Gessel (1975) reported on the treatment of 23 patients with chronic facial pain through a combination of EMG biofeedback from either the masseter or the frontalis and home practice in relaxation. In this group, 15 patients showed substantial alleviation of symptoms with this treatment.

Carlsson and Gale (1977) reported on the treatment of 11 patients with long-standing (at least three years) TMJ pain with EMG feedback from the masseter. All patients had had trials on at least two other forms of therapy and some as many as five different therapies. Patients received from 6 to 18 treatment sessions over 6–24 weeks. Results showed that 8 of 10 patients had lowered masseter EMG recordings. An evaluation of clinical status at follow-up (4–15 months posttreatment) by an independent expert showed 5 patients symptom-free, 3 much improved, 1 slightly improved, and 2 unchanged.

In a controlled-group outcome study, Dohrmann and Haskin (1976) (cited in Carlsson & Gale, 1977), treated 24 TMJ patients: 16 with EMG biofeedback and 8 with an attention–placebo condition. Of the 16, 12 were symptom-free or much improved at a one-year follow-up.

Comment

It appears that EMG biofeedback has demonstrated efficacy in the treatment of TMJ pain. This has been shown in at least three separate studies by different investigators. Results have held up for at least one year. From 50% to 75% of patients with long-standing TMJ difficulties have responded favorably to this type of treatment.

NEUROMUSCULAR REEDUCATION

Probably the oldest clinical application of biofeedback is in the area of neuromuscular reeducation, or the use of EMG feedback to assist patients to regain voluntary control of skeletal muscles. The normal voluntary control has been impaired by disease or trauma, such as the hemiplegia of the stroke victim. In almost all cases, EMG biofeedback is an adjunct to standard physical therapy.

Although with one exception, the work in this area is at the level of systematic case studies or single-group outcome studies, nevertheless the results are impressive because of the unusually long baselines during which the patient either has not spontaneously recovered function or has not responded to standard physical therapy.

Upper Extremity

In a study that was more a demonstration than a clinical treatment, Andrews (1964) reported that 17 of 20 patients suffering from hemiplegia of at least a year's duration were able to show improved upper extremity movement with only five minutes of feedback training. Brudny, Korein, Grynbaum, Friedmann, Weinstein, Sachs-Frankel, and Belandres (1976) reported on the treatment of 39 cases of upper extremity paralysis. EMG biofeedback of varying lengths led to improved functioning in 27 cases, with good transfer to everyday life over follow-ups of three months to three years.

Lower Extremity

Johnson & Garton (1973) treated 10 hemiplegics—none of whom had responded to standard physical therapy over the past year and all of whom wore a short leg-brace—with EMG biofeedback to regain quadriceps function and increase dorsiflexion. After initial training in the laboratory, all patients were switched to home training with a portable EMG biofeedback device. In this group, 7 of 10 had markedly improved dorsiflexion and 5 were able to walk without the brace.

In the only controlled-group outcome study in this area of clinical biofeedback, Basmajian, Kukulka, Narajan, and Takebe (1975) compared five weeks of standard physical therapy with five weeks of standard physical therapy and EMG biofeedback in a set of hemiplegic patients suffering from foot drop. Thus, biofeedback was an adjunct to the standard therapy. Results showed greater improvement in strength and range of motion for the patients receiving the biofeedback as well as greater improvement in gait. The gains were maintained at follow-ups of one to four months.

Spasmodic Torticollis

Brudny *et al.* (1976) summarized the results of the biofeedback treatment of a large series of patients with spasmodic torticollis. Treatment consisted primarily of teaching the patients simultaneously to relax the hypertrophied sternocleidomastoid muscle while increasing the EMG level of the atrophied side. Results showed significant improvement in the laboratory in 26 of 48 patients, with "substantial carryover" to the natural environment. Follow-ups of three months to three years revealed that 19 of the 26 improved patients had sucessfully maintained their improved status.

Comment

Although the sophistication of the experimental designs used in these studies is, with one exception, somewhat limited, nevertheless it does seem that EMG biofeedback may play an important role in the rehabilitation of patients with neuromuscular disorders. Certainly, the evidence to date would warrant more controlled comparisons of the type performed by Basmajian *et al.* (1975).

MIGRAINE HEADACHES

Migraine headaches are a form of vascular headache characterized by recurrent episodes of headache, varying in intensity, frequency, and duration which are usually unilateral in onset. Furthermore, they are frequently accompanied by nausea and irritability. The accepted pathophysiology is a two-phase process: initially, there is vasoconstriction of cranial and cerebral arteries; during the headache phase, there is vasodilation of these arteries, including the extracranial arteries. There follows a sterile inflammation of the arterial wall and vascular edema, which lead to the throbbing pain.

Temperature Biofeedback

The use of temperature biofeedback as a treatment for migraine headache was developed by a group at the Menninger Clinic. The initial "treatment package" consisted of autogenic training, relaxation training, and feedback of the difference in temperature between the fingertip and the forehead. After several sessions in the laboratory with the temperature feedback device, the patient was switched to practice at home with a portable device.

Although the initial report (Sargent, Green, & Walters, 1972) seems like a single-group outcome study, its quality is such as to make it an anecdotal case report. It is difficult to tell how many patients actually were helped by the treatment.

In a later study, Sargent, Green, and Walters (1973) reported on the treatment of 28 patients, 20 of whom had definite migraine headache. Of the 20 patients, 12 were improved as a result of the combined treatment package in this single-group outcome study.

In a more recent report, Solbach and Sargent (1977) reported follow-up data on 110 patients treated at the Menninger Clinic. Of the 74 who completed at least nine months of treatment, 55 (74%) were judged to be at least moderately improved or more (at least a 26% reduction of headache activity) at the end of treatment. Follow-up data showed trends toward improvement to be maintained.

Turin and Johnson (1976) presented data on seven migraineurs treated solely with temperature feedback training designed to teach the patients to warm their hands. After a four- to six-week baseline, biofeedback training was given for an average of nine weeks on a twice-per-week basis. Three of the seven had marked reductions in headache frequency. These three plus one more had reductions in medication use. Success was only marginally related to ability to warm the hands. No follow-up data were given for this small-scale single-group outcome study.

A controlled-group outcome evaluation of the combination of temperature biofeedback and autogenic training was completed by Andreychuk and Skriver (1975). After a six-week baseline of headache recordings, 11 migraineurs were assigned to each of three conditions: (1) temperature training plus autogenic training; (2) EEG alpha training; and (3) instruction in relaxation and self-hypnosis and regular practice of both. Treatment was once per week for 10 weeks.

The results showed significant improvement in *all three* groups, with no differential improvement. No follow-up data were given. Thus, while the efficacy of the temperature biofeedback–autogenic training combination was established, there remains the possibility that it was entirely an attention–placebo effect.

Another controlled-group outcome study of the biofeedback treatment of migraine headache was recently completed by the author and his colleagues (Blanchard, Theobald, Williamson, Silver, & Brown, 1978). After a one-month baseline of headache diary recordings, 30 patients selected by explicit inclusion and exclusion criteria to have exclusively or predominantly migraine headaches were randomly assigned from matched triads to one of three conditions: (1) temperature biofeedback training combined with some training in autogenic phrases; (2) progressive relaxation; or (3) a waiting-list controls, who continued to monitor headache activity. Patients in the first two conditions were instructed to practice daily and were seen twice per week for six weeks. At the end of six weeks, those patients in the waiting-list condition who still desired treatment were randomly assigned to either the biofeedback condition or the relaxation condition. Thus we conducted a controlled-group outcome evaluation of biofeedback versus another effective therapy.

Results showed a slight statistical advantage at the end of treatment of the expanded groups ($n = 13$ each) for relaxation over biofeedback on frequency, duration, peak intensity of headaches, and reduction in medication usage. However, there were no differences between the two conditions at follow-ups of one, two, or three months. At the one-month follow-up 9 of 13 patients from the relaxation condition were still headache-free ($n = 4$) or much improved ($n = 5$), as compared with 6 of 11 in the biofeedback condition (1 headache-free, 5 much improved).

Comment

Migraine headache is another disorder for which the Biofeedback Society of America claims demonstrated efficacy of biofeedback treatment. At this point, temperature biofeedback designed to teach patients to warm their hands, combined with regular practice of selected autogenic phrases, has been shown to be effective in single-group outcome and controlled-group outcome studies in reducing headache activity for sufferers of migraine. It has not been shown to be more effective than various forms of relaxation training, however, and, if anything, seems slightly inferior to the latter form of treatment.

No good explanation has been proposed for the physiological mechanism through which temperature biofeedback works. To my mind, given the comparable results in controlled comparisons with relaxation training, it would seem that it is either an elaborate way to teach patients to relax or else may involve an overall reduction in sympathetic arousal.

Cephalic Vasomotor Biofeedback

It has been noted for some time that the external cranial arteries of migraine sufferers have a more labile vasomotor response than in nonheadache patients (Delessio, 1972). Using an elaborate on-line computer analysis of vasomotor responding, Friar and Beatty (1976) treated 19 migraineurs in a controlled-group outcome study. The experimental group received feedback of temporal artery pulse amplitude and instructions to try to reduce it. The control group received feedback of pulse amplitude of the index finger. Treatment lasted for nine sessions.

Results showed significant reduction in temporal artery pulse amplitude for the experimental group on both a within-group and a between-group basis. There were some limited therapeutic effects: the experimental group had significantly fewer major migraine headaches (over three hours) as compared with its own pretreatment baseline and as compared at posttreatment with the control group. No follow-up data were available.

Feuerstein and Adams (1977) reported on the treatment of two migraineurs using cephalic vasomotor feedback training in a complex single-subject design. The purpose of the feedback training was to reduce the lability of the vasomotor response, that is, to reduce the frequency of very large and very small responses. Only one of the migraine sufferers demonstrated significant reduction in pulse amplitude during the feedback training. For this patient, headache duration and intensity *increased* during the vasomotor training to reduce cranial artery vasomotor responding. Although the rationale for this form of training is clearer than that for training patients to warm their hands, the clinical results are not as impressive. Biofeedback training can lead to changes in cephalic vasomotor responding. The clinical results in terms of reduced headache activity are not especially impressive at this point, despite, or perhaps because of, evaluation in controlled studies.

RAYNAUD'S DISEASE

Raynaud's disease is a functional disorder of the peripheral vascular system in which the patient suffers painful episodes of vasoconstriction in the hands and sometimes the feet. During an attack, the skin blanches and is cold to the touch. Attacks are usually precipitated by exposure to cold or by emotional upset. This is another condition for which the Biofeedback Society of America claims demonstrated efficacy of biofeedback treatment.

Temperature Biofeedback Training

With the exception of two cases treated with vasomotor feedback training by Schwartz (1972), all of the reported cases have involved temperature biofeedback training. Because of the relative rarity of this disorder, until recently all of the reports but one were of single patients or small groups of patients and at the level of systematic case studies.

One single-subject experiment was reported by Blanchard and Haynes (1975). In this case, it was shown that temperature biofeedback plus instructions to raise hand temperature were consistently more effective than instructions alone. During the course of 24 treatment sessions spread over four months, the patient's basal hand temperature increased by 12°F, and vasospastic episodes decreased. The benefits were partially maintained and followed up at seven months.

The state of knowledge in this field took a giant step forward with the completion of a controlled-group outcome study by Surwit, Pilon, and Fenton (1978). In this study, all patients were independently diagnosed as suffering from idiopathic Raynaud's disease. All received autogenic training designed to help them relax and warm their hands. Half also received temperature biofeedback training. For half of the patients, all treatment was in the laboratory; for the other half there were three group meetings and then all further training took place at home. The entire 2×2 experiment was then replicated on a second set of patients, who served as no-treatment controls during the first phase of the study.

Two factors stand out in the results. First, there were no differential effects of temperature biofeedback added to autogenic training over simple autogenic training, and there were no differential effects of laboratory versus home training. Thus, patients who received instruction in autogenic training and practiced at home did as well as patients who received the autogenic training and six laboratory-based temperature biofeedback training sessions. Second, the treated subjects did significantly better than the untreated subjects on a cold stress test and also had fewer vasospastic episodes. After treatment, the performance of the controls matched that of the treated subjects and replicated it in every way. Vasospastic episodes decreased from about two and a half per day prior to treatment to slightly more than one per day by the end of treatment.

Comment

Although temperature biofeedback seems to have some efficacy in the treatment of Raynaud's disease, it has been shown fairly conclusively to add nothing to a simpler treatment based on autogenic training and carried out at home. Thus, while there do seem to be psychological treatments for this disorder, temperature biofeedback should probably be reserved for those patients who do not respond to autogenic training.

CARDIAC ARRHYTHMIAS

One of the interesting paradoxes of biofeedback research is the great amount of basic research that has been published involving cardiac rate and the relatively infrequent clinical use of this response. By my count, by 1977 there were over 60 articles in the biofeedback literature on control of cardiac rate, and fewer than a dozen clinical applications of control of cardiac rate. An area where biofeedback training to teach control of cardiac rate has been used is in the treatment of cardiac arrhythmias, or irregular or abnormal cardiac rhythms.

Premature Ventricular Contractions (PVCs)

By far the best study in this area is a series of systematic case studies by Weiss and Engel (1971). Eight patients with well-documented and frequent PVCs were given essentially the same training program, designed to teach them to control their heart rate (HR). It was hypothesized that once the patients had learned control of the HR, this control could lead to a decrease in PVCs. The number of phases of training completed by each patient varied somewhat. All training took place while the patient was hospitalized.

The training sequence involved teaching the patients to increase their HR, decreases their HR, and then alternately increase and decrease it for brief periods. Next, the patient was taught to reduce the variability of the HR by holding it within a specified range. In this phase, patients also received direct information about the occurrence of PVCs due to the feedback arrangement. Finally, feedback was faded out while the patient kept his HR within the specified range as a way of teaching true "self-control" instead of feedback-assisted control. Three patients completed the entire training sequence, while two others had some of the feedback–fade-out training.

Five of eight patients had marked reduction in PVCs in the laboratory, while four of these showed reductions in outside, independent assessment over follow-ups of 3–21 months. Improvement was related somewhat to length of training.

Engel and Bleecker (1974) were able to replicate these results with another patient in a systematic case study. Independent confirmation of her improvement was obtained several times during a lengthy follow-up.

Very important independent confirmation of the efficacy of HR biofeedback in the treatment of PVCs was provided by Pickering and Gorham (1975). A woman with rate-dependent PVCs learned to control her HR and through this to increase markedly the basal HR at which her PVCs began. Pickering and Miller (1977) also noted two other patients with PVCs successfully treated by HR biofeedback by Pickering in Miller's laboratory.

Comment

Although the level of experimental design used in studies of the treatment of PVCs with biofeedback is fairly low, nevertheless the evidence does point to some possible efficacy for this procedure. What is needed, of course, is a small-scale con-trolled-group outcome study similar to Surwit *et al.*'s (1978) on Raynaud's disease. Even with relatively rare disorders, a well-controlled study can be done that can provide more definitive answers as to efficacy.

Sinus Tachycardia

The other cardiac arrhythmia that has received some attention from biofeedback researchers is sinus tachycardia, or abnormally high cardiac rate. Blanchard and his associates (Blanchard & Abel, 1976; Scott, Blanchard, Edmundson, & Young, 1973) have reported on three cases of sinus tachycardia treated with HR biofeedback in single-subject experiments. In each case, clinically meaningful reductions (that is, reduction to the normal range) in HR were obtained. However, because of the failure to obtain reversals in certain phases of the A-B-A designs, firm conclusions are not possible. Follow-up data revealed maintenance of the improvement in HR. Informal reports from two patients, S-1 in Scott *et al.* (1973) and the single-patient in Blanchard and Abel (1976), revealed marked improvement in certain areas, such as a return to work for a patient on disability benefits in the former case and cessation of "blackout" spells in the latter case.

Engel and Bleecker (1974) reported an independent confirmation of the value of HR biofeedback with sinus tachycardia. In a systematic case study, HR-lowering training was given and led to a reduction of HR to the normal range after a history of years in the elevated range.

Comment

Although the number of reported cases is small, there is some evidence for the efficacy of HR biofeedback in the treatment of two cardiac arrhythmias, PVCs and sinus tachycardia. In each instance, successful treatment has been replicated in other laboratories. The lack of more controlled work precludes definitive statements in this interesting area, however.

HYPERTENSION

Essential hypertension, or elevated blood pressure (BP) in the absence of demonstrable physical cause, is one of the two most researched ailments in the biofeedback literature. The other is muscle contraction headaches. The reasons for all of this research are probably the widespread nature of the disorder (estimates are that from 10% to 20% of the adult population in the United States suffer from hypertension) and some of the early reports of the successful control of BP in normotensive subjects (Shapiro, Tursky, Gershon, & Stern, 1969).

Direct Blood Pressure Feedback

Utilizing the constant cuff method of giving direct feedback of BP developed by the Harvard group (Tursky, Shapiro, & Schwartz, 1972), Benson, Shapiro, Tursky, and Schwartz (1971) treated seven hypertensive patients on an outpatient basis in a series of systemic case studies. A very good feature of this study was the prolonged baseline: patients were run until they showed no decrease in systolic BP for five consecutive sessions. Average length of baseline was 11 sessions. They were then run in the treatment condition until they showed no decrease in BP for five consecutive sessions. Treatment length averaged 22 sessions, with a range of 8–34.

The results were very favorable: average systolic BP decreased by 16.5 mm Hg from a stable baseline to the end of treatment, and five of seven patients showed a significant decrease in systolic BP. No follow-up data were obtained, nor were measures obtained of transfer to the natural environment. Nonetheless, these initial results were very promising, even if obtained in an uncontrolled study.

Schwartz and Shapiro (1973) attempted a replication of these results with another group of seven patients in a single-group outcome study in which patients received 5 baseline sessions and 15 daily treatment sessions. There was *no* overall decrease in diastolic BP. One patient showed a decrease of 14 mm Hg. Thus, the systematic replication was a failure.

In a later study by some of these same investigators, Surwit, Shapiro, and Good (1978) conducted a controlled-group outcome study comparing three treatments: (1) a combined feedback of systolic BP and HR; (2) feedback of frontal EMG; and (3) training in a passive-meditative form of relaxation called the relaxation reponse (Benson, 1975). Eight patients with verified borderline hypertension were assigned to each condition after two baseline sessions. Over the eight training sessions and a six-week follow-up, no significant reduction in systolic BP was found for any group, and no differential treatment effects were found. There was a small, but statistically significant, within-session decrease in systolic BP ($\overline{X} = 3.4$ mm Hg) found for all groups averaged over all treatment sessions.

Two other single-group outcome studies utilizing essentially the same constant cuff BP feedback system have been reported. Goldman, Kleinman, Snow, Bidus, and Korol (1975) treated seven hypertensives for nine sessions. No baseline measures were obtained. Results showed a slight (6 mm Hg) decrease in systolic BP.

In a much more elaborate single-group outcome study, Kristt and Engel (1975) obtained five weeks of self-monitored BPs on four diagnosed hypertensive patients before admitting them to the hospital. In the three-week hospital stay, the patients received elaborate training in increasing and decreasing BP with the aid of feedback. At the end of the hospitalization, all four patients showed decreases in BP and averaged decreases of 18 mm Hg systolic and 7.5 mm Hg diastolic. Patients continued to monitor BP at home during the two to three-month follow-up and continued to try to lower BP using what they had learned and a manual sphygmomanometer as feedback. Three of the four maintained their improvement.

While this study is excellent in terms of having good baseline and follow-up data and in-hospital demonstration of control of BP, it nevertheless has problems. The BP of most hypertensive patients decreases with hospitalization; thus, the role of biofeedback is unclear in the absence of a control group.

There have been two other reports of the treatment of hypertension using a similar beat-by-beat BP feedback system. Miller (1972) presented an elaborate systematic case study of the treatment of hypertension in a female patient. After 26 baseline sessions over six weeks, diastolic BP was decreased by 21 mm Hg (from 97 to 76) over 37 treatment sessions. Antihypertensive medication was also stopped with no increase in BP. In a later attempt with over 20 other hypertensive patients, Miller (1975) reported no replication of the success.

Comment

At this point, there is no well-controlled study with adequate baseline that shows that direct BP biofeedback on a beat-by-beat basis has any efficacy for the treatment of hypertension.

Two other research teams have reported treating hypertensive patients with direct BP feedback given on an intermittent, rather than a beat-by-beat, basis. Elder, Ruiz, Deabler, and Dillenkoffer (1973) assigned six inpatients to each of three conditions: intermittent BP biofeedback and social reinforcement, intermittent BP biofeedback, and monitoring of BP. After one baseline session, the patients received seven treatment sessions over a four-day period. Results showed no differences in systolic BP. The diastolic BP of the biofeedback plus social reinforcement group was reduced to 80% of baseline, while that of the biofeedback-only group dropped to 93% of baseline. The former change was significantly greater than that of the control group.

In an outpatient replication, Elder and Eustis (1975) treated 22 patients in a single-group outcome study with 20 sessions spread over 12 or 82 days. The average decrease in systolic BP of biofeedback training was about 8 mm Hg, while diastolic BP decreased about 6 mm Hg. Significant decreases were found in 9 of 22 participants. Thus, the very strong initial results of Elder failed to be replicated.

Blanchard, Young, and Haynes (1975) treated four hypertensives in single-subject experiments using an intermittent BP biofeedback procedure. After a four-session baseline, all four patients showed noticeable decreases in systolic BP averaging 26 mm Hg (range: 9–51 mm Hg). Follow-up after one to four weeks showed that three of four patients maintained about two-thirds of the decreases.

In a recently completed study, Blanchard, Miller, Abel, Haynes, and Wicker (1977) tested their intermittent BP biofeedback procedure in a controlled-group outcome study. Patients were assigned to BP biofeedback (n = 10), frontal EMG biofeedback (n = 9), or a self-relaxation condition (n = 9). After 4 baseline sessions, all patients received 12 treatment sessions and then were followed up for four and a half months. Results showed no change for the frontal EMG group. The BP biofeedback group showed a slight decrease (about 8 mm Hg, p = .07) in systolic BP, while the relaxation group showed a significant (p = .05) decrease (about 10 mm Hg) in systolic BP. The changes in diastolic BP were very small (1–2 mm Hg). The relaxation group also showed a significant decrease in BP as measured before and after treatment at a consulting physician's office. The gains manifested by the relaxation group dissipated during the follow-up, while those of the biofeedback group tended to be maintained.

Comment

In the field of the treatment of hypertension by direct feedback of BP, failure of replication seems to be the rule. Four separate research teams (Shapiro, Miller,

Elder, and Blanchard) have obtained good initial results, only to have relative failures on more extensive replication. The other two uncontrolled successes have not yet been replicated.

Despite the lack of generalized success with direct BP feedback, there are individuals who seem to be helped by these procedures. Although essential hypertension is sometimes represented as a monolithic entity, in fact, there are varieties of essential hypertension. It may be the case that the best strategy is to try to match the feedback technique to the particular hypertensive patient who can benefit. Research on individual differences could be useful here. As a general rule, however, direct BP biofeedback does not seem to have much utility.

Other Biofeedback Treatment of Hypertension

In addition to the attempts to treat hypertension with direct BP biofeedback, there have been several other attempts using other forms of biofeedback. In all of this work, the rationale seems to have been to reduce BP either through reducing sympathetic arousal or through reducing overall level of muscle tension.

Love and his associates (Love, Montgomery, & Moeller, 1974; Moeller & Love, 1974) treated hypertensives with a combination of frontal EMG biofeedback and other relaxation techniques in single-group outcome studies. In one study, five of six patients showed good results, and average decreases in BP were 18 mm Hg systolic and 12 mm Hg diastolic. In the second study (Love *et al.*, 1974), 27 of 40 patients completed the 16 weeks of treatment and showed decreases in BP of 15 mm Hg systolic and 13 mm Hg diastolic. Moreover, for the 23 who were available for an eight-month follow-up, both systolic and diastolic BPs were further reduced (6.5 mm and 4 mm Hg, respectively). However, controlled-group outcome evaluations of frontal EMG biofeedback alone by Surwit *et al.* (1978) and Blanchard *et al.* (1977) failed to show any particular effectiveness for this form of treatment.

Probably the most impressive work in the area of biofeedback and hypertension is that of Chandra Patel and her associates in England. In each of three separate studies, groups of 17–20 clearly hypertensive patients were used. Most were on antihypertensive medication. In the first two studies (Patel, 1973, 1975), a combination of biofeedback of galvanic skin response (GSR) and a set of yoga exercises involving passive relaxation and meditation were used in a treatment program lasting for 36 sessions spread over three months.

In the first study, a single-group outcome study, systolic BP was reduced by 25 mm Hg, diastolic BP was reduced by 14 mm Hg, and 16 of 20 patients showed significant improvement. In the second study, a controlled-group outcome study, similar reductions in BP were found in the experimental subjects. Very importantly, the benefits were maintained over a 12-month follow-up.

The third study (Patel & North, 1975) was more rigorously controlled, and treatment was shortened to 12 sessions over six weeks. (In addition to the GSR biofeedback, some EMG biofeedback was added, as were special instructions to aid in the transfer of the training to the natural environment.) All BP measurements were made by a "blind examiner." Again, comparable (26 mm systolic, 15 mm diastolic) decreases were found for the experimental group. Four months after the end of the initial phase of the study, the control subjects were given the treatment package to complete the half-crossover, replication design. They also showed significant decreases in BP with treatment (28 mm Hg systolic, 16 mm Hg diastolic). Further follow-up showed that the gains were maintained by both groups after treatment.

Comment

It certainly seems that Patel has developed a very realiable and effective "treatment package." Whether biofeedback plays a crucial role is not known. However, personal communications from Patel seem to indicate that the regular practice of relaxation and meditation are more important.

In any event, this treatment package seems well worth investigating further. A major question, especially in light of the replication difficulties of other investigators, is whether another investigator using Patel's methodology can obtain similar results.

All evidence seems to point to the beneficial effects of various forms of relaxation training for hypertension and to the relative lack of generalized efficacy of direct BP biofeedback.

EPILEPSY

One of the more novel clinical applications of biofeedback training is in the areas of seizure disorders. Sterman and his associates (Sterman, 1973; Sterman & Friar, 1972) intially described a procedure that involved teaching patients to increase the incidence of a particular EEG pattern, a 12–14 Hz rhythm recorded over the sensorimotor cortex. This particular band of activity was called the sensory motor rhythm (SMR).

Sterman's initial reports were systematic case studies and some informal single-subject experiments with a total of four patients who had frequent seizures that were poorly controlled by medication. As the patients learned to increase the incidence of SMR, the seizure frequency and intensity decreased. Discontinuation of treatment led to a return of seizures.

The exciting aspect of this work is that three other investigators in different parts of the country have replicated Sterman's work. Lubar and Bahler (1976) reported on the successful treatment of eight cases. Finley, Smith, and Etherton (1975) also replicated Sterman's work. Kaplan (1975) failed to replicate the beneficial effects of SMR training but did get improvement with a slightly different procedure.

Since the early work, Sterman (1977, personal communication) has focused less on specific SMR biofeedback training and more on analyzing irregularities in the spectral analysis of the total EEG and then trying to correct them. His approach seems to be to try to normalize the distribution of frequencies and the amount of energy in each frequency band. This approach certainly represents an advance over the clinical EEG and may provide a psychophysiological and behavioral basis for understanding and treating difficult seizure disorders. The area certainly warrants more widespread clinical trials of a controlled nature, especially since seizure disorders can have a psychological component.

ALPHA BIOFEEDBACK TRAINING

Next to HR biofeedback training, attempts to produce relatively high levels of alpha in the EEG through biofeedback have been the most popular research topic. However, while HR biofeedback has had some clinical applications, to date there have been no clear-cut studies showing a clinical benefit from alpha biofeedback training.

Glueck and Stroebel (1975) failed to find any clinical utility in alpha training for a psychiatric population. There have been some marginal reports but no meaningful data on attempts to treat alcoholism and drug abuse with alpha biofeedback. It could be that since the production of occipital alpha through biofeedback training seems to involve primarily an oculomotor strategy of "not looking" (Plotkin, 1976), there is little reason to expect it to help.

One ambitious attempt to use alpha biofeedback was a study on the treatment of chronic, continuous, unremitting pain by Melzack and Perry (1975). One group of patients received alpha biofeedback training, a second received hypnotic training, and the third a combination of the two. Only the group receiving the combination treatment (which was confounded, since the patients also received 50% more treatment sessions) showed any significant effect: a reduction within the treatment session only of the self-report of pain. Moreover, there were no comparisons of the changes in this group with changes in the other two groups, so we are left not knowing if there was a truly reliable result.

At this point, there are no good data to support the clinical treatment of any medical or psychological problem with alpha biofeedback. Perhaps later, research will show some utility.

ASTHMA

There have been several anecdotal reports and systematic case studies reporting slight improvement in some asthmatics treated by systems designed to measure and give feedback of changes in airway resistance (Feldman, 1976; Levenson, Manuck, Strupp, Blackwood, & Snell, 1974; Vachon & Rich, 1976). As yet, no controlled work has appeared on this methodology.

It has been known for some time that relaxation training can help asthmatics to have fewer attacks and manage their disease better overall (Alexander, 1972). Kotses and his associates (Kotses, Glaus, Crawford, Edwards, & Scherr, 1976) have successfully demonstrated that frontal EMG feedback training as a relaxation technique can have a similar beneficial effect.

In a controlled-group outcome study with asthmatic children, Davis, Saunders, Creer, and Chai (1973) assigned subjects to receive (1) frontal EMG biofeedback training and progressive relaxation training; (2) relaxation training alone; and (3) instructions to relax but no formal training. The results indicated that for mild asthmatics, the EMG feedback-assisted relaxation produced significantly greater reductions in airway resistance than for those in the control group (Group 3). Those receiving relaxation training alone showed some improvement but less than for Group 1. For the more severe asthmatics, neither treatment led to any change over that shown by the control subjects. Moreover, at a one-week follow-up, the advantage initially shown by the EMG-assisted relaxation group had disappeared.

Comment

Although the data suggest that frontal EMG-assisted relaxation may be more efficacious than straight progressive relaxation training, definitive conclusions must await more research. This does seem to be a promising area, however. Moreover, since frontal EMG as typically monitored reflects the muscle tension of the whole head, it may be that some direct relaxation of musculature involved in the airway is taking place.

FECAL INCONTINENCE

The last disorder for which the Biofeedback Society of America claims demonstrated efficacy is chronic fecal incontinence. Engel, Nikoomanesh, and Schuster (1974) reported on seven cases of this very socially debilitating disorder treated with brief biofeedback therapy. All patients had been regularly incontinent for several years. Through the use of an elaborate pressure transducer, the patients were taught to control and synchronize the internal and external anal sphincters. The external sphincter is a striate muscle normally under voluntary control.

Of the six patients who completed treatment, four were completely continent and the other two were much improved at follow-ups ranging from six months to five years. More recently, Cerulli, Nikoomanesh, and Schuster (1976) have reported on 40 cases of chronic fecal incontinence treated with this procedure. The results showed 28 cases as markedly improved.

Although no controlled-outcome studies have been done, as in the work on neuromuscular reeducation, the relatively long baselines and repeated failures of patients to respond to standard medical therapies give strong evidence of the efficacy of this procedure for this disorder.

OTHER DISORDERS

There have been scattered reports of the treatment of several other psychophysiological disorders with biofeedback, which I mention briefly here. In each instance, the work is at a very preliminary stage.

There have been several reports about demonstrating that feedback of stomach acid pH could lead to some reliable changes (Blanchard & Epstein, 1978; Welgan, 1974; Whitehead, Renault, & Goldiamond, 1975). However, as Blanchard and Epstein (1978) pointed out, the therapy is so noxious that it seems to have little practical value for ulcer patients.

Beaty (1976), working with patients with peptic ulcers, was able to show some benefit from relaxation training based on frontal EMG feedback. Furman (1973) reported good initial results in treating spastic colon or irritable bowel syndrome with feedback of bowel sounds. However, Weinstock (1976) failed to replicate these results.

There have been isolated reports of the value of biofeedback in treating hyperhidrosis (excessive sweating) (Rickles, 1978) and dermatitis (Haynes, 1976). There have also been reports of the value of biofeedback in treating dysmenorrhea (Tubbs & Carnahan, 1976). In another genetourinary disorder, Csillag (1976) has reported on the value of penile circumference biofeedback in treating impotent males.

CONCLUSIONS AND FUTURE DIRECTIONS

Biofeedback as a therapeutic modality and a field of research has become fairly well established during its brief lifetime of less than 20 years. The Biofeedback Society of America has, in its 10-year history, progressed from a small interest group to a professional society with over 1,200 members. It publishes its own journal, *Biofeedback and Self-Regulation.*

A major question that needs to be asked is, Does biofeedback have a future? Silver and Blanchard (1978), in a recent review, compared biofeedback and various forms of relaxation training across the whole spectrum of psychophysiological disorders and found "whenever direct comparisons have been made of biofeedback training and relaxation training, there is no consistent advantage for one form of treatment over the other." Thus, despite its alleged specificity in treating a variety of disorders, no advantage can be found in the psychophysiological disorders for biofeedback over the more generalized treatment of relaxation training.

There are, of course, areas where such comparisons have not been made and in fact make no sense: neuromuscular reeducation, treatment of epilepsy through alternating of EEG power spectrum, and treatment of fecal incontinence. In these areas, the specificity of biofeedback may prove to be of long-term utility. Certainly, in the two areas related to skeletal muscle regulation, biofeedback seems a useful adjunct.

Does the above analysis mean that there is no future for specific psychological treatment of medical disorders? Far from it. Biofeedback has led the way in showing that there are viable nonpharmacological and nonsurgical treatments for many traditional "medical" problems. It if proves to be the case that relaxation, generally construed, is the key therapeutic ingredient in most successful treatments, then we need to emphasize it. Moreover, we need more research to investigate its mode of action and to optimize its application. In this way, *behavoiral* approaches to medical problems can be given their due.

A final point concerns the place of biofeedback and relaxation training in the new "stress management" therapies described by Holroyd in this volume. It may be that some judicious mixture of relaxation and biofeedback along with some cognitive approaches may be the more practical and efficacious approach to the myriad of psychophysiological or stress-related disorders in today's medical practice. Perhaps, through an emphasis on primary prevention through relaxation training and self-management skills, we can have a healthier tomorrow. Only time and future research will tell.

SUMMARY

This chapter provides a summarization and critique of several problem areas in which biofeedback treatment has been reported. As noted in the introduction to the chapter, the strength of the conclusions one may draw about the efficacy of a biofeedback treatment for a particular disorder is dependent in part on the levels of the experimental design used in studies of the disorder.

The disorders reviewed can be roughly divided into two groups: (1) those for which biofeedback seems to have some demonstrated efficacy independent of relaxation aspects and (2) those for which comparisons of biofeedback and some form of relaxation training tend to show equal efficacy. Very brief summaries of the state of the art with the disorders reviewed follow.

For the problems of chronic fecal incontinence and epilepsy involving motor seizures, biofeedback has been shown to have real efficacy. As an adjunct to standard physical therapy, biofeedback seems to aid neuromuscular reeducation. Finally, there is promising but inconclusive evidence that biofeedback can be useful in problems of cardiac arrhythmia.

For muscle contraction headaches, migraine headaches, and Raynaud's disease, controlled studies have shown that biofeedback and relaxation training of various sorts are equally efficacious. In essential hypertension, there is a lack of consistent positive results for biofeedback treatment. Relaxation training seems to provide more consistent results.

In two other areas, asthma and myofacial pain, there is demonstrated efficacy in controlled studies for both biofeedback and relaxation training, but the two have not yet been compared in the same study.

In the end, some judicious combination of biofeedback, relaxation training, and cognitive therapy may provide a nonpharmacological alternative for many of today's stress-induced disorders.

REFERENCES

Alexander, A. B. Systematic relaxation and flow rates in asthmatic children: Relationship to emotional precipitants and anxiety. *Journal of Psychosomatic Research*, 1972, *16*, 405–410.

Andrews, J. M. Neuromuscular re-education of the hemiplegic with the aid of the electromograph. *Archives of Physical Medicine and Rehabilitation*, 1964, *45*, 530–532.

Andreychuk, T., & Skriver, C. Hypnosis and biofeedback in the treatment of migraine headache. *International Journal of Clinical and Experimental Hypnosis*, 1975, *23*, 172–183.

Bakal, D. A. Headache: A biopsychological perspective. *Psychological Bulletin*, 1975, *82*, 369–382.

Basmajian, J. V., Kukulka, C. G., Narajan, M. G., & Takebe, K. Biofeedback treatment of foot-drop compared with standard rehabilitation technique: Effects on voluntary control and strength. *Archives of Physical Medicine and Rehabilitation*, 1975, *56*, 231–236.

Beaty, E. T. Feedback-assisted relaxation training as a treatment for gastric ulcers. Paper presented at Seventh Annual Meeting of Biofeedback Research Society, Colorado Springs, Colo., 1976.

Benson, H. *The relaxation response*. New York: William Morrow, 1975.

Benson, H., Shapiro, D., Tursky, B., & Schwartz, G. E. Decreased systolic blood pressure through operant conditioning techniques in patients with essential hypertension. *Science*, 1971, *173*, 740–742.

Birk, L. (Ed.). *Biofeedback: Behavioral medicine*. New York: Grune & Stratton, 1973.

Blanchard, E. B. Behavioral medicine: A Perspective. In R. Williams & W. D. Gentry (Eds.), *Behavioral approaches to medical practice*. Cambridge, Mass.: Ballinger, 1977.

Blanchard, E. B., & Abel, G. G. An experimental case study of the biofeedback treatment of a rape-induced psychophysiological cardiovascular disorder. *Behavior Therapy*, 1976, *7*, 113–119.

Blanchard, E. B., & Epstein, L. H. Clinical applications of biofeedback. In M. Hersen, R. M. Eisler, & P. M. Miller (Eds.), *Progress in behavior modification*, Vol. 4. New York: Academic Press, 1977.

Blanchard, E. B., & Epstein, L. H. *A biofeedback primer*. Reading, Mass: Addison-Wesley, 1978.

Blanchard, E. B., & Haynes, M. R. Biofeedback treatment of a case of Raynaud's Disease. *Journal of Behavior Therapy and Experimental Psychiatry*, 1975, *6*, 230–234.

Blanchard, E. B., & Young, L. D. Clinical application of biofeedback training: A review of evidence. *Archives of General Psychiatry*, 1974, *30*, 573–589.

Blanchard, E. B., Young, L. D., & Haynes, M. R. A simple feedback system for the treatment of elevated blood pressure. *Behavior Therapy*, 1975, *6*, 241–245.

Blanchard, E. B., Miller, S. T., Abel, G. G., Haynes, M. R., & Wicker, R. The failure of blood pressure feedback in treating hypertension. Paper presented to meeting of AABT, Atlanta, Ga., Dec. 1977.

Blanchard, E. B., Theobald, D. E., Williamson, D. A., Silver, B. V., & Brown, D. A. Temperature biofeedback in the treatment of migraine headaches. *Archives of General Psychiatry*, 1978, *35*, 581–588.

Brown, B. B. *New mind, new body*. New York: Harper & Row, 1974.

Brudny, J., Korein, J., Grynbaum, B. B., Friedmann, L. W., Weinstein, S., Sachs-Frankel, G., & Belandres, P. V. EMG feedback therapy: Review of treatment of 114 patients. *Archives of Physical Medicine and Rehabilitation*, 1976, *57*, 55–61.

Budzynski, T., Stoyva, J., & Adler, C. Feedback-induced muscle relaxation: Application to tension headache. *Journal of Behavior Therapy and Experimental Psychiatry*, 1970, *1*, 205–211.

Budzynski, T. H., Stoyva, J. M., Adler, C. S., & Mullaney, D. J. EMG biofeedback and tension headache: A controlled outcome study. *Psychosomatic Medicine*, 1973, *6*, 509–514.

Butler, F. *Biofeedback: A survey of the literature*. New York: Plenum, 1978.

Carlsson, S. G., & Gale, E. N. Biofeedback in the treatment of long-term temporo-mandibular joint pain: An outcome study. *Biofeedback and Self-Regulation*, 1977, *2*, 161–172.

Cerulli, M., Nikoomanesh, P., & Schuster, M. M. Progress in biofeedback treatment of fecal incontinence. *Gastroenterology*, 1976, *70*, part Z, A-11/869.

Chesney, M. A., & Shelton, J. L. A comparison of muscle relaxation and electromyogram biofeedback treatments for muscle contraction headache. *Journal of Behavior Therapy and Experimental Psychiatry*, 1976, *7*, 221–225.

Cox, D. J., Freundlich, A., & Meyer, R. G. Differential effectiveness of electromyograph feedback, verbal relaxation instructions, and medication placebo with tension headaches. *Journal of Consulting and Clinical Psychology*, 1975, *43*, 892–899.

Csillag, E. R. Modification of penile erectile response. *Journal of Behavior Therapy and Experimental Psychiatry*, 1976, *7*, 27–30.

Dalessio, D. J. *Wolff's headache and other head pain*, 3rd ed. New York: Oxford University Press, 1972.

Davis, M. H., Saunders, D. R., Creer, T. L., & Chai, H. Relaxation training facilitated by biofeedback apparatus as a supplemental treatment in bronchial asthma. *Journal of Psychosomatic Research*, 1973, *17*, 121–128.

Diamond, S., & Franklin, M. Indications and contraindications for the use of biofeedback therapy in headache patients. Paper presented at the Biofeedback Research Society meeting, Colorado Springs, Colorado, February 1974.

Elder, S. T., & Eustis, N. K. Instrumental blood pressure conditioning in outpatient hypertensives. *Behaviour Research and Therapy*, 1975, *13*, 185–188.

Elder, S. T., Ruiz, Z. B., Deabler, H. L., & Dillenkoffer, R. L. Instrumental conditioning of diastolic blood pressure in essential hypertensive patients. *Journal of Applied Behavior Analysis*, 1973, *6*, 377–382.

Engel, B. T., & Bleecker, E. R. Application of operant conditioning techniques to the control of cardiac arrhythmias. In P. A. Obrist, A. H. Black, J. Brener, & L. V. DiCara (Eds.), *Cardiovascular psychophysiology*. Chicago: Aldine, 1974.

Engel, B. T., Nikoomanesh, P., & Schuster, M. M. Operant conditioning of rectosphincteric responses in the treatment of fecal incontinence. *New England Journal of Medicine*, 1974, *290*, 646–649.

Epstein, L. H., & Abel, G. G. An analysis of biofeedback training effects for tension headache patients. *Behavior Therapy*, 1977, *8*, 37–47.

Feldman, G. M. The effect of biofeedback training on respiratory resistance of asthmatic children. *Psychosomatic Medicine*, 1976, *38*, 27–34.

Feuerstein, M., & Adams, H. E. Cephalic vasomotor feedback in the modification of migraine headache. *Biofeedback and Self-Regulation*, 1977, *2*, 241–254.

Finley, W. W., Smith, H. A., & Etherton, M. D. Reduction of seizures and normalization of the EEG in a severe epileptic following sensorimotor biofeedback training. *Biological Psychology*, 1975, *2*, 195–209.

Friar, L. R., & Beatty, J. Migraine: Management by a trained control of vasoconstriction. *Journal of Consulting and Clinical Psychology*, 1976, *44*, 46–53.

Friedman, A. P. Headaches. In A. M. Freedman, H. I. Kaplan, & B. J. Sadock (Eds.), *Comprehensive textbook of psychiatry*, Vol. 2. Baltimore: Williams & Wilkins, 1975.

Furman, S. Intestinal biofeedback in functional diarrhea: A preliminary report. *Journal of Behavior Therapy and Experimental Psychiatry*, 1973, *4*, 317–321.

Gessel, A. H. Electromyographic biofeedback and tricyclic anti-depressants in myofascial pain-dysfunction syndrome: Psychological predictors of outcome. *Journal of American Dental Association*, 1975, *91*, 1048–1052.

Gessel, A. H., & Alderman, M. N. Management of myofascial pain dysfunction syndrome of the temporomandibular joints by tension control training. *Psychosomatics*, 1971, *12*, 302–309.

Glueck, B. C., & Stroebel, C. F. Biofeedback and meditation in the treatment of psychiatric illnesses. *Comprehensive Psychiatry*, 1975, *16*, 303–321.

Goldman, H., Kleinman, K. M., Snow, M. Y., Bidus, D. R., & Korol, B. Relationship between essential hypertension and cognitive functioning: Effects of biofeedback. *Psychophysiology*, 1975, *12*, 569–573.

Haynes, S. Personal communication, 1976.

Haynes, S. N., Griffin, P., Mooney, D., & Parise, M. Electromyographic biofeedback and relaxation instructions in the treatment of muscle contraction headaches. *Behavior Therapy*, 1975, *6*, 672–678.

Hutchings, D. F., & Reinking, R. H. Tension headaches: What form of therapy is most effective? *Biofeedback and Self-Regulation*, 1976, *1*, 183–190.

Johnson, H. E., & Garton, W. H. Muscle re-education in hemiplegia by use of EMG device. *Archives of Physical Medicine and Rehabilitation*, 1973, *54*, 320–325.

Kaplan, B. J. Biofeedback in epileptics: Equivocal relationship of reinforced EEG frequency to seizure reduction. *Epilepsia*, 1975, *16*, 477–485.

Kotses, H., Glaus, K. D., Crawford, P. L., Edwards, J. E., & Scherr, M. S. Operant reduction of frontalis EMG activity in the treatment of asthma in children. *Journal of Psychosomatic Research*, 1976, *20*, 453–459.

Kristt, D. A., & Engel, B. T. Learned control of blood pressure in patients with high blood pressure. *Circulation*, 1975, *51*, 370–378.

Levenson, R. W., Manuck, S. B., Strupp, H. H., Blackwood, G. L., & Snell, J. D. A biofeedback technique for bronchial asthma. Paper presented to meeting of Biofeedback Research Society, Colorado Springs, Feb., 1974.

Love, W. A., Montgomery, D. D., & Moeller, T. A. Working paper number 1. Unpublished manuscript. Nova University, Ft. Lauderdale, Fla., 1974.

Lubar, J. F., & Bahler, W. W. Behavioral management of epileptic seizures following EEG biofeedback training of the sensorimotor rhythm. *Biofeedback and Self-Regulation*, 1976, *1*, 77–104.

Melzack, R., & Perry, C. Self-regulation of pain: The use of alpha-feedback and hypnotic training for the control of chronic pain. *Experimental Neurology*, 1975, *46*, 452–469.

Miller, N. E. Postscript. In D. Singh & C. T. Morgan (Eds.), *Current status of physiological psychology: Readings*. Monterey, Calif.: Brooks-Cole, 1972.

Miller, N. E. Clinical applications of biofeedback: Voluntary control of heart rate, rhythm, and blood pressure. In H. I. Russek (Ed.), *New horizons in cardiovascular practice*. Baltimore: University Park Press, 1975.

Miller, N. E. Biofeedback and visceral learning. In *Annual Review of Psychology*, Vol. 29. Palo Alto, Calif.: Annual Reviews, 1978.

Moeller, T. A., & Love, W. A. A method to reduce aterial hypertension through muscular relaxation. Unpublished manuscript. Nova University, Ft. Lauderdale, Fla., 1974.

Orne, M. T. Address to Biofeedback Society of America, Albuquerque, N.M., March 1978.

Patel, C. H. Yoga and biofeedback in the management of hypertension. *Lancet*, 1973, *2*, 1053–1055.

Patel, C. H. 12-Month follow-up of yoga and biofeedback in the management of hypertension. *Lancet*, 1975, *1*, 62–67.

Patel, C. H., & North, W. R. S. Randomized controlled trial of yoga and biofeedback in management of hypertension. *Lancet*, 1975, *2*, 93–99.

Pickering, T., & Gorham, G. Learned heart-rate controlled by a patient with a ventricular parasystolic rhythm. *Lancet*, February 1, 1975, 252–253.

Pickering, T. G., & Miller, N. E. Learned voluntary control of heart rate and rhythm in two subjects with premature ventricular contractions. *British Heart Journal*, 1977, *39*, 152–159.

Phillips, C. The modification of tension headache pain using EMG biofeedback. *Behaviour Research and Therapy*, 1977, *15*, 119–129.

Plotkin, W. B. On the self-regulation of the occipital alpha rhythm: Control strategies, states of consciousness, and the role of physiological feedback. *Journal of Experimental Psychology: General*, 1976, *105*, 66–69.

Reinking, R. Follow-up and extension of "Tension headaches: What method is most effective?" Paper presented at the meeting of the Biofeedback Research Society, Colorado Springs, Colo., February 1976. (Abstract.)

Rickles, W. H. Treatment of a case of hyperhydrosis with vapor pressure feedback. In *Proceedings of the Biofeedback Society of America Ninth Annual Meeting*. Denver: Biofeedback Society of America, 1978, pp. 92–94.

Sargent, J. D., Green, E. E., & Walters, E. D. The use of autogenic feedback training in a pilot study of migraine and tension headaches. *Headache*, 1972, *12*, 120–125.

Sargent, J. D., Green, E. E., & Walters, E. D. Preliminary report on the use of autogenic feedback training in the treatment of migraine and tension headaches. *Psychosomatic Medicine*, 1973, *35*, 129–135.

Schwartz, G. E. Clinical applications of biofeedback: Some theoretical issues. In D. Upper & D. S. Goodenough (Eds.), *Behavior modification with the individual patient: Proceedings of third annual Brockton symposium on behavior therapy*. Nutley, N.J.: Roche, 1972.

Schwartz, G. E., & Shapiro, D. Biofeedback and essential hypertension: Current findings and theoretical concerns. In L. Birk (Ed.), *Biofeedback: Behavioral medicine*. New York: Grune & Stratton, 1973.

Scott, R. W., Blanchard, E. B., Edmundson, E. D., & Young, L. D. A shaping procedure for heart-rate control in chronic tachycardia. *Perceptual and Motor Skills*, 1973, *37*, 327–338.

Shapiro, D., Tursky, B., Gershon, E., & Stern, M. Effects of feedback and reinforcement on control of human systolic blood pressure. *Science*, 1969, *163*, 588–590.

Silver, B. V., & Blanchard, E. B. Biofeedback and relaxation training in the treatment of psychophysiological disorders: Or, are the machines really necessary? *Journal of Behavioral Medicine*, 1978, *1*, 217–239.

Solbach, P., & Sargent, J. D. A follow-up evaluation of the Menninger pilot migraine study using thermal training. *Headache*, 1977, *17*, 198–202.

Sterman, M. B. Neurophysiological and clinical studies of sensorimotor EEG biofeedback training: Some effects on epilepsey. In L. Birk (Ed.), *Biofeedback: Behavioral medicine*. New York: Grune & Stratton, 1973.

Sterman, M. B., & Friar, L. Suppression of seizures in an epileptic following sensorimotor EEG feedback training. *Electroencephalography and Clinical Neurophysiology*, 1972, *33*, 89–95.

Strobel, C. F., & Glueck, B. C. Biofeedback treatment in medicine and psychiatry: An ultimate placebo? In L. Birk (Ed.), *Biofeedback: Behavioral medicine*. New York: Grune & Stratton, 1973.

Surwit, R. S., Pilon, R. N., & Fenton, C. H. Behavioral treatment of Raynaud's disease. *Journal of Behavioral Medicine*, 1978, *1*, 323–335.

Surwit, R. S., Shapiro, D., & Good, I. M. Comparison of cardiovascular biofeedback, neuromuscular biofeedback and meditation in the treatment of borderline essential hypertension. *Journal of Consulting and Clinical Psychology*, 1978, *46*, 252–263.

Tubbs, W., & Carnahan, C. Clinical biofeedback for primary dysmenorrhea: A pilot study. Paper presented at the meeting of the Biofeedback Research Society, Colorado Springs, Colo., Feb. 1976.

Turin, A., & Johnson, W. G. Biofeedback therapy for migraine headaches. *Archives of General Psychiatry*, 1976, *33*, 517–519.

Tursky, B., Shapiro, D., & Schwartz, G. E. Automated constant cuff-pressure system to measure average systolic and diastolic blood pressure in man. *IEEE Transactions in Bio-Medical Engineering*, 1972, *19*, 271–276.

Vachon, L., & Rich, E. S. Visceral learning in asthma. *Psychosomatic Medicine*, 1976, *38*, 122–130.

Weinstock, S. A. The reestablishment of intestinal control in functional colitis. Paper presented at the meeting of the Biofeedback Research Society, Colorado Springs, Colo., Feb. 1976.

Weiss, T., & Engel, B. T. Operant conditioning of heart rate in patients with premature ventricular contractions. *Psychosomatic Medicine*, 1971, *33*, 301–321.

Welgan, P. R. Learned control of gastric acid secretions in ulcer patients. *Psychosomatic Medicine*, 1974, *36*, 411–419.

Whitehead, W. E., Renault, P. F., & Goldiamond, I. Modification of human gastric acid secretion with operant-conditioning procedures. *Journal of Applied Behavior Analysis*, 1975, *8*, 147–156.

Wickramasekera, I. Electromyographic feedback training and tension headache: Preliminary observations. *American Journal of Clinical Hypnosis*, 1972, *15*, 83–85.

7

Interactions between Drugs and Behavior Therapy

WILLIAM E. WHITEHEAD AND BARRY BLACKWELL

DRUGS VERSUS BEHAVIOR THERAPY: DEFINING THE PROBLEM

Both chemotherapy and behavior therapy are powerful technologies for treating behavioral disorders. Drug therapy, which was the first of these two to gain widespread application, revolutionized the treatment of the major psychoses. Major tranquilizers permit most psychotic patients to be cared for in their communities, and drugs make possible a much more humane treatment of hospitalized psychotic patients than was formerly possible. Psychotropic drugs have also contributed to the management of anxiety and depression in nonpsychotic patients.

Behavior therapy has also altered the pattern of mental health care delivery on a large scale. Behavioral approaches to the treatment of phobias and obsessive-compulsive disorders are regarded as superior to any alternative treatments available (Marks, 1975), and behavior therapy has contributed greatly to the treatment of hyperkinesis, eating disorders, and psychosomatic disorders. Behavioral strategies for treating other varieties of neurotic, depressed, and socially inadequate individuals are also gaining widespread acceptance.

In view of the fact that they are both powerful technologies for changing behavior, it is surprising that so few attempts have been made to study interactions between drug therapy and behavior therapy. They tend more often to be regarded as rival therapies, as illustrated by the following studies.

Rush, Beck, Kovacs,' and Hollon (1977) compared the efficacy of cognitive behavior therapy to imipramine in the treatment of chronically depressed outpatients, but these investigators did not include any groups that received both treat-

WILLIAM E. WHITEHEAD • Psychophysiology Laboratory, Departments of Psychiatry and Physical Medicine and Rehabilitation, University of Cincinnati, Cincinnati, Ohio 45267.   BARRY BLACK-WELL • Department of Psychiatry, Wright State University School of Medicine, Dayton, Ohio 45324.

ments. The results rather uniformly favored cognitive behavior therapy. Cognitive behavior therapy resulted in greater improvement on both self-rating and clinician ratings of depression, and the dropout rate was greater for pharmacotherapy.

Similarly, Solyom, Heseltine, McClure, Solyom, Ledwidge, and Steinberg (1973) compared several behavior therapies—aversion relief, systematic desensitization, and flooding—to treatment with phenelzine plus brief psychotherapy and to placebo plus brief psychotherapy in the treatment of phobias. No combinations of drug and behavior therapy were included. By the end of treatment, the behavior therapies and the phenelzine group were about equally effective, and all were superior to placebo plus brief psychotherapy. However, at two-year follow-up, the relapse rate was not over 10% for any of the behavior therapies, whereas all six patients treated with phenelzine who stopped the drug relapsed. The authors noted that the phenelzine group showed a more rapid improvement during treatment and suggested that phenelzine plus behavior therapy might be superior to either alone.

The results of these two studies are very gratifying to behavior therapists, but they fall short of providing the clinician with an adequate guide because it is obvious that combined treatment is almost as easy to provide as behavior therapy alone. In both cases, pharmacotherapy had some beneficial effects on the disordered behavior; it is possible that the effects of the two may be additive. Alternatively, the combination of drugs with behavior therapy may impair its effectiveness, and the clinician needs to know that as well.

Davison and Valins (1968) have in fact suggested that drug therapy may impair the effectiveness of psychotherapy or behavior therapy by causing the patient to attribute behavior change to an external agency, the drug. However, no negative interaction was observed in two studies that investigated attribution effects. Wilson and Thomas (1973) found that systematic desensitization worked equally well in snake-fearful college students whether the instructions attributed relaxation to the behavioral procedures or to a placebo pill. Johnston and Gath (1973) manipulated attribution to drug or to flooding procedures independently of whether diazepam or placebo was actually given. They concluded that diazepam enhanced the effectiveness of flooding in phobic patients independently of whether patients were instructed to attibute the improvement to a drug or not. Thus, the attribution of behavior change to a drug does not appear to significantly impair the effectiveness of behavior therapy.

At the preclinical level, there have been many attempts to study the interactions of behavioral and pharmacological techniques, but the interest has usually been in using drugs to understand behavior or in using behavioral probes to investigate drug action. For example, Weiss and Engel (1971) used anticholinergic and antiadrenergic drugs to study the mechanism by which their subjects controlled heart rate following biofeedback training and the mechanisms by which cardiac arrhythmias were produced. Cook and Davidson (1973, 1978) described behavioral tests that they used to screen new psychoactive compounds in animals and suggested that these animal behavioral tests permitted rather precise estimates of the probable clinical efficacy of these compounds. The growing number of books on behavioral pharmacology (e.g., Iversen & Iversen, 1975; Thompson & Pickens, 1971; Thompson & Schuster, 1968) also focus on the use of behavioral technologies to understand pharmacological mechanisms. Thus, there have been many preclinical investigations that have included both behavioral and pharmacological manipulations, but there have been few serious efforts to apply combinations of these two approaches to clinical problems apart from their use in aversion therapy.

One is tempted to attribute this situation to philosophical differences between the practioners of behavior therapy and of drug therapy. Clearly, there are such differences. Drug therapy is based on the implicit assumption that the most important determinants of behavior are biochemical events occurring inside the brain, whereas behavior modification is based on the explicit assumption that the critical determinants of behavior are environmental events occurring outside the skin. The philosophical gulf between these points of view may seem difficult to bridge, but, in fact, animal psychopharmacologists have been doing so successfully for many years.

The fundamental cause for segregation of drug therapy from behavior therapy is grounded in differences of professional backgrounds. Since the time of Flexner, traditional medical training has emphasized the classification of illnesses into categories, with emphasis on their biological causes. This classification has led, naturally, to the view that particular diseases should be treated with specific medical remedies. This reductionistic viewpoint has focused chiefly on diagnoses and syndromes rather than on discrete behaviors, with the consequent widespread use of drugs and the relative neglect of alternative strategies. The availability of powerful psychotropic drugs from the mid-1950s on contributed to this line of development.

The advent of psychological and social perspectives on illness susceptibility and the development of effective psychosocial treatment techniques are now resulting in a reappraisal of the shortcomings of a rigid biomedical model. George Engel (1977) has recently made the case for an expanded biopsychosocial model applicable to all disease.

In the field of mental illness, learning theory and its associated techniques for modifying behavior have also provided an impetus for reexamination of the older disease–drug model. Lasagna (1978) has reviewed the problems of attempting to match individual psychotropic drugs to a procrustean bed of disease nomenclature that itself dates from the early part of the century. In a previous review (Blackwell & Whitehead, 1975), we examined this issue with specific regard to the evaluation of antianxiety drugs, and we drew attention to the anomalous fact that psychotropic drugs were selected on the basis of specific behavioral end points in animals but were often evaluated in man and prescribed to patients for global and imprecise reasons.

Kornetsky and Markowitz (1978) recently reviewed the data on a variety of animal models used to predict the activity of drugs that are effective in the management of schizophrenia. A number of these models are derived directly from learning theory (Cook & Davidson, 1978). As might be expected, the closest attention to the relationship between behavior and drug action has been in the case of drug abuse, where the self-administration of drugs can be readily and appropriately interpreted in terms of reinforcement contingencies and where the bridge between animal experiments and human behavior is most credible (Woods, 1978). Finally, Seligman and Groves (1970) developed the model of "learned helplessness" in dogs and have made interesting extrapolations to depression and its drug treatment in humans.

Some years ago, Irwin (1968) proposed a rational framework for the development, evaluation, and use of psychotropic drugs based on their effects on observed behaviors rather than on classificatory labels. The fact that these suggestions failed to germinate may be related to both premature timing and lack of practical, clinical methodology. Since then, the rapid development of behavioral analysis, treatment, and evaluation techniques has created at least the tools for reassessing this problem.

That this remains to be done may be partly because of the divisive fact that learning theory and behavior therapy are viewed as the domain of the psychologist, while the right to prescribe drugs remains the unique prerogative of the psychiatrist. What clinical psychologist has not experienced a sense of frustration at having to refer a patient to a physician for medications in the midst of therapy, with the inevitable consequences of that move on the therapeutic alliance, and what psychiatrist can feel comfortable with the legal responsibility of prescribing medications to a patient whom he does not know on the recommendation of a psychologist who is not legally responsible for any adverse consequences? The issue is perpetuated because psychiatrists are rarely trained in behavior therapy techniques and tend, in the United States at least, to defer in the use of these techniques to psychologists, while psychologists receive little training in pharmacology.

One unfortunate result of the segregation of drug therapy and behavior therapy into rival professional groups is that combination therapies that may have advantages over either mode of therapy used alone are not available to the patient. These neglected possibilities are discussed futher below.

A more immediate problem is the very real possibility that, as a result of such professional differences, patients may receive inadequate or inappropriate treatment. For example, the drug treatment of schizophrenia, of certain categories of depression, and of mania is so well established that to withhold medications while treating these people behaviorally might be considered unethical. Similarly, the behavioral treatment of phobias and obsessive-compulsive disorders is so well established (e.g., Marks, 1975) that the treatment of these patients exclusively with paliative drugs would also be considered unethical by some.

The same kinds of dangers exist in the management of patients with psychophysiological disorders. For example, since the popularization of biofeedback, relaxation, and meditational techniques, patients with hypertension, peptic ulcer, and other disorders involving morbid pathophysiological processes have consulted unqualified practitioners of those techniques and requested these forms of treatment as a substitute for drug management of their symptoms. Often, biofeedback or relaxation techniques can be of real benefit to such patients, but there are obvious risks for the patient and the professional whom he consults (Blackwell, 1977). In some cases, the professional is being asked to substitute a treatment of unproven efficacy (such as biofeedback for hypertension) for a treatment of proven efficacy (drugs) in a disease that can be fatal. Such a professional may also be unprepared by his training to judge when, for example, blood pressure becomes high enough to make a stroke likely.

The opposite kind of risk also exists in the management of psychophysiological disorders. Patients with back pain or muscle dystonias such as torticollis are often operated on or treated exclusively with drugs when a trial of biofeedback treatment or other behavior modification procedures would clearly be indicated on the basis of the research literature. Also, a growing body of evidence (cf. Wooley, Blackwell, & Winget, 1978) indicates that some psychophysiological disorders are made worse by traditional patterns of medical management, which may involve the reinforcement of pathophysiological events. At best, strictly medical management of a psychophysiological disorder without attention to psychological determinants is often inadequate treatment.

The ideal solution to the problem we have tried to define above would involve training and licensing clinical psychologists to prescribe psychotropic drugs and training psychiatrists to do behavior therapy. In a time of scarce professional manpower, that solution might eventually be adopted, but, at present, economic pressures and professionalism appear more likely to result in a perpetuation of the current restrictions on prescribing privileges and of the limitation of training opportunities.

A more pragmatic approach to the problem is to demonstrate a need, if there is one, by research such as that reviewed below. If it can be shown that combinations of drugs and behavior therapy have advantages over either method of therapy used alone, people will find ways of providing both for their patients. It is possible for psychologists and physicians to collaborate on an equal footing—not on an employer–employee footing—as the authors have done for several years. Such collaboration has many advantages over going it alone because medical school and graduate school training differ in ways that are often complementary.

In the remainder of this chapter, we review the literature on interactions between drugs and behavior therapy. We propose that many, though not all, of the effects of psychotropic drugs may be conceptualized in terms familiar to learning theorists, such as *discriminative stimulus*, *reinforcing* or *aversive consequence*, and *potentiating variable*. These terms are defined in the next section. Conceptualizing the effects of drugs on behavior in this way not only helps to clarify the known interactions between drugs and behavior therapy but also suggests some new interactions that have not been investigated and that may have clinical value.

DEFINITIONS OF BEHAVIORAL TERMS

The terms of the behavioral schema that are used here to describe drug action are defined below. These are definitions derived from the operant and classical conditioning literature. They are related to one another as shown in Figures 1 and 2.

Discriminative stimuli, abbreviated S^D in Figure 1, are stimuli whose presence or absence influences the probability that behavior will occur. An example is a traffic light, which, when it is green, signals drivers to proceed but, when red, signals them to stop. Discriminative stimuli acquire the ability to influence the occurrence of behavior by a history of being consistently associated with differential reinforcement of the behavior. Thus, for example, green traffic lights have in the past signaled that not proceeding through an intersection will cause other drivers to beep and otherwise behave aggressively, whereas proceeding in the absence of a green light may be punished by a traffic ticket, an accident, or aggressive behavior on the part of other drivers. This history of differential reinforcement as signaled by the

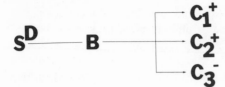

Figure 1. Operant conditioning paradigm. S^D = discriminative stimulus; B = behavior or response; C^+ = reinforcing consequence tending to increase subsequent response probability, C^- = punitive consequence tending to reduce subsequent response probability.

traffic light may continue to influence behavior even at 2:00 A.M., when the consequences are unlikely actually to be applied.

Of some importance to our analysis of drug action later on is the concept of stimulus fading. This term refers to the fact that one can shift control of behavior from one kind of discriminative stimulus to another, perhaps more subtle stimulus, as follows. Suppose that a disruptive elementary school student has been referred to a special education teacher, and she has taught him to sit still and attend to lessons for acceptable periods of time by rewarding him for longer and longer periods of quiet sitting. However, the behavior that is emitted alone with the special education teacher does not generalize to the crowded classroom with the regular teacher. We would begin the transfer of stimulus control by introducing the regular teacher into the situation in which the special education teacher controls the behavior and then in steps have the regular teacher take over the delivery of reinforcement. We might then introduce other children into the situation, a few at a time, and move the training session back to the regular classroom with the special education teacher still attending. We have now faded in the stimuli we want to control the behavior, so we begin to fade out the original discriminative stimulus—the special education teacher—in the same gradual way. It is possible that a few shortcuts could be made in this sequence, but the principle of transfer of stimulus control by means of fading stimuli in and out is illustrated by the example.

Behavior, abbreviated B in the diagram, is any arbitrarily defined piece of behavior that can be made publicly observable. Thus, proceeding through an intersection can be arbitrarily isolated from the sequence of behaviors involved in driving across town, so that the effects of applying differential consequences to this behavior can be studied.

Consequences, abbreviated C in the diagram, are any events that, when they are made to occur or are systematically postponed contingent on a behavior, alter the future probability of occurrence of the behavior. A positive consequence or reinforcer is any event that increases the probability of a behavior when it is presented contingent on the behavior, as when praise for doing well on a test increases the probability of studying. A negative consequence or punishment is any event that decreases the probability of a behavior that it follows, as when receiving a traffic ticket decreases the probability of driving faster than the speed limit. Consequences may also control behavior when their removal or postponement is made contingent on the behavior. Thus, loss of privileges (a positive consequence) is used to punish behavior in institutional settings, and escape from or avoidance of feelings of guilt or anxiety (negative consequences) reinforce handwashing in the compulsive patient.

In Figure 1, behavior is shown as being maintained by three different consequences, two of which are positive and one of which is negative. This relationship is intended to convey that naturally occurring human behaviors are likely to be influenced by multiple consequences that may exert conflicting potential influences. The probability that the behavior will recur (or that its frequency or intensity will be altered) reflects the algebraic sum of these differing influences. (Perhaps a more accurate metaphor might be to represent the effects of a complex reinforcement history on behavior in terms of vector addition, but usually we do not know enough about the reinforcement history to assign relative weights to the different consequences.)

Potentiating variables are any factors that influence the potency of positive and negative consequences independently of the schedule of reinforcement, such as depriving an animal of food to make food a more potent reinforcer or reducing stimulus input to make novelty a more effective reinforcer. Manipulations in the other direction are also possible. One can feed an animal to satiety to decrease the likelihood of his working for food, and one can administer an analgesic to decrease the effect of pain on behavior.

Pavlovian *conditional stimuli*, abbreviated CS in Figure 2, are similar to the Skinnerian notion of discriminative stimuli. A conditional stimulus is a biologically neutral stimulus that acquires the ability to elicit some behavior by a process of classical conditioning. The conditional stimulus is paired with some unconditional stimulus (US in Figure 2), which produces a reflex response (UR in Figure 2). After several such pairings, the conditional stimulus presented by itself will elicit the conditional reflex response (CR in Figure 2). An example of a conditional stimulus is the word *lemon*, which causes an increase in salivation in many people because in the past it has been repeatedly paired with the taste of lemon, which elicits reflex salivation.

Conditional stimuli differ from discriminative stimuli in the way in which they come to control responding. Discriminative stimuli are stimuli in the presence of which certain behaviors have been differentially reinforced or punished in the sense in which these terms are meant in operant conditioning. Conditional stimuli have acquired their ability to control responding by being paired consistently with other potent stimuli that elicit reflex responses. No response need even occur so long as the temporal relationship between the conditional stimulus and an unconditional stimulus like the lemon is preserved. Another difference is that, as a general rule, discriminative stimuli control overt skeletal muscle responses, whereas Pavlovian conditional stimuli control visceral or affective responses. There are, however, exceptions to this generalization.

Pavlovian *unconditional stimuli* are stimuli that have the ability to elicit reflexively some response as described above. They are most comparable to conse-

CONDITIONING TRIAL

CS + US ➡ UR

Figure 2. Classical conditioning paradigm. CS = conditional stimulus; US = unconditional stimulus; UR = unconditioned (reflex) response; CR = conditioned response.

TEST TRIAL

CS ➡ CR

quences in the operant learning model, except that they strengthen responses that they precede rather than responses that they follow. Also, the relationship between the unconditional stimulus and the response is biologically determined and invariable, whereas the operant consequence can be used to strengthen any arbitrary response. For example, money could not serve as an effective unconditioned stimulus to elicit reflex salivation, although money could serve as an operant reinforcer to increase the probability of salivation if it were systematically given immediately following any occurrences of salivation.

Rescorla and Solomon (1967) and Trapold (1971), among others, have argued that classical conditioning should be regarded as the conditioning of a motivational state rather than as the conditioning of a specific response. When a stimulus that has been previously paired with electric shock is superimposed on an operant shock avoidance schedule, the rate of responding increases, whereas a stimulus previously used as a safety signal to indicate that shock will not occur decreases the rate of avoidance responding when it is superimposed on an operant avoidance schedule. Thinking of classical conditioning as the conditioning of motivational states is a useful way of conceptualizing the use of drugs in aversion therapy.

DRUGS AS DISCRIMINATIVE STIMULI

There have been a number of experiments, primarily in animals, showing that drug-produced sensations may serve as discriminative stimuli. Drug-produced stimuli show remarkable similarities to exteroceptive stimuli such as lights and sounds in terms of the way they affect behavior, as described below.

Interest in the stimulus properties of drugs stems largely from the dramatic phenomenon called *state-dependent learning* (Overton, 1968). *State-dependent learning* refers to the fact that behaviors that are learned in a drugged state may be forgotten in the drug-free state but may recur when the subject is again drugged. *State-dependent learning* is obviously a misnomer, since the same learning could occur under either drugged or drug-free conditions; it is state-dependent performance that is being discussed, and that is the term that we will use.

The usual way of demonstrating state-dependent performance is in an experiment in which one group of subjects learns under drug and is tested under drug, a second group learns under drug and is tested without drug, a third group learns while drug-free and is tested while drug-free, and a fourth group learns while drug-free and is tested while drugged. The hypothesis of state-dependent performance is confirmed if performance is superior when training and testing are done under the same conditions (drug to drug and drug-free to drug-free) compared to the groups in which training is done under different conditions from testing (drug to drug-free and drug-free to drug).

This phenomenon is illustrated in an experiment by Goodwin, Powell, Bremer, Haine, and Stern (1969) in which medical students served as subjects, and in which the drugged state was produced by ingestion of 8–10 ounces of 80-proof vodka one hour prior to experimental sessions. The drug-free state was produced by ingesting soft drink before the session. Learning tasks included avoidance of a noxious tone, a word association task, a rote learning task, and picture recognition. Training and testing for recall occurred on consecutive days. Recall was significantly better when tested under training conditions compared to tests done under different conditions for the first three tasks, thus supporting the state-dependent performance hypothesis.

A similar study showing that state-dependent performance effects may also occur with marijuana intoxication was reported by Hill, Schwin, Powell, and Goodwin (1973). These investigators trained their subjects on a visual avoidance task, a word association task, and recall of sequences of words and objects. Subjects were experienced marijuana users. A state-dependency effect was reported for the rote learning task and for recall of the ordered series of objects. The other tasks showed no state-dependent effect. There are also reports of state-dependent effects for amobarbital and methylphenidate. These and other studies of state-dependent performance in humans, including some which yielded negative results, have been reviewed by Altman, Albert, Milstein, and Greenberg (1977).

Anecdotal reports have attributed a great deal of importance to state-dependent performance. There are references to dissociated states of consciousness produced by alcohol, marijuana, and several drugs with abuse potential. State-dependent performance is used to account for belligerence and other socially inappropriate behaviors as well as amnesia for events during a drugged state. Ross and Schwartz (1974) argued that the state-dependent performance phenomena contribute to the process of becoming addicted because drugs that produce state-dependent performance are frequently abused (Overton, 1973). Overton (1968) has suggested that because of this phenomenon, behavior change learned during psychotherapy may not be well maintained if the psychotherapy has been combined with drug therapy.

The phenomena of state-dependent performance have often been attributed to the dissociated states of consciousness that are produced by the drug. It is argued that there is little transfer of learning between different drug states. However, this explanation does not take into account that there is excellent transfer of some types of learning from the drug-free to the drugged state—the subject does not forget how to walk or talk, for example. The lack of transfer is limited to new learning, and there is usually poorer transfer from the drugged to the undrugged state than vice versa. Moreover, once state-dependent performance is established, one can decrease the dose in steps and demonstrate what amounts to a generalization gradient. Therefore, it is more parsimonious to explain state-dependent performance as an instance of the stimulus control of behavior by drug-produced cues than as an instance of how different states of consciousness are independent of one another.

Experiments that are used to study discriminative stimulus properties of drugs employ a different experimental design than those based on the state-dependent performance hypothesis. As in studies of stimulus control by external stimuli (tones and lights), some arbitrary response is reinforced following injection of the drug and not reinforced following placebo injections. Following multiple trials of both kinds, the subject is tested under extinction conditions, and the drug dose may be varied to examine stimulus generalization.

An example of the kind of experiment used to study stimulus control by drugs is the study by Overton (1971) in which rats were reinforced by escape from shock in a

T maze. The correct choice depended on whether the session had been preceded by an injection of pentobarbital or placebo. Drug and placebo alternated on successive days. The outcome measure was the proportion of animals making the correct choice on the first trial of a session. (If the rat cannot distinguish drug from placebo, it tends always to make errors on the first trial because it always emits the response that was reinforced on the previous day.) In the experiment being described, Overton compared the discriminability of four different doses of pentobarbital (5, 10, 15, and 20 mg/kg) from placebo, using a different group of subjects for each dose.

Several aspects of this experiment are worth noting. First, all doses of pentobarbital except 5 mg/kg were reliably differentiated from placebo after less than 16 training sessions, and high doses were associated with significantly earlier differential control than low doses, indicating that high doses are easier to differentiate than low doses. In other studies, Overton showed that stimulus control of T-maze behavior is acquired more rapidly by 15 mg/kg pentobarbital versus placebo than by light stimuli (7-W light versus 150-W light).

A partial listing of drugs that produce discriminative stimulus control and an estimate of their relative efficacy is given in Table 1, which is taken from Overton (1971). The class of drugs that produces the most rapid stimulus control is the group of anesthetic drugs that at preanesthetic doses function as sedative tranquilizers. Ethyl alcohol is included in this group. It is interesting to note that the major tranquilizers that have potent CNS effects are at best weak discriminative stimuli. Also, there is an apparent correlation between the abuse potential of drugs and their potency as discriminative stimuli. This correlation has not been adequately explained.

Overton (1971) noted that although different doses of the same drug can be discriminated, there is a common stimulus dimension involved in each of the stimulus classes in Table 1. Thus, one can find doses of pentobarbital and ethyl alcohol that are not distinguishable from each other, although both are reliably distinguished from placebo. However, this stimulus equivalence is not observed between drug classes in Table 1. Thus, pentobarbital and atropine are easily distinguished at all doses that can be discriminated from placebo. Lal (1976) noted that aspirin has conditional discriminability; it is difficult to discriminate from placebo for normal subjects but is readily discriminated by arthritic subjects.

To summarize the foregoing discussion of the discriminative stimulus properties of drugs, it is apparent that drug-produced cues can serve as discriminative stimuli controlling behavior, that they have many of the formal characteristics of exteroceptive stimuli, and that drug-produced cues are relatively potent stimuli compared to exteroceptive stimuli. This discussion suggests that state-dependent performance is an instance of the discriminative stimulus properties of drugs.

It has been suggested that stimulus control accounts for some of the differences between the intoxicated and the drug-free states for alcohol, marijuana, and other drugs used socially. Obviously, stimulus control does not account for all such differences, because there are direct effects of these drugs on behavior. However, to the extent that there are qualitative diffferences between the drug experiences of different drug users (experienced versus naive, etc.), one may infer that these effects are due to the discriminative stimulus properties of the drugs. This inference suggests

Table 1. Centrally Acting Drugs Tested for Discriminative Control[a]

Strong control	Moderate	Weak
Anesthetics	*Antimuscarinic drugs*	*Phenothiazines*
Pentobarbital 10–20	Atropine 20–200	Chlorpromazine 4
Phenobarbital 60–80	Scopolamine 1–300	Acepromazine 8
Secobarbital 15–20	Benactyzine 10–50	Perphenazine 5
Na barbital 150	Ditran 5–60	Prothipendyl 12
Amobarbital 30		
Chloral hydrate 150	*Nicotinic drugs*	*Dibenzazepines*
Ethyl alcohol 1000–3000	Nicotine 1–4	Imipramine 20
Paraldehyde 300	Lobeline 40	
Progesterone 125	Antagonist: Mecamylamine	*Relatively inactive drugs*
Hydroxydione 25		Pryilamine 50
Ethyl carbamate	*Narcotics*	Phenoxybenzamine 10
Ether	Morphine 9–26	Physostigmine 1
Nitrous oxide		Dilantin 175
Antagonist: Bemegride	*Antinicotinic drugs*	
	Mecamylamine 10–30	
Minor tranquilizers		
Librium 30	*Convulsants*	
Meprobamate 200	Metrazol 30	
	Bemegride 7.5	
	Other drugs	
	Amphetamine 1–5	
	Mescaline 50	
	Acetylcholine (in dogs)	
	Epinephrine (in dogs)	
	Norepinephrine (in dogs)	
	Erythroidine (in dogs)	

[a] *NOTE:* Tested dose levels are given beside each drug in mg/kg for i.p. injection in the rat. The ordering according to relative effectiveness is only approximate and refers to the maximally effective tested dose of each drug. From D. A. Overton. Discriminative control of behavior by drug states. In T. Thompson and R. Pickens (Eds.), *Stimulus properties of drugs.* New York: Appleton-Century-Crofts, 1971, pp. 87–110.

that the origins of such drug experiences lie in the history of differential reinforcement rather than in pharmocological activity or in differences between states of consciousness.

The discriminative stimulus properties of drugs have been used in three categories of clinical applications, namely, those in which the intent is to decrease or control intake of a drug such as alcohol, applications in which phobic patients are treated with combinations of drugs and systematic desensitization, and applications in which drugs are used to induce amnesia for painful medical procedures. In the first instance, a straightforward stimulus discrimination training procedure is used.

Lovibond and Caddy (1970) gave alcoholics various alcoholic beverages and taught them to discriminate their blood alcohol levels by providing feedback with a breath analyzer. The authors reported that subjects quickly learned to discriminate accurately and continued to be able to do so, with occasional feedback, after training. This discrimination training was one part of a treatment program intended to establish self-control over drinking, as compared to the usual treatment goal of establishing total abstinence. The results of the combined treatment program were encouraging in that 85% were "improved" at 6 months after treatment and 59% were still rated improved at 12 months following treatment. However, a high dropout rate made the outcome data inconclusive.

Later Silverstein, Nathan, and Taylor (1974) investigated blood alcohol discrimination training as the primary approach to establish self-control over social drinking. These investigators found that their four subjects could learn to estimate their blood alcohol levels more accurately than before training, but their accuracy decreased rapidly when feedback was discontinued. Also, only one of four subjects exhibited controlled drinking after discharge, and he appeared not to rely on perception of blood alcohol level to control his drinking.

Strickler, Bigelow, Lawrence, and Liebson (1976) incorporated blood alcohol level discrimination training into a self-control program that was largely successful: subjects improved in accuracy of estimation, and two of three subjects maintained controlled drinking during six months of follow-up. Also, Caddy and Lovibond (1976) reported a second study in which they incorporated blood-alcohol-level discrimination training into a successful program for establishing self-control over drinking.

These studies suggest that training in the discrimination of blood alcohol levels may be a useful part of a treatment program for establishing self-control over drinking, but the data also suggest that discrimination training alone is not an adequate treatment. The relative contribution of discrimination training to these treatment procedures has not yet been systematically studied.

Systematic desensitization in the treatment of phobias has been reported by some investigators to be facilitated by short-acting barbiturates such as methohexitone (Friedman & Lipsedge, 1971; Mawson, 1970; Razani, 1974) and propranidid (Silverstone & Salkind, 1973). Also, treatment of phobias by flooding has been reported to be facilitated by thiopental (Hussain, 1971) and by diazepam (Johnston & Gath, 1973; Marks, Viswanathan, Lipsedge, & Gardner, 1972; McCormick, 1973). These studies are reviewed in more detail in the section on potentiating variables, but it should be noted here that the positive interactions between drugs and behavior therapy may be due in part to the tendency of these drugs to establish discriminative stimulus control over behavior. Thus, positive interactions have been observed only when drugs were used that have strong discriminative stimulus properties and only when the treatment procedures are arranged so that behavior therapy overlaps the waxing and waning of conditioned fears.

The use of drugs to produce amnesia for painful surgical procedures or endoscopies is another type of clinical application of the discriminative stimulus properties of drugs. Several studies have shown that lorazepam given as a premedication for surgery results in an antegrade amnesia for events occurring within a few hours following drug administration. For this purpose, lorazepam is superior both to diazepam (Fragen & Caldwell, 1976) and to pentobarbital (Blitt, Petty, Wright, & Wright, 1976). This use of the stimulus properties of drugs to isolate painful memories would be most useful where a painful medical procedure must be frequently repeated, such as in the treatment of burns.

Although the techniques described above seem to exhaust the existing behavior modification procedures that make use of drugs as discriminative stimuli, several other possibilities can be suggested that future research might address. Since drugs are known to be powerful discriminative stimuli, there is a potential role for drugs wherever stimulus control programs might ordinarily be used.

One category of clinical problems in which stimulus control programs are frequently used is the elimination of "bad habits" such as cigerette smoking, frequent or excessive alcohol intake, disruptive behavior in the classroom, or anti-social behavior. The analysis of behaviors like these usually suggests (1) that they are under the stimulus control of several events in the environment (e.g., smoking after meals, smoking when drinking coffee), and (2) that they produce some immediate reinforcing consequence, but (3) that they produce a delayed aversive consequence. Assuming that one has a reasonable program for bringing the remote consequences to bear on the behavior, the problem becomes one of disrupting existing stimulus control, and this is best done by changing the environment or by introducing a novel stimulus. It is for this reason that individuals who are attempting to make major changes in their behavior, involving high-frequency behaviors, are encouraged to alter their environments or to enter a special hospital environment. One might use for this purpose drug-produced cues whose discriminative stimulus properties are potent enough to produce the phenomena referred to as *state-dependent performance*.

As an example, suppose that one is consulted by an exhibitionist who wants to change. After analyzing the environmental stimuli that control the behavior and its reinforcing consequences and planning an intensive desensitization program, combined perhaps with some training in alternative social skills, one could put the patient on significant doses of a drug like pentobarbital simply to disrupt the existing stimulus control of the inappropriate behavior and thereby facilitate behavior change. One would want fairly quickly to discontinue or fade out the drug because novel stimuli that do not in fact have differential consequences attached to them quickly lose their ability to disrupt ongoing behavior. However, the drug could be reintroduced for short periods of time on several occasions, such as in situations in which the exhibitionistic behavior is particularly likely to recur.

For some problem behaviors it would be unnecessary or even detrimental to introduce drugs into the behavior change program because this represents an extra step; the behavior may change quite rapidly without the drug. However, some high-frequency habits, such as compulsive rituals and obsessive thoughts, are slow and difficult to change; it would be worthwhile to experiment with combining drugs with behavior modification procedures in these cases. Note that the type of drug one might use is different when the intent is to alter the stimulus control of behavior rather than to reduce anxiety. One would want to use drugs with potent discriminative stimulus properties.

Another kind of clinical problem for which stimulus control procedures are frequently used is the establishment of new habits or the sharpening of stimulus control over existing behaviors. Studying and eating are instances of behaviors that one may want to bring under strong stimulus control. Assertive social behaviors, such as sticking up for one's rights or simply speaking in social situations, are instances of behaviors that one may want to establish. One might use short-acting drugs to establish rapid stimulus control over these behaviors and then, once the behaviors are established, use fading procedures to transfer this stimulus control to appropriate environmental stimuli.

As an example of this kind of application, suppose one is consulted by a patient with uncontrolled eating behavior and serious obesity. One might decide as a first step to let the patient eat anytime he wished but to give a short-acting drug such as thiopental with easily discriminable stimulus properties before any food intake and have the patient avoid eating in the absence of this stimulus. This program should bring eating behavior rapidly under control of this stimulus. One might then restrict the stimulus to appropriate occasions and link it to natural environmental cues, such as sitting at a table with others. As a last step, one would fade out the drug.

In a similar way, one can make use of the stimulus properties of a drug in combination with its other properties. For instance, minor tranquilizers appear to disinhibit behaviors that are ordinarily suppressed because of a history of punishment, and this action may be unrelated to the discriminative stimulus properties of the drug (Cook & Davidson, 1978). One might train a severely inhibited patient to emit new social behaviors while under the influence of diazepam, use the diazepam to cause the new behaviors to be emitted in appropriate social settings, and then fade out the drug gradually. One could attack insomnia similarly by using hypnotics with strong discriminative stimulus properties and then fading the drug, provided there is not already a long history of hypnotic drug use.

The discriminative stimulus properties of drugs have been incorporated into behavior therapy in only two areas: the training of alcoholics to discriminate blood alcohol levels and the use of minor tranquilizers to facilitate the behavioral treatment of phobias. In both areas, the stimulus properties of drugs appear to contribute to positive interactions between drugs and behavior therapy. The use of drugs to produce amnesia for painful events does not directly involve behavior therapy, but drugs may be used to prevent the development of phobic aversions to medical procedures. We have suggested that there are other clinical problems in which the stimulus control of behavior needs either to be strengthened (e.g., eating) or disrupted (e.g., smoking) and that the potent stimulus properties of drugs could be incorporated into behavior change programs in these areas.

DRUGS THAT DIRECTLY AFFECT BEHAVIOR

There are several important classes of drugs that produce useful changes in behavior by mechanisms that are not easily conceptualized in behavioral terms. These include the major tranquilizers, the tricyclic antidepressants, and the stimulants used to treat hyperactivity. We have chosen to discuss these together under the heading of direct effects of drugs on behavior. This phrase implies nothing about the actual physiological mechanisms of action of these drugs but is used simply to point out that neither stimulus control nor consequential control of behavior seems involved in their action.

It is not the purpose of this review to discuss interactions between drugs and nonbehavioral modes of psychotherapy. Studies of these possible interactions have been recently reviewed by Hollon and Beck (1978) and by Schooler (1978). Their reviews suggest that for the treatment of schizophrenia, major tranquilizers are more effective than a variety of nonbehavioral psychotherapies. Such psychotherapeutic treatment has not been shown capable either of shortening hospitalization or of reducing the relapse rate after discharge, although psychotherapy does appear to improve the social adjustment of discharged patients who have not relapsed. One study (Goldstein, Rodnick, Evans, & May, 1975) reported a tendency (not statistically significant) for discharged schizophrenic patients treated with a combination of drugs and psychotherapy to relapse at a lower rate than patients treated with drugs alone, but the preponderance of studies suggest that there are neither positive nor negative interactions between drugs and psychotherapy; the effect of both is equal to the effect of drugs alone.

On the other hand, there is increasing evidence to indicate a positive interaction between drugs and nonbehavioral psychotherapy in the management of neurotic depression. Weissman (1978) reviewed published and ongoing studies on this topic and concluded that there is merit to combined treatment because drug therapy and psychotherapy modify different aspects of depression (symptoms and social functioning, respectively). Weissman also suggested that drugs render depressed patients more amenable to psychotherapy, which would represent a positive interaction, but the evidence for such an interaction is indirect.

The best study of possible interactions between behavior therapies and major tranquilizers in schizophrenic patients is the excellent study by Paul, Tobias, and Holly (1972). Fifty-two chronic schizophrenic patients were assigned to two treatment units. In one of these, a token economy program was used to increase social skills and instrumental skills and to decrease bizarre behaviors. In the other unit, the same staff employed milieu therapy in which the focus was upon group cohesiveness, group pressure, and group problem-solving. The goal of the milieu therapy was also to increase social and instrumental skills and to decrease bizarre behaviors. Half the patients in each treatment unit were continued on the same dose and type of medication they had been on at referral, and half were switched abruptly to placebo. Low to moderate doses of major tranquilizers, often combined with tricyclic antidepressants, were typical of the medications these patients were on. Neither the treatment staff nor the patient evaluators knew that some of the patients were switched to placebo.

Over 17 weeks of treatment, patients in both treatment units showed a significant increase in adaptive behaviors and a significant decrease in the occurrence of bizarre behaviors. Differences between milieu therapy and social learning therapy were apparently found but were not reported in detail. There was no significant main effect for the drug nor any significant interaction between drug and type of treatment. In short, low to moderate doses of major tranquilizers had no discernible effect when examined in patients receiving an apparently quite powerful "social-environmental treatment." This finding contrasts with most studies reviewed by Hollon and Beck (1978) and Schooler (1978), which found no effect of psychotherapy and a reliable effect of major tranquilizers. The one weakness of the Paul *et al.*'s (1972) study is that the drug doses investigated were low to moderate.

Liberman (1976) reported a single-case study that examined interactions between chlorpromazine and a time-out contingency in the control of delusional speech in a schizophrenic woman. Although there was no drug-free baseline prior to the introduction of the behavioral program, the author showed that removing and reinstating the time-out contingency controlled the occurrence of delusional speech in this woman, and that withdrawal of medication had no effect. No interaction between the drug and the behavioral program was apparent.

McConahey and Thompson (1971) reported on interactions between behavior therapy and chlorpromazine in institutional retarded women. Behavior therapy improved the social skills of these women, and addition of chlorpromazine yielded no further improvements.

These three studies of major tranquilizers and behavior therapy are in agreement with studies of phenothiazines and psychotherapy in showing no interaction between the psychological and the pharmacological intervention, but they differ from the psychotherapy studies in suggesting that behavior therapy is more effective than pharmacotherapy in some types of schizophrenia. However, the limitations of the available studies in terms of the doses used and the sample sizes studied do not permit one to place confidence in the apparent superiority of behavior therapy over drug therapy.

Christensen and Sprague (1973) reported a study that appeared to demonstrate a positive interaction between a stimulant, methylphenidate, and a behavior modification program in the treatment of hyperactive children. These children were of normal intelligence. The 12 subjects were divided into a drug group (0.3 mg/kg methylphenidate in a single dose prior to each session) and a placebo group on the basis of parental permission for medication. Behavior modification involved awarding points exchangeable for money for reduced activity in the seat, but the program did not include social reinforcement. Both groups improved relative to baseline, and the drug group improved more than the placebo group. Moreover, when the behavioral contingency was reversed for one session, seat activity increased in the placebo group but not in the drug group. This finding suggested that both treatments were effective and that their effects were additive. However, there were two serious methodological problems, which render these results inconclusive: group assignment was not random and apparently not blind. Also, the two groups were diverging during the baseline prior to the intervention, suggesting that some of the differences during treatment may have been unrelated to treatment.

Subsequently, Christensen (1975) reported a more definitive study of this issue. Sixteen retarded, hyperactive children were entered in a 12-week study using a within-subjects design. This design involved a 2-week baseline, a 4-week behavior modification phase, a 2-week reversal (reinstatement of baseline conditions), and another 4-week behavior modification phase. Each 4-week block of behavior modification included 2 weeks of methylphenidate (0.3 mg/kg given 1.5 hours before sessions) and 2 weeks of placebo. Behavior modification involved giving tokens and social reinforcement for paying attention, working hard, completing work, and doing work correctly. Results showed that behavior modification reduced hyperactivity and increased on-target behavior with no drug–placebo differences. Thus, the results of the Christensen and Sprague (1973) study were not replicated.

Shafto and Sulzbacher (1977) reported a study of a single hyperactive child in which they manipulated different doses of methylphenidate and a behavior modification program involving food and praise contingent on appropriate play. The behavioral contingency reduced hyperactivity more reliably than the drugs, and no interactions between drug therapy and behavior modification were observed.

Wulbert and Dries (1977) reported another single-case study of the interactions between methylphenidate (10 mg four times a day) and a contingency management system in which tokens were given for "hands down" and for accuracy in memory tasks. The mother gave tokens at home for cooperative play with others and for compliance with her requests. Results indicated that in the clinic, the drug had no effect on ritualistic behavior or accuracy in the memory tasks, whereas reinforcement contingencies affected both. At home, where the same behavioral contingency was always maintained by the mother, the drug significantly reduced aggressive behavior but significantly *increased* ritualistic behavior. There was no generalization from clinic to home environment, which is disturbing, and no evidence of an interaction between drug treatment and contingency management. The differences between home and clinic data were not adequately explained. Possible explanations include that the mother's home behavior modification program was not rigorously carried out and/or that the experimenters unwittingly biased their data against finding a drug–placebo difference.

An unpublished study by Gittelman-Klein, Klein, Abikoff, Katz, Gloisten, and Kates (1976), which is reviewed by Hollon and Beck (1978), is consistent with these studies in showing no interaction between drugs and behavior therapy. Thirty-six hyperactive children were treated with methylphenidate only (10–60 mg/day), behavior therapy plus methylphenidate, or behavior therapy plus placebo. All treatments yielded pre–post improvements. Unlike previous studies, these investigators found drug only and drug plus behavior therapy both to be superior to behavior therapy alone, and combined therapy was not different from drug alone.

Except for the Christensen and Sprague (1973) study, which had methodological problems, these studies are consistent in showing no interaction between behavior therapy and drug therapy in treating hyperactivity. These data do not provide an adequate basis for judging the relative efficacy of methylphenidate and behavior modification. Differences in studies are probably accounted for by differences in drug dosage and in the skill with which behavior modification was implemented.

Several studies have appeared that deal with combinations of behavior therapy and antidepressant or beta-blocker drugs in the treatment of phobias or obsessive-compulsive disorders. The rationale for these combinations is different from the rationale for combining minor tranquilizers with behavior therapy: the antidepressants and beta-blockers (e.g., propranolol) block the panic reactions that occur in many phobics and that tend to disrupt behavioral treatment programs (Marks, 1969), whereas the minor tranquilizers are used because they are presumed to lower the general level of anxiety. The antidepressant and beta-blocker studies are reviewed below.

Amin, Ban, Pecknold, and Klinger (1977) studied six phobic patients and six patients with obsessive-compulsive neurosis in a 24-week study. Groups of four patients were treated with clomipramine (a tricylic antidepressant) plus behavior therapy (consisting of relaxation training and systematic desensitization), with clomipramine plus mock behavior therapy, or with placebo plus behavior therapy. Patients' rating of their target symptoms over the entire trial showed no statistically significant improvements for the total population of 12 subjects and no differences between groups, but clinicians' global ratings favored the combined treatment group followed by the behavior-therapy–only group over the clomipramine-only group. There were several dropouts. These data contribute relatively little to an understanding of the interaction between drugs and behavior therapy since no treatment was effective for the target symptoms.

Zitrin, Klein, Lindemann, Tobak, Rock, Kaplan, and Ganz (1976) published an interim report in which imipramine and placebo treatments were compared in groups of phobics receiving behavior therapy or supportive therapy. Preliminary results indicated that imipramine was superior to placebo, but there was no support for the hypothesis that behavior therapy was different from supportive therapy. Consequently, no interaction between drug and behavior therapy was evident. However, the study was less than half completed at the time of the report.

Lipsedge, Hajioff, Huggins, Napier, Pearce, Pike, and Rich (1973) studied combinations of iproniazid, a monoamine oxidase inhibitor, and systematic desensitization. Although 71 patients were entered into the study and the design was rather ambitious, results of the study were inconclusive. Iproniazid tended to be better than placebo for reducing anxiety as rated by clinicians but not for reducing avoidance behavior. Only on self-ratings of anxiety was there a significant interaction between drug and behavior therapy: iproniazid plus systematic desensitization was rated *less* effective than placebo plus systematic desensitization. Other studies of monoamine oxidase inhibitors in phobic patients have also reported that discontinuation of the drug leads to a return of symptoms even when patients have been encouraged to expose themselves to the phobic situation (Solyom et al., 1973; Tyrer, Candy, & Kelly, 1973). Marks (1976) reviewed many of these studies and summarized other unpublished studies not readily available in the United States.

Hafner and Milton (1977) studied the interaction between flooding and propranolol, a beta-blocker drug that prevents many peripheral physiological indications of anxiety, in the treatment of 23 agoraphobics. The propranolol group did significantly worse than the placebo group following treatment: the drug group spent less time traveling alone and improved less on a measure of general symptoms. The authors speculated that this negative interaction was due to waning of the drug's effect during the last hour of the flooding session. However, this explanation is opposite to the explanation offered by Marks et al. (1972) for the facilitation of flooding by diazepam; they argued that diazepam is effective only if the flooding session does overlap the waning phase of the drug's effect on the body.

The literature on interactions between behavior therapy and drugs that directly modify behavior in the treatment of schizophrenia, hyperactivity, and agoraphobia is rather consistent in suggesting that there is either no interaction or a negative interaction. The only studies reporting positive interactions were the Christensen and Sprague (1973) study of methylphenidate in hyperactive children and the Amin et al. (1977) study of clomipramine. Both these studies were of questionable generality since the former study was not replicated by Christensen (1975) and the Amin *et al.* study showed no effect of any treatment on target symptoms.

This lack of interaction between behavior therapy procedures and drugs that directly affect behavior contrasts sharply with other areas reviewed in this chapter: drugs that have discriminative stimulus properties or reinforcing properties or other properties outlined here typically do interact with behavioral contingencies even though the resulting interactions are not always practical treatment procedures. One can see a parallel between this situation and the statement by Gantt (1953) that classical conditioning occurs only in situations in which the unconditional stimulus acts on sensory nerve endings and thus through the nervous system, and that classical conditioning does not occur when the unconditional stimulus acts directly on the end organ without the mediation of the nervous system. The drugs we have discussed in this section have a site of action within the central nervous system, but they are like Gantt's unconditionable stimuli in that they appear to have only weak sensory stimulus properties at the doses used here (cf. the section "Drugs as Discriminative Stimuli" and Table 1). Perhaps only the afferent or stimulus properties of drugs enable them to interact with behavioral contingencies.

DRUGS AS REINFORCING CONSEQUENCES

A reinforcer in behavioral terms is anything which increases the future probability of the occurrence of any response that precedes it. There can be little doubt that many drugs fit this definition (Crowley, 1972). C. R. Schuster and others (e.g., Pickens & Thompson, 1971; Woods & Schuster, 1971) have developed experimental paradigms in which animals self-administer intravenous infusions of various drugs by pressing a lever. This model is used to compare various drugs for abuse potential. Similar experimental arrangements have been set up for humans, as illustrated by Schuster, Smith, and Jaffe (1971) and by Bigelow, Griffiths, and Liebson (1977). The latter investigators had subjects ride an exercise bicycle in order to earn tokens that could be exchanged for ethanol drinks.

Experiments such as these reveal some similarities and some differences between drug reinforcers and ordinary food or water reinforcers. In common with food reinforcers, one observes extinction phenomena: high rates of responding followed by a disappearance of responding when a saline solution is substituted for the drug, or simply a disappearance of responding when drug infusions are made to be independent of responding (i.e., noncontingent). Responding for drugs can be maintained on various schedules of reinforcement (e.g., fixed ratio, fixed interval, variable interval), and the distribution of responses is similar to that observed with food or water. However, rates of responding are often lower, and responses are spaced so as to maintain a relatively constant rate of drug infusion. Beyond a certain minimal dose, response rate decreases with increasing dose per injection. Another difference between stimulant drug reinforcers and conventional reinforcers is that animals (Pickens & Thompson, 1971) and man typically alternate long periods of drug abstinence (e.g., several days) with long periods of drug intake. Also, animals given unlimited access to stimulant self-administration will stop eating, lose large amounts of weight, and ultimately die. (This suppression of appetite by stimulants is made use of in diet medications.)

Studies reviewed by Woods and Schuster (1971) indicate that the reinforcing properties of opiates are not attributable to physical dependency since self-administration occurs at doses too low to produce dependency. Woods and Schuster also note that naloxone, a narcotic antagonist, eliminates responding for opiates.

Experiments on the use of drugs as punishing consequences confound operant punishment procedures with classical conditioning procedures because the purpose is usually to decrease drug intake by pairing drug intake with the administration of a second drug that makes the subject ill. This approach is illustrated by the study by Farrar, Powell, and Martin (1968), who gave curare to alcoholic human subjects after they had drunk alcohol, in an unsuccessful attempt to decrease drug intake. This kind of application is discussed in the section on classical conditioning.

The range of drugs that have been shown to have reinforcing properties include the opiates morphine, methadone, and codeine (Woods & Schuster, 1971); the stimulant drugs amphetamine, caffeine, cocaine, fencamfamine, methamphetamine, methylphenidate, nicotine, phenmetrazine, pepradrol, and tranylcypromine (Pickens & Thompson, 1971); and the sedative drugs ethanol, pentobarbital, and diazepam (Griffiths, Bigelow, & Liebson, 1976). For humans, marijuana and hallucinogens such as LSD and mescaline also appear to act as reinforcers (Crowley, 1972). Most of the entries in this list are of little value to behavior therapists because of ethical and toxic considerations, but a few of them have been incorporated into behavior change programs, either intentionally or unintentionally.

Cigarettes have often been used as reinforcers for behavior change in institutional settings. For example, Goldiamond (1968) used cigarettes as well as other rewards to reinforce study behavior in delinquent adolescents, and Liberman (1976) used cigarettes to increase the frequency of socially appropriate behaviors in a psychotic woman. Cigarettes and coffee have been used as reinforcers in various self-control programs for outpatients. For example, Todd (1972) used coffee breaks to reinforce the utterance of positive self-statements in a depressed patient. There are few systematic data on the effectiveness of these stimulant drugs as reinforcers relative to other reinforcers because they are considered functionally equivalent to other classes of reinforcers by extrapolation from the Premack principle. Some authors have found them to be potent and convenient reinforcers to use in outpatient self-control programs, especially in frequent coffee or tea drinkers. However, one must pay attention to the special characteristics of drug reinforcers: subjects tend to ingest them frequently but at a steady rate so as to maintain a constant rate of drug intake.

It is reported that rum was used contingently to control behavior in the British navy in the last century, and experiments demonstrate that alcohol is an effective reinforcer of behavior in some humans (Bigelow *et al.*, 1977). It is a toxic substance, however, and therefore its usefulness is limited. On the other hand, it is socially condoned and is widely used. One could justify using it in the same way that coffee and cigarettes are used as adjuncts to outpatient self-control programs. Patients who already use alcohol with some frequency (but are not alcoholics) could be counseled to make their drinking contingent on other low-frequency behaviors that they wish to increase (such as talking to a member of the opposite sex or behaving assertively).

Other experimental applications of drugs as reinforcers include the following. Kurland, Unger, Shaffer, and Savage (1967) gave LSD to chronic alcoholics following a series of counseling sessions in which the patients emitted a number of positive intention statements. Since the therapist decided when the patient was ready for the LSD experience, Liberman (1976) has labeled this a use of drugs as reinforcers even though the investigators were inclined to interpret their procedure in terms of exposure to an alternative state of consciousness. The preliminary results of this study were promising but not conclusive. The remaining example is not a study but a proposal published by Rosenberg (1973). He indicated that he would try to use marijuana as a reinforcer for taking Antabuse in chronic alcoholics.

As the foregoing discussion suggests, drugs are powerful reinforcers of behavior, but their applications to behavior change have been relatively few and weak because reinforcing drugs are by definition abused drugs, and most abused drugs are not socially acceptable. In some cases, social acceptability is based on the potential of these drugs to produce physical dependency or toxic effects, but in other cases, such as marijuana, the evidence of physical dependency and toxicity do not appear to justify keeping these drugs illegal. Marijuana may eventually join caffeine, and to a lesser extent ethanol and nicotine, as drugs that may appropriately and effectively be used to reinforce behavior change. Caffeine, nicotine, and ethanol have, in the opinion of the authors, been underutilized as agents of behavior change in neurotic outpatients.

DRUGS AS POTENTIATING VARIABLES

Potentiating variables include all the factors that modify the effectiveness of consequences for controlling behavior. Food deprivation and satiation are examples of nonpharmacological potentiating variables. There are three broad classes of drugs that also act as potentiating variables, namely, analgesics, narcotic antagonists, and minor tranquilizers.[1] Analgesics modify the perceived intensity of painful stimuli, and narcotic antagonists render narcotics ineffective by replacing them at nerve endings. Based on the evidence that is reviewed below, it appears that minor tranquilizers such as the benzodiazepines and barbiturates also attenuate the control of behavior by aversive consequences and enhance the effectiveness of positive reinforcers.

The experimental task that has been most useful for distinguishing minor transquilizers from other classes of drugs in animals is the conflict-avoidance schedule (Cook & Davidson, 1973, 1978). This task consists of two components that alternate. During part of the experimental session, the animal subject is reinforced with food for pressing a lever; during other parts of the session, the animal is both

---

[1] Research reviewed by Stein (1978) indicates that drugs that alter brain norepinephrine and dopamine also alter the rat's behavior of pressing a lever to produce electrical stimulation of the brain. Stein interpreted these data as showing that the motivational and reinforcing properties of electrical self-stimulation (i.e., potentiating variables) are altered by these drugs. The relevance of this research to reinforcers other than brain stimulation has not been demonstrated, however, and for this reason, Stein's work is not included in this section.

rewarded with food and punished with electric shock for pressing the lever. Typically, the shock suppresses but does not eliminate responding during the second (food plus shock) component. Minor tranquilizers selectively increase the rate of responding by the animal in the conflict component, the amount of the increase being proportional to the dose or to the potency of the drug. Other classes of drugs do not exhibit this selective action. Major tranquilizers such as chlorpromazine reduce responding in both components of the schedule, and stimulants such as amphetamine increase responding in both schedule components.

Minor tranquilizers can be shown to have similar effects on conflict behavior—behavior that is both punished and rewarded—in humans. Lehmann and Ban (1971) showed that minor tranquilizers increased the length of time human subjects would hold down a key when depressing it produced both money reward and electric shock, and Beer and Migler (1975) found that diazepam increased the number of lever presses made by human subjects when such lever presses were rewarded with money and punished with electric shock.

Noting that there were both technical and ethical problems associated with the use of electric shock in humans, we have experimented with a different type of conflict. In two separate sessions, we asked subjects to hold their breath for as long as possible and paid them at a rate of two cents per second for doing so. They did this immediately before and at one-, two-, and three-hour intervals after taking either diazepam (10 mg) or placebo. As predicted, breath-holding time was significantly increased following diazepam compared to placebo. Moreover, the breath-holding measure was a more sensitive measure of drug action than a self-report measure of subjective anxiety. For these reasons, we felt that this simple test might have value as a preclinical screening measure of minor tranquilizers under development.

Minor tranquilizers also can be shown to increase more clinically meaningful behavior that appears to have been suppressed by a history of aversive consequences. Whitehead, Blackwell, and Robinson, (1978) showed that diazepam increased the approach of phobic subjects to the animal of which they were phobic more than did placebo, and Silverstone (1973) showed that diazepam and lorazepam decreased phobic anxiety more than did placebo.

People apparently recognize and make use of the tendency of alcohol to release behaviors that are inhibited in conflict situations. Vogel-Sprott (1972) summarized studies showing that alcohol intake increases in both animals and humans under stressful circumstances; and an experiment by Miller, Hersen, Eisler, and Hilsman (1974) suggests that alcoholic humans, but not social drinkers, increase alcohol intake following a stressful interview. Winstead, Anderson, Eilers, Blackwell, and Zaremba (1974) showed that when diazepam is prescribed on an as-needed (prn) schedule, it is taken primarily at times of maximum social interaction, presumably because social interactions are stressful.

In addition to their effects on behavior that has been suppressed by punishment, minor tranquilizers have other interesting behavioral effects that must be taken into account in interpreting their behavioral mechanism of action. These compounds increase the amount of quinine-tainted milk drunk by rats and also increase the amount of untainted milk drunk by rats who have already drunk to satiety. These compounds have also been reported to increase responding in extinction if the drug is given in the early phases of extinction of a formerly food-reinforced response in rats (Margules & Stein, 1967). However, no increases in responding are observed if the drug is given late in extinction. Similar phenomena have been reported anecdotally in humans. Minor tranquilizers increase food intake, and DiMascio, Shader, and Harmatz (1967) reported increases in hostility in people taking minor tranquilizers.

These phenomena, taken together with the effects of the minor tranquilizers on behavior suppressed by punishment, have led some writers to characterize the minor tranquilizers as agents that disinhibit behavior that has been suppressed for any reason. However, other data suggest that this interpretation is inaccurate. Rats are capable of learning a discrimination while in a drug state produced by benzodiazepines as rapidly as they do when undrugged, and they are capable of reversal learning in which the go and no-go signals are reversed (Sachs, Weingarten, & Klein, 1966). Both discrimination learning and reversal learning involve inhibition of responses to a cue that has been associated with their occurrence in the past, so inhibition appears not to be impaired by these drugs. Barrett (1977) reported other studies that are inconsistent with a disinhibition hypothesis. He noted that chlordiazepoxide, pentobarbital, and ethanol increased the rate of food-reinforced responding in rats but decreased the rate of a response maintained by shock avoidance. Amphetamine, on the other hand, increased the rate of both kinds of behavior, and morphine decreased the rate of both kinds of behavior.

An alternative explanation, which better accounts for the data discussed above, is that minor tranquilizers act as potentiating variables to diminish the effectiveness of aversive consequences such as electric shock on behavior and to enhance the effectiveness of appetitive consequences on behavior. In the clinical situation, the aversive consequences might be conceptualized as including the displeasure of a peer or a spouse; attenuation of the fear of this consequence by minor tranquilizers might result in an individual's engaging in previously suppressed social interactions. These might be socially desirable (assertive) or undesirable (hostile) behaviors, depending on the existing behavioral repertoire of the individual and the social setting.

Minor tranquilizers appear to give this effect by a mechanism different from that of analgesics. Analgesics reduce the perceived intensity of noxious stimuli, whereas minor tranquilizers appear to affect the motivational or emotional properties of the reinforcing or punishing stimulus at a step removed from the stimulus itself. For example, Cook and Davidson (1973) showed that the disinhibiting effects of minor tranquilizers on conflict behavior in rats were not reproduced by lowering the intensity of electric shock; lowering the intensity altered behavior more slowly and apparently less sensitively than minor tranquilizers. Similarly, Chapman and Feather (1973) showed that diazepam increased the tolerance of human subjects to pain but did not affect the subject's ability to distinguish between painful stimuli of different intensities and did not raise the threshold for labeling the stimuli as painful.

Several investigators have reported that the treatment of phobias by systematic desensitization is facilitated by methohexitone (Brady, 1966; Friedman & Lipsedge, 1971; Mawson, 1970; Razani, 1974) or by propranidid (Silverstone & Salkind, 1973). Use of these drugs is said to reduce the number of sessions required to treat phobias. In addition, there have been several reports that flooding as a treatment of phobias is facilitated by thiopental (Hussain, 1971) or by diazepam (Johnston & Gath, 1973; Marks *et al.*, 1972; McCormick, 1973). Taken together, these experiments provide compelling support for a positive interaction between minor tranquilizers and behavior therapy.

There have, however, been conflicting reports. Yorkston, Sergeant, and Rachman (1968) did not find a facilitation of systematic desensitization by metohexitone, and Hussain (1971) found no benefit for systematic desensitization with thiopental. Hussain suggested that his inexperience with the technique of systematic desensitization may have contributed to his failure to show an effect of drug. Hafner and Marks (1976) failed to replicate the earlier study by Marks *et al.* (1972) in which diazepam facilitated flooding; and Whitehead, Robinson, Blackwell, and Stutz (1978) found no difference between diazepam and placebo in the treatment of small-animal phobias. Switching from flooding individuals to flooding groups may have accounted for the failure of Hafner and Marks (1976) to find a drug effect, and Whitehead *et al.* (1978) suggested that use of a chronic dose regimen (5 mg three times daily) instead of a single dose before each session may have accounted for their results for the reasons discussed below.

Although the human studies have usually shown an interaction between minor tranquilizers and behavior therapy, animal studies of the extinction of conditioned fears by means of response prevention (which is comparable to flooding) have usually failed to show any effect of minor tranquilizers on the rate of extinction of the conditioned fear (Christy & Reid, 1975; Cooper, Coon, Mejta, & Reid, 1974; Kamano, 1968, 1972; Voss, Mejta, & Reid, 1974). Paradoxically, two studies have indicated that amphetamine, a stimulant, facilitates the extinction of conditioned fears in rats, whereas chlorpromazine, amobarbital, and chlordiazepoxide do not (Christy & Reid, 1975; Cooper *et al.*, 1974).

It is evident that only further experimentation can resolve the differences in these experimental results. However, we tentatively advance the following hypotheses: it appears that short-acting barbiturates are superior to long-acting drugs for both systematic desensitization and flooding. When diazepam, a long-acting drug, is used, its effectiveness seems to relate to whether the flooding session occurs during the waning phases of the drug's effects. Thus, Marks *et al.* (1972) found flooding during the waning diazepam effect to be superior to flooding during the peak effect; so also did McCormick (1973). This effect could also account for the failure of Whitehead *et al.* (1978) to find a drug effect when diazepam was given on a schedule that was intended to maintain constant blood levels of the drug. The animal data may also be accounted for in this way, since experimental sessions with animals are typically shorter than 30 minutes and are therefore not likely to extend into the waning phases of the drugged state.

It should not be surprising that minor tranquilizers facilitate the extinction of phobias only when the waxing and waning of the drugged state overlaps active behavior therapy because the effects of these drugs on phobic anxiety are known to be reversible. Thus, diazepam and lorazepam reduce phobic anxiety only temporarily, and the phobic anxiety returns when the drug wears off (Silverstone, 1973).

The available experimental literature seems consistent with the hypothesis that the facilitation of flooding or systematic desensitization is related to two properties of these drugs: (1) their ability to act as potentiating variables, thereby reducing temporarily the control of phobic avoidance behavior by its consequences, and (2) the ability of these drugs to act as discriminative stimuli. As potentiating variables, these drugs must act to enable the fearful subject to approach or confront the feared object more quickly or more closely, thereby permitting new learning to occur. Because these drugs tend to act as discriminative stimuli controlling new learning, it may be essential to include stimulus fading procedures by having the behavioral contingencies overlap the waxing and waning of the drugged state. This method has the effect of enhancing the transfer of new learning in the drugged state to the drug-free state.

It is not clear whether the discriminative stimulus properties of the minor tranquilizers are essential to their facilitation of behavior therapy or whether these properties are simply an inconvenient obstacle to the transfer of learning from the drugged state to the nondrugged state. It should be possible to design experiments to distinguish between these possibilities.

The implication of the experimental literature for clinical practice in the treatment of phobias is to suggest that short-acting barbiturates may be of more value than long-acting drugs such as diazepam or chlordiazepoxide. These data also suggest that minor tranquilizers should be given immediately before or during the therapy session rather than being prescribed on a regular schedule such as three times daily.

In contrast to minor tranquilizers, interactions between analgesics and behavior therapy have not been investigated in any systematic way, yet analgesics have the same behavioral properties as minor tranquilizers: they may act as potentiating variables and as discriminative stimuli. Analgesics are commonly used in hospital physical therapy programs when pain is likely to interfere with the physical rehabilitation program. Use of analgesics is typically restricted to patients with acute pain (e.g., acute neck and back pain, postsurgical and postfracture patients, and patients with recent spinal cord injuries), and analgesics are used early in treatment and are discontinued as quickly as possible (Rusk, 1977). Occasionally, a tranquilizer such as chlordiazepoxide may be used along with the analgesic. Burn patients present special problems because their treatment is usually quite painful and may continue over a period of months. Burn patients are often given Demerol, Talwin, or morphine prior to physical therapy, and these may be combined with tranquilizers (Middaugh, 1978). These applications represent positive interactions between specialized behavioral therapy programs and drugs used as potentiating variables.

The only other therapy program known to us that makes use of a possible interaction between analgesics and behavior therapy is Fordyce's (1976) treatment of chronic pain patients. Fordyce found these patients to be using excessive amounts of analgesics and tranquilizers, and he set as a goal of treatment that patients should increase the amount of activities they could engage in despite the pain and should decrease the amount of medication taken. This goal was accomplished by placing the patients on a graded-activities program and by gradually reducing the amount of analgesics and tranquilizers given them. The drug fading procedure involved putting all their medications into a "pain cocktail," which included a placebo syrup, and then gradually decreasing the amount of active drug in the mixture. The patient was aware that the medications would be gradually decreased in this way but did not know when the changes were actually made. Although not based on a controlled experiment, this treatment regimen appears to involve a positive interaction between drugs and behavior therapy. We believe that this interaction is explained by the ability of analgesics to act as potentiating variables.

Narcotic antagonists are another category of drug that acts as a potentiating variable and that may be useful in combination with behavior therapy procedures. Narcotic antagonists such as nalorphine render opiates inactive. Their administration to monkeys who are pressing a bar to self-administer opiates results eventually in a decrease in responding (Woods & Schuster, 1971). It has been proposed that we make use of this property of nalorphine to treat human drug addicts. However, practical problems have arisen with this treatment approach: many patients refuse to take nalorphine. Also, nalorphine causes withdrawal symptoms if given to an addict who has not already been withdrawn from physical dependency. Its usefulness may be restricted to highly motivated patients engaged in self-control programs, where nalorphine may help to control the immediate temptation to take drugs. However, there are attempts to develop long-lasting injectable narcotic antagonists or implantable, slow-release devices to extend the usefulness of nalorphine treatment to the larger body of narcotic addicts.

To summarize, animal and human experiments have shown that analgesics and minor tranquilizers may act as potentiating variables that reduce the effectiveness of aversive consequences on behavior and, in the case of minor tranquilizers, may also increase the effectiveness of positive reinforcers. Experimental studies suggest that minor tranquilizers facilitate the treatment of phobias when short-acting drugs are used and when the behavior therapy procedures are made to overlap the waxing and waning of the drug's effects. Physical rehabilitation practices and Fordyce's (1976) program for treating chronic pain patients suggest positive interactions between analgesics and behavioral treatment procedures. Observations on the effects of narcotic antagonists suggest that they may also facilitate the behavioral treatment of narcotic addiction.

CLASSICAL CONDITIONING: DRUGS AS PAVLOVIAN CONDITIONAL STIMULI AND AS PAVLOVIAN UNCONDITIONAL STIMULI

Animal studies have shown that several drugs may act as unconditional stimuli in the sense that the behavioral and physiological effects of the drugs can be transferred to other stimuli with which they have been paired. For example, Perez-Cruet (1971) reported that pairing injections of bulbocapnine with a tone led to the occurrence of conditioned heart-rate changes, Pickens and Dougherty (1971) demonstrated classical conditioning of the increases in activity produced by amphetamine injections in rats, and Goldberg (1971) reviewed evidence of the classical conditioning of the morphine abstinence syndrome produced by injections of nalorphine. Bykov (1957) reported on the classical conditioning of the effects of morphine, nitroglycerin, strophanthin, epinephrine, and acetylcholine by various Russian investigators.

Cook, Davidson, Davis, and Kelleher (1960) have shown that drugs may also act as Pavlovian conditional stimuli. These investigators paired injections of epinephrine, norepinephrine, and acetylcholine with electric shock to the hind leg of dogs and demonstrated conditioning of the leg-flexion response to the drug infusion alone.

Several experimental treatment paradigms have made use of the conditional stimulus properties of abused drugs to produce conditioned aversions to these drugs. The earliest experiments used drugs such as lithium carbonate or apomorphine to produce nausea (e.g., Liberman, 1968). In a typical application, the nausea-producing drug is given, and then the alcoholic patient is instructed to drink alcohol at about the time the drug is expected to cause nausea. This procedure produced some encouraging results but was felt to be unreliable because of individual differences in the time course of the nausea-producing drug and in susceptibility to its effects. Practitioners of aversion therapy then turned to electric shock because it was a more easily controlled unconditional stimulus to pair with alcohol (Franks, 1966), but the modest treatment results achieved have not seemed to justify the ethical objections to shocking patients, and aversion therapy by means of electric shock is not frequently done.

Currently, there is much interest in the use of disulfiram (Antabuse) in the treatment of alcoholism (e.g., Bigelow, Strickler, Liebson, & Griffiths, 1976). This is a drug that has little effect on its own, but when alcohol is subsequently ingested, it causes nausea. It is unclear whether this effect should be classified as punishment of an operant response (drinking) or whether it might better be classified as classical conditioning in which the alcohol acts as a conditional stimulus that is paired with an aversive unconditional stimulus. From a procedural point of view, however, disulfiram is a nearly ideal drug for aversion therapy since it ensures that the aversive consequences will immediately and reliably follow the alcohol ingestion even outside the therapy setting. Disulfiram has been shown to be an effective adjunct in the behavioral treatment of highly motivated alcoholics; it helps the alcoholic to plan ahead of time to resist the temptation of drinking in situations in which he has difficulty with self-control. However, its efficacy in the treatment of the poorly motivated alcoholic patient, who may simply refuse to take it, has not been established. The National Institute of Alcoholism and Drug Abuse is currently sponsoring a multicenter clinical trial of disulfiram treatment of alcoholism.

Some clinical applications that make use of the ability of drugs to act as unconditional stimuli have been referred to above. These have all capitalized on the aversive properties of drugs. An application that makes use of a specific unconditioned stimulus effect of a drug is the program reported by M. Schuster (1977) for the treatment of constipation associated with megacolon in children. Schuster treated these chronically constipated children by having them go into the bathroom for 10 minutes every morning regularly after breakfast. The gastrocolic reflex caused by eating after a fast increases the probability of a natural bowel movement at this time. If now bowel movement occurs naturally for two days, the child is given a suppository or other unconditional stimulus for eliciting a bowel movement on the second day. This regimen usually results in naturally occurring bowel movements within two or three weeks.

To summarize, the use of drugs as Pavlovian conditional and unconditional stimuli has resulted in effective behavior therapy procedures. Aversion therapy appears to be effective only in highly motivated patients because poorly motivated patients avoid exposing themselves to the aversive consequences. Within the group of patients motivated to achieve self-control over drinking, disulfiram has advantages over other aversion therapies because it can be used by the patient in the natural environment to assist him in resisting the temptation to drink, and disulfirm ensures an effective and reliable relationship between alcohol ingestion and immediate aversive consequences.

SUMMARY

There have been few attempts to study combinations of drugs with behavioral therapy apart from their use in aversion therapy, despite the fact that drugs and behavior therapy are both regarded as powerful technologies for producing behavior change. We have suggested that the lack of interest in drug–behavior therapy interactions is a consequence of professional differences between psychologists and psychiatrists.

This chapter has shown that many of the properties of drugs may be conceptualized in terms familiar to learning theorists, such as *discriminative stimulus* and *reinforcing stimulus*. Treating drugs in this way and reviewing the available literature on drug–behavior therapy interactions, we have concluded that drugs may interact positively with behavior therapy techniques only when they act as stimuli themselves or when they modify the way in which stimuli are perceived. Thus, positive interactions are observed when drugs are used as discriminative stimuli (e.g., the discrimination of blood alcohol levels in the treatment of alcoholism), when drugs are used as reinforcing stimuli (e.g., the use of coffee or cigarettes to increase low-probability behavior in self-control programs), when drugs are used as potentiating variables to modify the effects of a reinforcer (e.g., minor tranquilizers in the treatment of phobias), and when drugs are used as Pavlovian conditional or unconditional stimuli (e.g., in aversion therapy for alcoholism). However, drugs do not produce positive interactions when they do not act as stimuli but affect behavior directly. For example, in the treatment of hyperkinetic children, methylphenidate and reinforcement contingencies each yield positive treatment effects, but they do not appear to interact in any positive way: the effect of both together is no greater than the effects of either separately.

Although the pharmacological and behavioral treatments of schizophrenia, depression, and hyperkinesis do not produce additive effects, neither do they interfere with one another; it is safe to combine the two treatment approaches. In the treatment of panic reactions in agoraphobics, however, there is some evidence that antidepressants and beta-blocker drugs may impair the effectiveness of behavior therapy.

Our review of these studies of interactions between drugs and behavior therapy suggests to us that drugs should be selected by different criteria when they are to be combined with behavior therapy rather than being prescribed for conventional drug therapy. Drugs should be selected that have potent stimulus properties or potent reinforcing or aversive qualities, and short-acting drugs are to be preferred to long-acting ones.

ACKNOWLEDGMENTS

This chapter owes much to a generous grant from Hoffman-La Roche, Inc., who supported the authors during a period when much of the conceptualization occurred. Preparation of the manuscript was completed while the first author was a guest worker at the Laboratory for Behavioral Sciences, Gerontology Research Center (Baltimore), National Institute on Aging, and the Baltimore City Hospitals.

REFERENCES

Altman, J. L., Albert, J., Milstein, S. L., & Greenberg, I. Drugs as discriminative events in humans. In H. Lal (Ed.), *Discriminative stimulus properties of drugs*. New York: Plenum, 1977.

Amin, M. M., Ban, T. A., Pecknold, J. C., & Klinger, A. Clomipramine and behavior therapy. Paper presented at the Joint U. K.–Canada Scientific Symposium on Obsessive Compulsive Neuroses and Phobic Disorders, Montreal, 1977.

Barrett, J. E. Drug effects and the control of behavior. Paper presented at the Fourth Annual Meeting of the Midwestern Association for Behavioral Analysis, Chicago, 1977.

Beer, B., & Migler, B. Effects of diazepam on galvanic skin response and conflict in monkeys and humans. In A. Sudilovsky, S. Gershon, & B. Beer (Eds.), *Predictability in psychopharmacology: Preclinical and clinical correlations*. New York: Raven Press, 1975.

Bigelow, G., Strickler, D., Liebson, I., & Griffiths, R. Maintaining disulfiram ingestion among outpatient alcoholics: A security-deposit contingency contracting procedure. *Behaviour Research and Therapy*, 1976, *14*, 378–381.

Bigelow, G. E., Griffiths, R. R., & Liebson, I. A. Pharmacological influences upon human ethanol self-administration. In M. M. Gross (Ed.), *Alcohol intoxication and withdrawal—IIIb*. New York: Plenum, 1977.

Blackwell, B. Hypertension: Medicate or meditate? *American Heart Journal*, 1977, *93*, 262–265.

Blackwell, B., & Whitehead, W. E. Behavioral evaluation of antianxiety drugs. In A. Sudilovsky, S. Gershon, & B. Beer (Eds.), *Predictability in psychopharmacology—Preclinical and clinical correlations*. New York; Raven, 1975.

Blitt, C. D., Petty, W. C., Wright, W. A., & Wright, B. Clinical evaluation of injectable lorazepam as a premedicant: The effect on recall. *Journal of Anesthesia and Analgesia*, 1976, *55*, 522–525.

Brady, J. P. Brevital-relaxation treatment of frigidity. *Behaviour Research and Therapy*, 1966, *4*, 71–77.

Bykov, K. M. *The cerebral cortex and the internal organs*, trans. W. H. Gantt. New York: Chemical Publishing, 1957.

Caddy, G. R., & Lovibond, S. H. Self-regulation and discriminated aversive conditioning in the modification of alcoholics' drinking behavior. *Behavior Therapy*, 1976, *7*, 223–230.

Chapman, L. R., & Feather, B. W. Effects of diazepam on human pain tolerance and pain sensitivity. *Psychosomatic Medicine*, 1973, *35*, 330–340.

Christensen, D. E., Effects of combining methylphenidate and a classroom token system in modifying hyperactive behavior. *American Journal of Mental Deficiency*, 1975, *80*, 266–276.

Christensen, D. E., & Sprague, R. L. Reduction of hyperactive behavior by conditioning procedures alone and combined with methylphnidate (Ritalin). *Behaviour Research and Therapy*, 1973, *11*, 331–334.

Christy, D., & Reid, L. Methods of deconditioning persisting avoidance: Amphetamine and amobarbital as adjuncts to response prevention. *Bulletin of the Psychonomic Society*, 1975, *5(2)*, 175–177.

Cook, L., & Davidson, A. B. Effects of behaviorally active drugs in a conflict-punishment procedure in rats. In S. Garattini, E. Mussini, & L. O. Randall (Eds.), *The benzodiazepines*. New York: Raven, 1973.

Cook, L., & Davidson, A. B. Behavioral pharmacology: Animal models involving aversive control of behavior. In M. A. Lipton, A. DiMascio, & K. F. Killam (Eds.), *Psychopharmacology: A generation of progress*. New York: Raven, 1978.

Cook, L., Davidson, A., Davis, D. L., & Kelleher, R. T. Epinephrine, norepinephrine, and acetylcholine as conditioned stimuli for avoidance behavior. *Science*, 1960, *131*, 990–991.

Cooper, S., Coon, K., Mejta, C., & Reid, L. Methods of deconditioning persisting avoidance: Amphetamine, chlorpromazine, and chlordiazepoxide as adjuncts to response prevention. *Physiological Psychology*, 1974, *2*, 519–522.

Crowley, T. J. The reinforcers for drug abuse: Why people take drugs. *Comprehensive Psychiatry*, 1972, *13*, 51–62.

Davison, G. C., & Valins, S. On self-produced and drug-produced relaxation. *Behaviour Research and Therapy*, 1968, *6*, 401–402.

DiMascio, A., Shader, R. I., & Harmatz, J. Psychotropic drugs and induced hostility. *Psychosomatics*, 1967, *10*, 46–47.

Engel, G. L. The need for a new medical model: A challenge for biomedicine. *Science*, 1977, *196*, 129–136.

Farrar, C. H., Powell, B. J., & Martin, L. K. Punishment of alcohol consumption by apneic paralysis. *Behaviour Research and Therapy*, 1968, *6*, 13–16.

Fordyce, W. E. Behavioral concepts in chronic pain and illness. In P. O. Davidson (Ed.), *The behavioral management of anxiety, depression and pain*. New York: Brunner/Mazel, 1976.

Fragen, R. J., & Caldwell, N. Lorazepam premedication: Lack of recall and relief of anxiety. *Journal of Anesthesia and Analgesia*, 1976, *55*, 792–796.

Franks, C. M. Conditioning and conditioned aversion therapies in the treatment of the alcoholic. *International Journal of Addiction*, 1966, *1*, 61–98.

Friedman, D. E., & Lipsedge, M. S. Treatment of phobic anxiety and psychogenic impotence by systematic desensitization employing methohexitone-induced relaxation. *British Journal of Psychiatry*, 1971, *118*, 87–90.

Gantt, W. H. The physiological basis of psychiatry: The conditional reflex. In J. Wortis (Ed.), *Basic problems in psychiatry*. New York: Grune & Stratton, 1953.

Gittelman-Klein, R., Klein, D. F., Abikoff, H., Katz, S., Gloisten, M. C., & Kates, W. Relative efficacy of methylphenidate and behavior modification in hyperkinetic children: An interim report. Unpublished report, 1976. Summarized by S. D. Hollon & A. Beck. Psychotherapy and drug therapy: Comparison and combinations. In S. L. Garfield & A. E. Bergin (Eds.), *Handbook of psychotherapy and behavior change: An empirical analysis* (2nd ed.). New York: Wiley, 1978.

Goldberg, S. R. Nalorphine: Conditioning of drug effects on operant performance. In T. Thompson & R. Pickens (Eds.), *Stimulus properties of drugs*. New York: Appleton-Century-Crofts, 1971.

Goldiamond, I. Programs, paradigms, and procedures. In H. L. Cohen, I. Goldiamond, J. Filipczak, & R. Pooley (Eds.), *Training professionals in procedures for the establishment of educational environments: A report on the CASE Training Institute*. Silver Spring, Md.: Educational Facility Press, Institute for Behavioral Research, 1968.

Goldstein, M. J., Rodnick, E., Evans, J., & May, P. R. A. In M. Greenblatt (Ed.), *Drugs in combination with other therapies*, New York: Grune & Stratton, 1975.

Goodwin, D. H., Powell, B., Bremer, D., Haine, H., & Stern, J. Alcohol and recall: State dependent effects in man. *Science*, 1969, *163*, 1358–1360.

Griffiths, R. R., Bigelow, G., & Liebson, I. Human sedative self-administration: Effects of temporal and dose manipulations. *Journal of Pharmacology and Experimental Therapeutics*, 1976, *197*, 488–494.

Hafner, R. J., & Marks, I. M. Exposure *in vivo* of agoraphobics: Contributions of diazepam, group exposure and anxiety evocation. *Psychological Medicine*, 1976, *6*, 71–88.

Hafner, J., & Milton, F. The influence of propranolol on the exposure in vivo of agoraphobics. *Psychological Medicine*, 1977, *7*, 419–425.

Hill, S. Y., Schwin, R., Powell, B., & Goodwin, D. W. State-dependent effects of marijuana on human memory. *Nature*, 1973, *243*, 241–242.

Hollon, S. D., & Beck, A. Psychotherapy and drug therapy: Comparison and combinations. In S. L. Garfield & A. E. Bergin (Eds.), *Handbook of psychotherapy and behavior change: An empirical analysis* (2nd ed.). New York: Wiley, 1978.

Hussain, M. Z. Desensitization and flooding (implosion) in the treatment of phobias. *American Journal of Psychiatry*, 1971, *127*, 1509–1514.

Irwin, S. A rational framework for the development, evaluation, and use of psychoactive drugs. *American Journal of Psychiatry*, 1968, *124* (Supplement), 1–19.

Iversen, S. D., & Iversen, L. L. *Behavioral pharmacology*. New York: Oxford University Press, 1975.

Johnston, D., & Gath, D. Arousal levels and attribution effects in diazepam-assisted flooding. *British Journal of Psychiatry*, 1973, *123*, 463–466.

Kamano, D. K. Joint effect of amobarbital and response prevention on avoidance extinction. *Psychological Reports*, 1968, *22*, 544–546.

Kamano, D. K. Using drugs to modify the effect of response prevention on avoidance extinction. *Behaviour Research and Therapy*, 1972, *10*, 367–370.

Kornetsky, C., & Markowitz, R. Animal models of schizophrenia. In M. A. Lipton, A. DiMascio, & K. F. Killam (Eds.), *Psychopharmacology: A generation of progress*. New York: Raven, 1978.

Kurland, A. A., Unger, S., Shaffer, J. W., & Savage, C. Psychedelic therapy utilizing LSD in the treatment of the alcoholic patient: A preliminary report. *American Journal of Psychiatry*, 1967, *123*, 1202–1209.

Lal, H. General characteristics of discriminative stimuli produced by drugs. *Psychopharmacology Communications*, 1976, *2*, 305–309.

Lasagna, L. The disease model and neuropsychopharmacology. In M. A. Lipton, A. DiMascio, & K. F. Killam (Eds.), *Psychopharmacology: A generation of progress*. New York: Raven, 1978.

Lehmann, H. E., & Ban, T. A. Effects of psychoactive drugs on conflict avoidance behavior in human subjects. *Activita Nervosa Superior*, 1971, *13*, 82–85.

Liberman, R. Aversive conditioning of drug addicts: A pilot study. *Behaviour Research and Therapy*, 1968, *6*, 229–231.

Liberman, R. P. Behavior therapy for schizophrenia. In L. J. West & D. E. Flinn (Eds.), *Treatment of schizophrenia: Progress and prospect*. New York: Grune & Stratton, 1976.

Lipsedge, M. S., Hajioff, J., Huggins, P., Napier, L., Pearce, J., Pike, D. J., & Rich, M. The management of severe agoraphobia: A comparison of Iproniazid and systematic desensitization. *Psychopharmacologia*, 1973, *32*, 67–80.

Lovibond, S. H., & Caddy, G. Discriminated aversive control in the moderation of alcoholics' drinking behavior. *Behavior Therapy*, 1970, *1*, 437–444.

McConahey, O. L., & Thompson, T. Concurrent behavior modification and chlorpromazine therapy in a population of institutionalized mentally retarded women. *Proceedings of the 79th Annual Convention of the American Psychological Association*, 1971, pp. 761–762.

McCormick, W. O. Declining-dose drug desensitization for phobias. *Canadian Psychiatric Association Journal*, 1973, *18*, 25–32.

Margules, D. L., & Stein, L. Neuroleptics vs. tranquilizers: Evidence from animal behavior studies of mode and site of action. In H. Brill, J. O. Cole, P. Deniker, H. Hippius, & P. B. Brady (Eds.), *Neurophychopharmacology: Proceedings of the Fifth International Congress of the Collegium Internationale Neuro-psychopharmacologicum*. New York: Excerpta Medica Foundation, 1967.

Marks, I. Behavioral treatments of phobic and obsessive-compulsive disorders: A critical appraisal. In M. Hersen, R. M. Eisler, & P. M. Miller (Eds.), *Progress in Behavior Modification*, Vol. 1. New York: Academic, 1975.

Marks, I. "Psycholopharmacology": The use of drugs combined with psychological treatment. In R. L. Spitzer & D. F. Klein (Eds.), *Evaluation of psychological therapies: Psychotherapies, behavior therapies, drug therapies, and their interactions*. Baltimore: Johns Hopkins University Press, 1976.

Marks, I. M. *Fears and phobias*. New York: Academic, 1969.

Marks, I. M., Viswanathan, R., Lipsedge, M. S., & Gardner, R. Enhanced relief of phobias by flooding during waning diazepam effect. *British Journal of Psychiatry*, 1972, *121*, 493–506.

Mawson, A. B. Methohexitone-assisted desensitization in treatment of phobias. *Lancet*, 1970, *1*, 1084–1086.

Middaugh, S. Personal communication, 1978.

Miller, P. M., Hersen, M., Eisler, A. M., & Hilsman, G. Effects of social stress on operant drinking of alcoholics and social drinkers. *Behaviour Research and Therapy*, 1974, *12*, 67–72.

Overton, D. A. Dissociated learning in drug states (state dependent learning). In D. H. Efron (Ed.), *Psychopharmacology: A review of progress 1957–1967*. Washington, D.C.: U.S. Department of HEW, Publication No. 1836, 1968.

Overton, D. A. Discriminative control of behavior by drug states. In T. Thompson & R. Pickens (Eds.), *Stimulus properties of drugs*. New York: Appleton-Century-Crofts, 1971.

Overton, D. A. State-dependent learning produced by addicting drugs. *Psychopharmacology Bulletin*, 1973, *9*, 29–31.

Paul, G. L., Tobias, L. L., & Holly, B. L. Maintenance psychotropic drugs in the presence of active treatment programs: A "triple-blind" withdrawal study with long-term mental patients. *Archives of General Psychiatry* 1972, *27*, 106–115.

Perez-Cruet, J. Drug conditioning and drug effects on cardiovascular conditional functions. In T. Thompson & R. Pickens (Eds.), *Stimulus properties of drugs*. New York: Appleton-Century-Crofts, 1971.

Pickens, R., & Dougherty, J. A. Conditioning of the activity effects of drugs, In T. Thompson & R. Pickens (Eds.), *Stimulus properties of drugs*. New York: Appleton-Century-Crofts, 1971.

Pickens, R., & Thompson, T. Characteristics of stimulant drug reinforcement. In T. Thompson & R. Pickens (Eds.), *Stimulus properties of drugs*. New York: Appleton-Century-Crofts, 1971.

Razani, J. Treatment of phobias by systematic desensitization: Comparison of standard vs. methohexital-aided desensitization. *Archives of General Psychiatry*, 1974, *30*, 291–293.

Rescorla, R. A., & Solomon, R. L. Two-process learning theory: Relationships between Pavlovian conditioning and instrumental learning. *Psychological Review*, 1967, *74*, 151–182.

Rosenberg, C. M. Marijuana reinforcement of disulfiram use in the treatment of alcoholism. *Psychopharmacology Bulletin*, 1973, *9*(3), 25.

Ross, S. M., & Schwartz, C. W. State-dependent learning and its implications for treatment of drug-abusers. *Psychiatric Quarterly*, 1974, *48*, 368–373.

Rush, A. J., Beck, A. T., Kovacs, M., & Hollon, S. Comparative efficacy of cognitive therapy and pharmacotherapy in the treatment of depressed outpatients. *Cognitive Therapy and Research*, 1977, *1*, 17–37.

Rusk, H. A. *Rehabilitation Medicine*. St. Louis: Mosby, 1977.

Sachs, E., Weingarten, M., & Klein, N. W., Jr. Effects of chlordiazepoxide on the acquisition of avoidance learning and its transfer to the normal state and other drug conditions. *Psychopharmacologia*, 1966, *9*, 17–30.

Schooler, N. R. Antipsychotic drugs and psychological treatment in schizophrenia. In M. A. Lipton, A. DiMascio, & K. M. Killam (Eds.), *Psychopharmacology: A generation of progress*. New York: Raven, 1978.

Schuster, C. R., Smith, B. B., & Jaffe, J. H. Drug abuse in heroin users: An experimental study of self-administration of methadone, codeine, and pentazocine. *Archives of General Psychiatry*, 1971, *24*, 359–362.

Schuster, M. M. Constipation and anorectal disorders. *Clinics in Gastroenterology*, 1977, *6*, 643–658.

Seligman, M. E., & Groves, D. P. Nontransient learned helplessness. *Psychonomic Science*, 1970, *19*, 191–192.

Shafto, F. & Sulzbacher, S. Comparing treatment tactics with a hyperactive preschool child: Stimulant medication and programmed teacher intervention. *Journal of Applied Behavior Analysis*, 1977, *10*, 13–20.

Silverstein, S. J., Nathan, P. E., & Taylor, H. A. Blood alcohol level estimation and controlled drinking by chronic alcoholics. *Behavior Therapy*, 1974, *5*, 1–5.

Silverstone, J. T. Lorazepam in phobic disorders: A pilot study. *Current Medical Research and Opinion*, 1973, *1*, 272–275.

Silverstone, J. T., & Salkind, M. R. Controlled evaluation of intravenous drugs in the specific desensitization of phobias. *Canadian Psychiatric Association Journal*, 1973, *18*, 47–53.

Solyom, L., Heseltine, G. F. D., McClure, D. J., Solyom, C., Ledwidge, B., & Steinberg, G. Behaviour therapy versus drug therapy in the treatment of phobic neurosis. *Canadian Psychiatric Association Journal*, 1973, *18*, 25–32.

Stein, L. Reward transmitters: Catecholamines and opioid peptides. In M. A. Lipton, A. DiMascio, & K. F. Killam (Eds.), *Psychopharmacology: A generation of progress*. New York: Raven, 1978.

Strickler, D., Bigelow, G., Lawrence, C., & Liebson, I. Moderate drinking as an alternative to alcohol abuse: A non-aversive procedure. *Behaviour Research and Therapy*, 1976, *14*, 279–288.

Thompson, T., & Pickens, R. *Stimulus properties of drugs*. New York: Appleton-Century-Crofts, 1971.

Thompson, T., & Schuster, C. R. *Behavioral pharmacology*. Englewood Cliffs, N.J.: Prentice-Hall, 1968.

Todd, F. J. Coverant control of self-evaluative responses in the treatment of depression: A new use for an old principle. *Behavior Therapy*, 1972, *3*, 91–94.

Trapold, M. A. Unconditioned stimulus functions of drugs: Interpretations. II. In T. Thompson & R. Pickens (Eds.), *Stimulus properties of drugs*. New York: Appleton-Century-Crofts, 1971.

Tyrer, P. J., Candy, J., & Kelly, D. H. W. Phenelzine in phobic anxiety: A controlled trial. *Psychological Medicine*, 1973, *3*, 120–124.

Vogel-Sprott, M. Alcoholism and learning. In B. Kissin & H. Begleiter (Eds.), *The biology of alcoholism: Vol. 2. Physiology and behavior*. New York: Plenum, 1972.

Voss, E., Mejta, C., & Reid, L. Methods of deconditioning persisting avoidance: Response prevention and counterconditioning after extensive training. *Bulletin of the Psychonomic Society*, 1974, *3*, 345–347.

Weiss, T., & Engel, B. T. Operant conditioning of heart rate in patients with premature ventricular contractions. *Psychosomatic Medicine*, 1971, *33*, 301–321.

Weissman, M. M. Psychotherapy and its relevance to the pharmacotherapy of affective disorders: From ideology to evidence. In M. A. Lipton, A. DiMascio, & K. F. Killam (Eds.), *Psychopharmacology: A generation of progress*. New York: Raven, 1978.

Whitehead, W. E., Blackwell, B., & Robinson, A. Effects of diazepam on phobic avoidance behavior and phobic anxiety. *Biological Psychiatry*, 1978, *13*, 59–64.

Whitehead, W. E., Robinson, A., Blackwell, B., & Stutz, R. M. Flooding treatment of phobias: Does chronic diazepam increase effectiveness? *Journal of Behavior Therapy and Experimental Psychiatry*, 1978, *9*, 219–225.

Wilson, G. T., & Thomas, M. G. W. Self- versus drug-produced relaxation and the effects of instructional set in standardized systematic desensitization. *Behaviour Research and Therapy*, 1973, *11*, 279–288.

Winstead, D. K., Anderson, A., Eilers, M. K., Blackwell, B., & Zaremba, L. Diazepam on demand: Drug seeking behavior in psychiatric inpatients. *Archives of General Psychiatry*, 1974, *30*, 349–351.

Woods, J. H. Behavioral pharmacology of drug self-administration. In M. A. Lipton, A. DiMascio, & K. F. Killam (Eds.), *Psychopharmacology: A generation of progress*. New York: Raven, 1978.

Woods, J. H., & Schuster, C. R. Opiates as reinforcing stimuli. In T. Thompson & R. Pickens (Eds.), *Stimulus properties of drugs*. New York: Appleton-Century-Crofts, 1971.

Wooley, S., Blackwell, B., & Winget, C. A learning theory model of chronic illness behavior: Theory, treatment, and research. *Psychosomatic Medicine*, 1978, *40*, 379–401.

Wulbert, M., & Dries, R. The relative efficacy of methylphenidate (Ritalin) and behavior-modification techniques in the treatment of a hyperactive child. *Journal of Applied Behavior Analysis*, 1977, *10*, 21–31.

Yorkston, N. J., Sergeant, H. G. S., & Rachman, S. Methohexitone relaxation for desensitizing agoraphobic patients. *Lancet*, 1968, *2*, 651–653.

Zitrin, C. M., Klein, D. F., Lindemann, C., Tobak, P., Rock, M., Kaplan, J. H., & Ganz, V. H. Comparison of short-term treatment regimens in phobic patients: A preliminary report. In R. L. Spitzer & D. F. Klein (Eds.), *Evaluation of psychological therapies: Psychotherapies, behavior therapies, drug therapies and their interactions*. Baltimore: Johns Hopkins University Press, 1976.

8
Stress, Coping, and the Treatment of Stress-Related Illness

KENNETH A. HOLROYD

> One's lifestyle, including patterns of eating, exercise, drinking, coping with stress, and use of tobacco and drugs, together with environmental hazards, are the major known modifiable causes of illness in America today. Medical care, on which we spend so much has, in comparison, only a weak effect on health. (Haggerty, 1977)

> Men as a rule find it easier to depend on healers than to attempt the more difficult task of living wisely. (Dubos, 1961)

Disease patterns in Western countries have shifted dramatically in the last century. In 1900, the leading causes of death tended to be infectious diseases; however, by mid-century they had become chronic diseases. For example, in 1968, the likelihood of dying from an infectious disease was one-sixth what it was in 1900, but the death rate from heart disease had increased by 268%. Current predictions indicate that over 80% of the male children born this year will eventually die of chronic diseases (Glazier, 1973). Moreover, chronic diseases are on the increase among the young as well as the old (Erhardt & Berlin, 1974; National Center for Health Statistics, 1977).

These figures reflect the impressive gains that have been made in the treatment of acute illness and the control of communicable disease. Unfortunately, they also reflect the failure of our medical care system to control disorders that result largely from the lifestyle variables described by Haggerty. When prevention or treatment requires changes in these areas, our medical care system, which is largely crisis-oriented, often proves impotent.

The present chapter focuses on one of the most controversial of these lifestyle variables, the individual's response to stress and its role in disease. Stress research

KENNETH A. HOLROYD • Department of Psychology, Ohio University, Athens, Ohio 45701. Support for the preparation of this chapter and some of the research reported here were provided by a grant from the Ohio University College of Osteopathic Medicine.

and behavior therapy appear to be converging; as the dependence of stress responses on cognitive processes becomes increasingly clear, behavior therapists are increasingly focusing on the cognitive processes underlying behavior change. As a result, developments in stress research may have important implications for behavioral medicine. In this chapter, some of these implications are discussed, and the value of a cognitive–behavioral approach to stress-related illness is explored.

STRESS AND DISEASE: CONCEPTUAL PROBLEMS

One reason confusion surrounds the stress concept is that it has been formulated in several ways, and these different formulations suggest distinct research questions and approaches to the problems of stress and disease. There appear to have been three main types of formulations: (1) most frequently, stress refers to a certain class of environmental events that are likely to impose unusual demands upon the individual; (2) alternately, stress refers to the individual's response to such demands; (3) finally, stress has been conceptualized in relational terms as a certain type of transaction with the environment.

Stress as an Environmental Event

Stress most commonly refers to an environmental event or crisis that is thrust upon the individual, taxing available resources and requiring unusual responses from the individual. Thus, obviously disruptive events, such as tornados, earthquakes, or fires (Birnbaum, Coplon, & Scharff, 1976); imprisonment (Spaulding & Ford, 1976), military combat (Bourne, 1969); the death of a family member (Parkes, 1972); the birth of a child (Dyer, 1976); change of residence (Levine, 1976); and physical injury and disability (Hamburg, Hamburg, & DeGoza, 1953), are referred to as stressful events, and individuals experiencing such events are regarded as being "stressed".

The approach to stress and disease that is most consistent with this conceptualization of stress as an environmental event is the research on the relationship between life events and disease stimulated by Holmes and Rahe (Holmes & Masuda, 1974; Rabkin & Struening, 1976). This research developed out of the finding that individuals can reliably provide estimates of the degree of adaptation required by specific life events (Holmes & Rahe, 1967). For the most part, research to date has focused on determining if the occurrence of events requiring greater adaptation (stressful events) will increase the likelihood of subsequent bodily disease. As several reviewers have noted (e.g., Lazarus & Launier, 1978), this research strategy is analogous to the stimulus–response (S–R) approach within psychology in that no references are made to variables mediating between environmental events and illness outcomes.

In spite of the growing number of studies reporting relationships between stressful life events and illness (see Holmes & Masuda, 1974, and Rabkin & Struening, 1976, for references), methodological problems limit the overall conclusions that can be drawn from this work. The life events questionnaires that are employed as independent variables have been criticized for yielding unreliable scores, at least for some populations (Sarason, 1975), and for including items (e.g., changes in sleeping and eating habits) that are as likely to reflect the presence of illness as the occurrence of an event that is independent of illness (Hudgens, 1974). The dependent measures of illness that have been employed, such as self-reports of illness or medical self-referral, have also been criticized as reflecting variables other than the actual presence of illness, particularly when the illnesses consist largely of minor respiratory problems, influenza, colds, etc. (Mechanic, 1972, 1974). Thus, truly prospective studies of serious illness that control some of these sources of error may find no significant relationship between stressful events and illness (Faire & Theorell, 1977; Hinkle, 1974). Even when relationships are found, they are typically small in magnitude. For example, in a study of 2,500 naval enlisted men aboard three heavy cruisers, correlations between life change scores and subsequent illness reports did not exceed .16 (Rahe, 1974). In a recent review of this literature, Rabkin and Struening (1976) concluded, "In practical terms . . . life event scores have not been shown to be predictors of the probability of future illness" (p. 1015).

An increasing number of investigators appear, at least implicitly, to be recognizing that a strong relationship between life events and illness is unlikely to be found if the way the individual interprets and copes with events is ignored. This trend is evident in current distinctions that are being made among life events. It has been suggested that positive events (Kellam, 1974), or events that induce psychophysiological strain (Garrity, Marx, & Somes, 1977), or involve a sense of mastery (Mechanic, 1974), or are unanticipated, or are not within the individual's control (Dohrenwend & Dohrenwend, 1974) should be distinguished from other life events; or even that events that are desired or anticipated but do not occur (Gersten, Langner, Eisenberg, & Orzek, 1974) contribute to illness. Furthermore, researchers are increasingly suggesting that the resources available to an individual for coping with environmental change and physiological arousal, as well as the occurrence of stressful events, must be evaluated if useful predictions are to be obtained (Antonovsky, 1974; Mattila & Solokangas, 1977; Mechanic, 1974; Rabkin & Struening, 1976; Rahe & Ransom, 1978). For example, in a methodological review of this work, Mechanic (1974) recommended that "as our research develops we need to give greater attention to such variables as coping skills and supportive relationships that may intervene between the occurrence of life events and the initiation of illness" (p. 92).

A recent review of epidemiological research examining the social variables associated with disease has similarly concluded that the impact of environmental events can be understood only in the context of the resources that are available for coping with them (Cassel, 1975, 1976). A study of pregnancy and birth complications by Nuckolls, Cassel, and Kaplan (1972) illustrates the way in which a consideration of coping resources might increase the predictive utility of life event questionnaires. In this study, neither a measure of stressful events (Holmes & Rahe, 1967) nor an index of psychosocial coping resources assessing variables such as the woman's perception of her ability to cope with pregnancy and delivery and the support available from husband, family, and community was related to medical complications. However, when these factors were considered jointly, a strong relationship emerged. Of the women with high life-change scores but low coping-resource scores, 90% had one or more complications, while only 33% of the women with equally high life-change scores, but high coping-resource scores, exhibited similar complications. Thus, the influence of stressful life events on health was evident only when resources for coping with these events were not available. It would seem reasonable to expect that a consideration of the way coping resources are employed would further clarify the effects of stressful life events on health because individuals are likely to differ in the way they employ and utilize available resources for coping with stress.

Stress as a Response

Stress has also been conceptualized, most commonly within the biological sciences, as a physiological response of the organism (e.g., Cannon, 1932; Selye, 1974). Thus, Selye's (1956, 1974, 1976) purely physiological definition of stress as the "nonspecific response of the body to any demand made upon it" has profoundly influenced a generation of investigators. Selye has argued for some time that there is a coordinated syndrome of physiological responses, termed the *general adaptation syndrome*, that is elicited by any demand or stress to which the organism is exposed. He has further argued that it is the prolonged or repeated elicitation of the general adaptation syndrome, or defects in this coordinated pattern of responses, that lies at the root of a large number of stress-related disorders, including cardiovascular and renal diseases, hypertension, peptic ulcers, migraine headaches, and numerous others.

It is only recently that the influential role of psychological processes in determining the physiological stress responses identified by Selye is beginning to be recognized. Because injurious agents (such as bacteria, toxins, and physical mutilation) are typically employed to elicit stress responses, Selye's research has eloquently documented the role of the pituitary–adrenal cortical axis in the organism's response to a wide variety of physical demands, but it has provided little information concerning psychological variables that might influence this response. However, recently Mason (1968, 1971, 1974; Mason, Maher, Hartley, Mougey, Perlow, & Jones, 1976) has convincingly argued that the stress responses identified by Selye are typically mediated by psychological variables. Mason has reviewed an impressive body of evidence indicating that psychological influences are among the most potent stimuli known to affect pituitary–adrenal cortical activity (1968, 1971), and he presented additional data indicating that a number of physical stressors fail to elicit adaptive hormonal responses when emotional distress that typically accompanies their administration is eliminated (1971, 1975). Mason concluded that the stress responses that Selye has identified are typically elicited by the organism's appraisal of "threatening or unpleasant factors in the life situation as a whole" (1971, p. 327).

Weiss has also documented the role of psychological factors in the development of the "stress ulcers" that were originally identified as part of the alarm stage of the general adaptation syndrome. In an ingenious series of experiments, Weiss (1972, 1977) has shown that ulceration is more profoundly influenced by variables such as the predictability and controllability of the stressor, the presence of conflict, and the availability of coping responses than by mere exposure to the stressor. For example, when stimulus conditions are arranged so the animals make aggressive coping responses, they show considerably less ulceration than when they do not make these responses, even though the responses have no effect on the stressor (electric shock). In summarizing this work, Weiss (1977) concluded that "psychological factors can be even more important than a physical stressor in determining the severity of gastric pathology" (p. 267).

More recently, Selye seems to have modified his original formulation by distinguishing two types of stress: the "pleasant stress of fulfillment and victory," which is *eustress* desirable, is distinguished from the "self-destructive distress of failure, frustration, *distress* hatred, and the passion for revenge" (1974, pp. 133–134). As Lazarus (1976) has noted, Selye has failed to make clear whether these two types of stress are distinguished by their psychological or their physiological characteristics. However, it is clear that Selye has been asserting that psychological variables (attitudes, values, motivations) influence the individual's response to stress, either by short-circuiting the general adaptation syndrome or by minimizing the physical ravages of this syndrome when it occurs, or both. In fact, Selye (1978) has indicated that by adopting the right attitude, "one can convert a negative stress into a positive one" (p. 63). *appraisals*

To the extent that physiological stress responses are elicited and controlled by psychological influences, or the effects of these responses on health are mediated by psychological variables, stress-related diseases have a significant psychological component. It then becomes crucially important to identify these psychological factors and to determine, as a prominent endocrinologist has noted, "What psychological mechanisms is this person using at this moment as he reacts to this life event?" (Mason, 1970, p. 434). This brings us to a third formulation of stress.

Transactional Approach

The third approach, and the one that is adopted here, explicitly focuses on those mediating psychological processes that have been included only as an afterthought in the previous two formulations. Here stress refers, most generally, to a transaction between a system (individual, biological, or social) and its environment, so that the adaptive resources of the system are taxed or strained (Lazarus, 1966; Lazarus & Launier, 1978). Thus, at the individual level, stress is not defined solely by the adaptive demands confronting an individual (e.g., Holmes & Rahe), or solely in terms of the individual's response to these demands (e.g., Selye), but by both factors and, most importantly, by the cognitive processes mediating them. The basic assumption of this approach is that these mediating processes profoundly influence the physiological state of the organism and, thus, the development of stress-related disorders.

Some years ago, Wolff (1950) presented a rudimentary transactional model of stress, emphasizing cognitive appraisals of threat and adaptive physiological response patterns.[1] According to this formulation, stress diseases result when appraisals of threat repeatedly elicit stereotyped patterns of physiological response, appro-

[1] Although Wolff conceptualized stress in a number of ways over the years (Hinkle, 1974), he came to agree that stress was present "when the adaptive mechanisms of the living organism—in this instance, man—are taxed or strained" (Wolf & Goodell, 1968, p. 252).

priate to physical threats but ineffective in coping with the interpersonal or symbolic threats actually confronting the individual. Wolff argued that physiological adjustments, such as the increased peripheral resistance occurring in essential hypertension, although representing an appropriate response to physical threat, are debilitating because they are repeatedly evoked in response to social or symbolic demands.

Although the details of his theoretical formulations have been questioned, Wolff and his associates (Grace, Wolf, & Wolff, 1951; Wolf, 1965; Wolf, Cardon, Shepard, & Wolff, 1950; Wolf & Goodell, 1968; Wolff, Wolf, & Hare, 1950) provided a valuable service by demonstrating that psychosocial stimuli are capable of eliciting physiological changes that mimic or reproduce pathological responses associated with specific disease states (e.g., gastric hyperacidity and hypermotility, tachycardia, hypertension, and numerous others). For example, in one group of studies employing stress interviews, the interviewer either interacted with the patient in a supportive manner or responded skeptically and introduced anxiety-arousing topics in an A-B-A design. This interview procedure proved capable of eliciting a variety of symptoms in susceptible individuals, including migraine, asthma, hay fever, eczema, and cardiospasms, and of increasing blood pressure and cholesterol level. In a second series of studies, patients' diaries, their verbal reports, or physicians' judgments were employed to evaluate relationships between psychological stress and physical symptoms. These indices of psychological distress were associated with disorders ranging from hypertension, cardiovascular disease, and diabetes to eczema, glaucoma, and rhinitis. Although these studies often failed to meet current methodological standards, they demonstrated that a wide variety of physiological responses and psychosomatic symptoms could be influenced by psychological stress.

Unfortunately, Wolff largely ignored the ways in which psychological means of coping with threat can influence stress responses. In fact, patients' cognitive and behavioral responses to the stress interviews were seldom described; only physiological data were presented. More recent conceptual analyses of stress have increasingly sought to understand the psychological processes that are employed to manage stress (e.g., Folkins, 1970; Haan, 1977; Lazarus & Launier, 1978; Murphy & Moriarty, 1976; Weisman & Worden, 1976).

In what is perhaps the best articulated of these formulations, Lazarus and his co-workers (Lazarus, 1966, 1976; Lazarus & Launier, 1978) have suggested that psychological influences on stress responses can be conceptualized in terms of interactions between appraisal and coping processes. *Appraisal* refers to ongoing evaluations of events in terms of their significance for the person's well-being (primary appraisal) or in terms of the available resources or options that the individual possesses for responding (secondary appraisal). *Coping* refers to activity that is designed to manage or control stress.

Lazarus's framework allows the mediating cognitive and behavioral processes to be categorized in a number of useful ways. For example, effective coping strategies for managing harm that has already occurred can be distinguished from those that are effective in governing responses to anticipated threat. Similarly, coping responses directed toward altering the environment can be distinguished from those serving to regulate the individual's emotional state; and different modes of coping, such as direct action, information seeking, and inhibition of action, can be systematically distinguished from one another and studied (Lazarus & Launier, 1978). Furthermore, treatment procedures can be designed to alter these appraisal and coping processes, and their effects on stress responses and stress-related symptoms can be evaluated (e.g., Holroyd, Andrasik, & Westbrook, 1977).

This formulation suggests at least three ways that dysfunctional patterns of coping with environmental demands might contribute to illness. By increasing the frequency, intensity, or character of the individual's stressful transactions with the environment, physiological regulatory processes might be disrupted (Schwartz, 1977). This disregulation could trigger symptoms in otherwise susceptible individuals or sufficiently alter the tissue state of the organism so as to be of primary etiological significance, as has been hypothesized in the case of coronary heart disease (Glass, 1977). Second, certain patterns of coping might directly expose the body to injurious physical agents, such as alcohol, tobacco smoke, or allergens. Finally, ways of coping with the symptoms of illness, such as minimizing their seriousness (e.g., Gentry, 1975; Pranulis, 1975) or persisting in attempts to cope with disability (Kinsman, Dahlem, Spector, & Staudenmayer, 1977), can influence the course of the illness and/or the medical care that is received.

PSYCHOPHYSIOLOGY OF STRESS

A few environments may be so profoundly debilitating, both physically and psychologically, that they impair the health of almost anyone who is exposed to them. Thus, there is some evidence of the long-term health consequences of internment in concentration camps during World War II (e.g., Eitinger & Strom, 1973). Extremely stressful work environments may also elicit physiological stress responses from most workers (Frankenhaeuser, 1976) and impair the health of a substantial number of individuals exposed to them (Cobb & Rose, 1973). The identification and modification of such toxic environments should be a top priority so that people are not faced with the choice between unemployment or ill health.

When environmental demands are less salient, stressful transactions are shaped as much by the individual as by the environment (Bandura, 1977; Mischell, 1973). Appraisals of internal and external demands and attempts to cope with these demands then profoundly influence stress responses. Of course, these psychological variables are probably also capable of influencing physiological stress responses in situations where environmental threats are salient (e.g., life threatening combat; Bourne, 1969). However, in everyday situations, where environmental demands are likely to be ambiguous and complex, psychological factors are likely to be of paramount importance.

Two general types of hypotheses have been offered concerning the influence of psychological variables on physiological stress responses. On one hand, the patterning of physiological stress responses has been regarded as largely biologically determined. According to this view, psychological threats elicit preprogrammed biological reaction patterns, such as the fight or flight reaction or the general adaptation syndrome. However, biological vulnerabilities, and not psychological vulnerabilities, determine the particular disorder that results when the stereotyped defensive reaction is repeatedly elicited. This hypothesis has been presented in various forms by Selye (1956), Cannon (1936), and Wolff (1950).

An alternate hypothesis holds that the patterning of physiological stress responses is dependent upon the specifics of the individual's interaction with the environment. According to this view, stress responses are shaped in significant ways by psychological variables: certain patterns of psychological responses are expected to be associated with specific physiological response patterns and thus predispose the individual to develop certain disorders but not others. This hypothesis has been articulated in various forms by Mason (1975) and Lazarus (1977).

Early attempts to evaluate these hypotheses tended to focus exclusively on emotional responses to stress. Findings from these studies have tended to support the first hypothesis; neither autonomic nor hormonal measures have proved capable of reliably distinguishing different stress emotions (Lacey, 1967; Oken, 1967). These results have led many investigators to conclude that attempts to relate specific psychological variables to identifiable stress responses are probably fruitless.

However, recent evidence suggests that when cognitive and behavioral rather than emotional responses to stress are examined, specific patterns of coping may be associated with identifiable patterns of physiological response. For example, Obrist (1976) has reviewed evidence indicating that during passive coping, such as occurs during classical aversive conditioning, the heart appears to be under vagal control, while blood pressure is dominated by vascular processes. However, during active coping, such as occurs during shock avoidance, the heart is under sympathetic control, and cardiac influences on blood pressure become dominant. In this case, different coping responses are associated with different underlying physiological mechanisms. Obrist (1976) further suggested that active coping, with its attendant cardiovascular mobilization, is likely to be implicated in stress-related cardiovascular disorders, while passive coping, with its associated vagal excitation, might be implicated in the development of gastrointestinal lesions.

Lacey (1967) has also disputed the view that the autonomic nervous system responds in a uniform manner to stress. He has reviewed evidence indicating that the patterning of activity reflects the specific "intended interaction between the organism and its environment" (p. 25) and not simply a more general state of arousal. In his own work, Lacey has shown that the heart-rate response is bidirectional: decreases in heart rate and vasoconstriction in the skeletal muscles are associated with attempts to detect stimuli, even those that are potentially threatening, whereas heart-rate increases and vasodilation are associated with the rejection of environmental stimuli (e.g., Lacey, Kagan, Lacey, & Moss, 1963; Lacey & Lacey, 1978). This response pattern thus reflects attentional activity and not simply arousal. Other autonomic nervous system end organ reactions, such as the electrodermal response, may similarly reflect both cognitive coping activity and arousal (e.g., Kilpatrik, 1972). The implications of these findings seem clear: autonomic responses to stress are, to some extent, patterned in accordance with the demands confronting the organism and the coping responses that these demands generate. This relationship between the patterning of autonomic response and coping activity is discussed in more detail in Holroyd and Appel (1979).

The way the individual copes with environmental demands also appears to shape hormonal responses to stress (Katz, Weiner, Gallagher, & Hellman, 1970; Wolff, Friedman, Hofer, & Mason, 1964). Thus, clinical observations of the parents of leukemic children indicate that 17-OHCS levels are sensitive to differences in the coping strategies adapted by parents (Wolff *et al.*, 1964). Parents who deny or minimize the implications of medical information may effectively maintain low 17-OHCS levels. If these strategies are disrupted, however, they may show sudden changes in hormone level. Similarly, variables such as the amount of control exerted over stressor stimuli and the availability of a coping response have been found to influence catecholamine responses to stress (Frankenhaeuser, 1976; Frankenhaeuser & Rissler, 1970; Weiss, Glazer, & Pohorecky, 1976). In particular, plasma and urinary norepinephrine levels remain elevated in individuals actively coping with a stressor (Frankenhaeuser, 1971; Frankenhaeuser & Rissler, 1970; Weiss, Stone, & Harrell, 1970), while substantial depletions in brain norepinephrine appear to occur when an individual responds with helplessness (e.g., Weiss *et al.*, 1976). In a review of the implications of recent work in endocrinology for psychosomatic medicine, John Mason (1975) has concluded that

> the new knowledge that highly complicated psychological influences are superimposed upon the hormonal machinery for endocrine regulation raises the possibility that disorders of bodily function may result when the more complex, and probably more fallible, psychological machinery preempts, disrupts, or otherwise works at odds against the simpler, lower-level, hormonal machinery of endocrine regulation. (p. 576)

Mason has also presented evidence for some time indicating that the patterning of the neurohormonal responses is influenced by the nature of the individual's interaction with the environment (e.g., Mason, 1968, 1971, 1975; Mason *et al.*, 1976). Rather than monitoring the levels of one or two hormones, he has simultaneously assessed changing levels of as many as nine hormones in situations where humans or animals are exposed to stress. Results from these studies indicate that hormone levels do not change in unison but change in different temporal sequences and in different relationships to one another in response to different stressors. On the basis of these findings, Mason has argued that different types of stressful transactions are probably associated with characteristic hormonal profiles, which may, in turn, predispose individuals to develop certain stress disorders and not others. Mason (1970) has therefore argued that research on the patterning of neurohormonal responses to stress may shed light not only on the neurohormonal precursors to stress disorders but also on the associated psychological and behavioral risk factors.

Of course, stress responses are not likely to be uniquely determined by the coping processes that are called into play in managing stressful transactions; there is a limited plasticity to these responses. Nonetheless, the above findings suggest that self-regulatory or coping processes may be capable of sufficiently altering the physiological state of the organism so as to predispose the individual to specific stress disorders. It is only recently, however, that attempts to identify such psychological predisposing factors have begun to prove successful.

PSYCHOLOGICAL FACTORS IN DISEASE

Early Theories: Personality and Psychosomatic Disorder

During the 1950s a variety of hypotheses were proposed concerning psychological characteristics that rendered individuals vulnerable to stress-related disorders (Hamilton, 1955). Within psychoanalysis, hypotheses were formulated in terms of psychological conflicts (Alexander, 1950), maternal dynamics (Gerard, 1953; Spitz, 1951), unconscious symbolism (Garma, 1950), and physiological regression (Margolin, 1953). Hypotheses were also formulated in terms of attitudes (Grace & Graham, 1952), chronic emotional states (Mahl, 1950), and personality types (Dunbar, 1935). Although different terminologies were used, these hypotheses were quite similar in form; in each instance, specific personality variables were hypothesized to predispose individuals to develop certain psychosomatic symptoms.

Support for etiological hypotheses of this sort requires prospective research, where psychological characteristics are assessed in healthy individuals, and the utility of these assessments in predicting the subsequent development of disease is evaluated (Weiss, 1977). Unfortunately, the prospective research that would be necessary to establish specific personality characteristics as risk factors for particular psychosomatic disorders has not been reported. In fact, only one well-controlled prospective study—evaluating a modified version of Alexander's conflict theory—has appeared since these hypotheses were formulated. This study (Weiner, Thaler, Reiser, & Mirsky, 1957) and a subsequent replication (Cohen, Silverman, Waddell, & Zuidema, 1961) are critiqued in the chapter by Whitehead, Fedoravicius, Blackwell, and Wooley in this volume.

Although there has been little prospective research, a large number of investigators have examined the personality correlates of different psychosomatic disorders. In general, the research has failed to support the psychosomatic hypotheses formulated during the 1950s. Current reviews of the personality correlates of tension and migraine headache (Bakal, 1975), duodenal ulcer (Yager & Weiner, 1971), essential hypertension (Davies, 1971), and coronary heart disease (Mordkoff & Parsons, 1968) have reached similar conclusions: when trait or psychodynamically based assessment procedures are employed, there is no convincing evidence of personality characteristics specific to these disorders. Not only are the personality characteristics of individuals suffering from different psychosomatic disorders often quite similar, but studies reporting differences are usually methodologically flawed. For example, in his review, Graham (1972) noted that only a few studies controlled for experimenter bias by employing experimentally blind interviewers or evaluators. Other problems have typically included the use of clinical evaluations of doubtful reliability (e.g., Alexander, 1953) and psychiatric referrals, who differ significantly from the more general population of individuals with psychosomatic disorders (e.g., Robinson, 1964).

More than two decades have passed since personality variables were systematically proposed as etiologically significant factors in psychosomatic disorders. However, there is still no reliable evidence indicating that either trait or psychodynamically based assessment procedures are capable of identifying personality variables that are pathogenic for specific psychosomatic disorders. As a result, the psychosomatic hypotheses formulated during the last few decades appear less tenable than they did when they were proposed, and interest in these formulations appears to be declining (Lipowski, 1977; Wittkower, 1977).

On the other hand, the utility of behavioral assessment procedures for identifying psychological factors contributing to stress-related disorders has yet to be systematically evaluated. Recent research on the coronary-prone behavior pattern suggests that results with behaviorally focused assessment procedures may be quite different than those obtained with traditional assessment procedures.

Recent Developments: The Coronary-Prone Behavior Pattern

Type A or coronary-prone behavior has most commonly been assessed by means of a standardized stress interview that is designed to elicit a representative sample of the behavior of interest. These behaviors are characterized as chronically hurried, intensely competitive, and frequently aggressive or hostile, characteristics that are assumed to be revealed more clearly in the subject's overt behavior (e.g., bodily movement, explosive accentuations of speech, interruptions of the interviewer) than in the content of the subject's responses to interview questions. Recently, a convenient self-administered questionnaire inquiring about specific behavior (e.g., "Do you ever set quotas for yourself at work or at home?") or typical reactions of others to the individual's behavior (e.g., "Has your spouse or some friend ever told you that you eat too fast?") has been developed. Although both assessment techniques have been shown to successfully predict the occurrence of coronary heart disease in large-scale predictive studies, prediction may be somewhat better with the added information available from the interview (Rowland & Sokol, 1977; Scherwitz, Berton, & Leventhal, 1977; Schucker & Jacobs, 1977). Since both the questionnaire and the stress interview focus on specific overt behaviors, it is not surprising that the coronary-prone behavior pattern is only weakly associated with performance on standardized personality tests (Caffrey, 1968; Glass, 1977; Rosenman, Rahe, Borhani, & Feinleib, 1974).

In spite of the fact that Type A behavior has only recently been studied systematically, a considerable body of research has associated this behavior pattern with coronary heart disease. A recent review cites 21 studies, including 8 prospective studies, that related the coronary-prone behavior pattern to some manifestation of coronary heart disease (Jenkins, 1976). For example, in one well-controlled prospective study, 3,154 men employed in 10 California companies were examined yearly for 8½ years. Men who exhibited Type A behavior at the beginning of the study showed twice the rate of new coronary heart disease and were five times more likely to have a second myocardial infarct during the follow-up period than men not exhibiting Type A behavior. Moreover, multiple regression analysis revealed that this effect could not be explained by the influence of other associated risk factors (e.g., serum lipids, blood pressure, and cigarette smoking). In fact, Friedman (1977) has recently argued that most of the major risk factors "may arise from, and certainly are aggravated by, the prior existence of Type A behavior" (p. 1).

At present, it appears that the pathogenic effects of the coronary-prone behavior pattern may be limited to coronary heart disease (Kenigsberg, Zyzanski, Jenkins, Wardwell, & Licciardello, 1974) and, more specifically, that different components of this behavior pattern may be related to different manifestations of this disorder (e.g., Jenkins, Zyzanski, & Rosenman, 1978). However, the occurrence of other disorders in individuals exhibiting this behavior pattern has not been studied in detail. It is thus possible that the behavior pattern is associated with other disorders as well (Friedman, 1969; Glass, 1977). In any case, consistent findings of well-controlled studies associating Type A behavior with coronary heart disease stand in sharp contrast with the apparent inability of traditional assessment techniques to identify personality variables associated with this disorder (Mordkoff & Parsons, 1968).

The resources of the psychological laboratory are increasingly being employed in more fine-grained analyses of the coronary-prone behavior pattern. Recent studies have shown that the pressured, competitive, and hostile behaviors associated with this behavior pattern are exhibited in a predictable manner in a variety of laboratory situations (Burnam, Pennebaker, & Glass, 1973; Carver, Coleman, & Glass, 1976; Glass, 1977; Glass, Snyder, & Hollis, 1974); that these behaviors are elicited by laboratory stress (Dembroski & MacDougall, 1978; Glass, 1977; Krantz, Glass, & Snyder, 1974) and real-life stress (Howard, Cunningham, & Rechnitzer, 1976); and that they are associated with elevated cardiovascular (Dembroski, MacDougall, & Shields, 1977) and neurohormonal (Friedman, Byers, Diamant, & Rosenman, 1975) stress responses.

Drawing largely on his own research, Glass (1977) has argued that this behavior pattern can be understood as a characteristic "style of responding to environmental stress which is appraised as a threat to the individual's sense of control" (p. 164). In a series of studies, he has provided evidence indicating that the coronary-prone behavior pattern is characterized by exaggerated attempts to control stressful stimuli that are followed by excessive helplessness when coping behaviors are ineffective. Glass (1977) further suggested that the dramatic fluctuations in catecholamine levels (particularly norepinephrine and epinephrine) associated with this coping behavior serve as the intermediary process whereby responses to stressful events induce biochemical and pathogenic phenomena leading to coronary heart disease. This formulation thus associates a specific style of coping with stress with a specific mediating pattern of physiological responses that contribute to pathogenic events for coronary heart disease.

Although additional research will be required before this formulation of the coronary-prone behavior pattern can be evaluated, this analysis is valuable because it focuses our attention on specific factors that render this behavior pattern costly to the individual's health. The development of systematic therapeutic interventions for stress-related disorders will probably be dependent upon such careful functional analysis of stress responses.

Additional research is also needed on stress-related behavior patterns that might be associated with disorders other than coronary heart disease. For example, we do not understand why some young people exhibiting labile hypertension subsequently develop essential hypertension while other, apparently similar individuals do not. It is reasonable to expect that certain types of repeatedly stressful transactions with the environment may be a contributing factor. An increased understanding of these interactions would facilitate both the identification and the preventive treatment of individuals at risk for hypertension.

TREATMENT

Biofeedback research has dominated the literature on the behavioral treatment of psychosomatic disorders in recent years (Price, 1974; Price, Gaas-Abrams, & Browder, 1977). For the most part, controlled-outcome research has been limited to the evaluation of biofeedback therapy and relaxation training. Since this literature has been amply reviewed (Blanchard, this volume; Blanchard & Epstein, 1978; Blanchard & Young, 1974; Miller, 1978; Shapiro & Surwit, 1976), the present discussion will emphasize some of the limitations of biofeedback and argue that an alternate treatment approach designed to alter the way individuals cope with daily life stresses may be more useful than biofeedback procedures in many instances.

Biofeedback

A great deal of the current interest in biofeedback appears to derive from the hope that this technology can be used effectively in the treatment of psychosomatic disorders (Birk, 1973; Shapiro & Surwit, 1976). This hope assumes that biofeedback can be used to teach people to control symptom-related physiological responses in the situations outside the laboratory where problems typically occur (Blanchard & Epstein, 1978). Although, in at least one instance, it has been suggested that training might alter the organism in such a way that symptoms would be automatically inhibited (Sterman, 1974), at present there is limited support for this contention (Mostofsky & Balaschak, 1977). It thus appears that effective symptom control generally requires that the client actively modify symptom-related physiological responses in the situations where these responses typically occur.

If stress reactions are highly dependent upon cognitive and behavioral responses to environmental demands, it is likely to prove difficult to control specific physiological responses without more comprehensively altering the individual's interaction with the environment. Often people are simply unable to control specific physiological reactions while they engage in transactions with the environment that generate the very responses they are attempting to control. In such instances, symptoms may more effectively be modified indirectly by altering environmental demands or cognitive and behavioral responses to these demands (Miller, 1976; Schwartz, 1977).

Problems that are likely to be encountered in the treatment of stress-related symptoms with biofeedback can be illustrated with the example of a 34-year-old secretary treated for chronic tension headache. In this instance, careful monitoring revealed that this woman's headaches inevitably began in the afternoon on the days she was at work, although they often continued into the evening, preventing her from sleeping without the aid of medication. An analysis of the situations in which the headaches occurred revealed that she was unable to allow herself to leave work uncompleted. As a result, she became increasingly tense and worried as the working day neared an end whenever work remained. In addition, her frantic attempts to finish work were frequently exploited by others, who delegated her additional "top-priority" tasks. Increasingly severe headache symptoms toward the end of the day elicited only additional worry that the pain might prevent her from completing any remaining work.

This woman was able to exercise considerable control over frontalis muscle activity in the laboratory, but she was apparently unable to do so at work because she feared that taking time to relax was a sign of laziness and would interfere with her work. Only when these stringent performance expectations were questioned and the costs of her behavior carefully pointed out was she able to adopt a reasonable pace of work, even though all her work might not be completed. As she changed her behavior, her headaches gradually declined and disappeared.

Although the effective elements of treatment are not evident in a case study of this sort, it does appear that the manner in which this woman coped with the demands she perceived in her work environment not only contributed to her tension headaches but prevented her from employing the skills learned in biofeedback training.

A recent analysis of the precipitants of childhood asthma also illustrates the way coping behavior and symptoms are often intertwined. Weiss (1977) noted that episodes of asthma are more often elicited indirectly by the child's coping behavior than more directly by emotional arousal. For example, a child who is sensitive to peer rejection may engage in strenuous athletic activities in an attempt to gain peer approval, even though this behavior aggravates the child's asthma. In this instance, biofeedback procedures designed to modify airway resistance may be of little use if the child cannot resist engaging in the physical activity that precipitates the attacks.

Self-regulation of other physiological responses is equally likely to be disrupted by stressful transactions outside the laboratory. For example, researchers have frequently reported that reductions in blood pressure attained in the laboratory are readily disrupted by extralaboratory stress (Miller, 1969; Schwartz, 1973). When this occurs, biofeedback training by itself may prove to be of limited therapeutic benefit.

In some instances, biofeedback training may be effective because it indirectly induces patients to alter their interactions with the environment, not because it enables them to directly control problematic physiological responses. Thus, Holroyd and Andrasik (1978b) have suggested that clients receiving electromyographic feedback for tension headaches often control their headaches by altering cognitive and behavioral responses to stressful situations rather than by directly reducing muscle tension levels. In such cases, biofeedback training is probably effective because it sensitizes clients to tension-eliciting situations and motivates them to find alternative ways of coping with them. When biofeedback works in this manner, there may be little relationship between the ability to directly control muscle tension and headache improvement (Epstein & Abel, 1977; Holroyd *et al.*, 1977).

A recent study of the treatment of tension headache provides support for this contention (Andrasik & Holroyd, 1978). Headache sufferers received feedback for either increasing or decreasing frontalis muscle activity, or they received feedback from an inelevant muscle group (forearm flexor), so that frontalis muscle activity remained constant. Although clients showed appropriate changes in muscle tension (increase, decrease, or no change) both during and following treatment, all clients were led to believe that they were learning to reduce their tension levels. Clients in all three treatment groups showed substantial reductions in headache activity relative to a wait-list control group, irrespective of the actual feedback they received. Interview data further suggested that clients in all the groups controlled their headaches by changing the way they coped with headache-eliciting situations.

Most of the research that will be necessary to evaluate the effectiveness of biofeedback as a treatment for psychosomatic disorders remains to be done (Miller & Dworkin, 1977; Shapiro & Surwit, 1976). Existing research does indicate that clients will need to alter their cognitive and behavioral responses to environmental demands if gains attained in the laboratory are to be extended to other situations (Lynn & Freedman, 1979). It is therefore crucial that treatment procedures be developed that focus on altering cognitive and behavioral responses to stress, in addition to physiological responses.

Stress-Coping Training

Whenever symptoms are aggravated or maintained by stressful transactions with the environment, it would appear reasonable to focus treatment not only on specific physiological stress responses but also on the cognitive and behavioral variables that influence these stress responses. Clients could be taught to monitor stressful transactions with the environment and to identify cognitive and behavioral components of their stress responses so that more effective ways of coping with relevant interactions can be employed.

As a result of recent trends not only within behavior therapy but within psychology as a whole, behavioral treatment approaches have increasingly taken into account the cognitive processes influencing responses to environmental events (Mahoney, 1974; Meichenbaum, 1977). Learning and therapeutic change are being conceptualized in cognitive and information-processing rather than conditioning terms (Bandura, 1977; Estes, 1975; Murray & Jacobson, 1979), and current therapeutic interventions focus as much on the client's appraisal of events as on the environmental events themselves (Goldfried & Davison, 1976; Meichenbaum, 1977). Consequently, research on stress and coping has converged nicely with recent developments in behavior therapy; as the dependence of stress responses on cognitive processes becomes increasingly clear, therapeutic procedures for modifying these processes are becoming increasingly available.

Recently, Donald Meichenbaum had presented guidelines for the application of behavioral treatment procedures to the problem of stress management (Meichenbaum, 1976, 1977; Meichenbaum, Turk, & Burnstein, 1975). He has suggested that effective training must (1) be sufficiently flexible so that it can be adapted to changing environmental demands and individual needs; (2) provide cognitive strategies or plans to facilitate the assimilation of potentially threatening events and information; and (3) provide graduated practice in the use of the coping strategies that are provided. This cognitive–behavioral approach to stress management has been termed *stress inoculation training* (Meichenbaum, 1976), since its goal is to increase the individual's ability to resist the pathological effects of stress.

Although such treatment procedures have yet to be extensively incorporated into the treatment of stress-related illness, there is a growing literature on their use in the treatment of other anxiety- and stress-related dysfunctions. Recent reviews of this literature (DiGuseppe & Miller, 1977; Goldfried, 1977; Mahoney & Arnkoff, 1978; Meichenbaum, 1977) can now refer to over 100 outcome studies primarily focusing on the management of stress-related emotions such as anxiety (e.g., Holroyd, 1976; Meichenbaum, 1972), anger (Novaco, 1975), fear (e.g., Girodo, 1979; Meichenbaum, 1971), depression (e.g., Rush, Beck, Kovacs, & Hollon, 1977) and pain (e.g., Turk, 1978, 1979).

Since these stress emotions play a prominent part in theoretical accounts of psychosomatic disorders and are reliably reported to accompany the onset of psychosomatic symptoms (Luborsky, Docherty, & Penick, 1973), this research can provide guidelines for the application of stress-coping treatments to stress-related illness. Recent books (Beck, 1976; Ellis & Grieger, 1977; Foreyt & Rathjen, 1978; Kendall & Hollon, 1979; Mahoney, 1974; Meichenbaum, 1977), and review articles (DiGuseppe & Miller, 1977; Goldfried, 1977, 1979; Mahoney & Arnkoff, 1978; Turk, 1979,a,b) provide excellent summaries of this research; therefore, only studies that are of particular relevance to the treatment of stress-related illness are discussed here.

Although the specific treatment procedures that have been employed vary somewhat from study to study, the major treatment components appear to be relatively consistent across studies. Generally:

1. An explanation is provided for the client's problem that encourages the client to attribute maladaptive stress responses to relatively specific cognitive and behavioral deficiencies rather than to external stimuli or complex inner dispositions. Since clients typically attribute their stress responses to external pressures or global personal inadequacies, the therapeutic task is to convincingly present an alternative framework for viewing the client's problem, one that emphasizes those cognitive and behavioral variables that are potentially under the client's control. Didactic examples, as well as more personal illustrations from both the client's and the therapist's experience, may be employed to illustrate the various ways specific beliefs, thoughts, or behavior might exacerbate the client's stress responses.

2. Instruction is provided in the monitoring of stress responses so that the client learns to identify specific eliciting stimuli and ongoing cognitive and behavioral responses to stress. The therapeutic task is to assist the client in identifying patterns of covert and overt events that regularly precede, accompany, and follow stressful interactions. The client is typically instructed to record the details of stressful interactions so that eliciting events and cognitive and behavioral responses to these events can be identified. Usually, the client also imaginally reviews these or other potentially stressful situations, describing aloud his or her thoughts and reactions, so that relationships between cognitive and emotional responses can be identified.

3. Didactic instruction, modeling, and graduated practice are employed to teach clients alternate ways of coping with stressful situations. Usually, clients are encouraged to employ signs of impending distress as a signal to engage in cognitive or behavioral strategies that are designed to alter the stressful interaction or to manage the client's emotional responses. Strategies may primarily involve changes in behavior (e.g., more assertive behavior or withdrawal from the situation) or changes in the client's cognitive responses (e.g., changes in interpretation or internal dialogue). Although these strategies are initially suggested by the therapist, the therapeutic goal is to enable the client to develop effective problem-solving skills for managing everyday life stresses without therapeutic assistance.

Modifying Stress-Related Emotional Responses

Anger. Novaco's (1975) recent adaptation of stress inoculation training to the treatment of chronic anger problems is of interest for two reasons. First, psychosomatic formulations of certain disorders (e.g., essential hypertension) have emphasized the etiological significance of chronic problems with anger. Second, situations arousing frustration or anger are frequently reported as preceding the onset of psychosomatic symptoms (Luborsky *et al.*, 1973). Thus, methods for teaching the effective self-regulation of anger might usefully be integrated into treatment programs for some stress-related illness. Also, support for the stress-coping approach to the management of anger has been provided by recent laboratory research implicating cognitive processes in anger reduction (Green & Murray, 1975).

Novaco's formulation of anger emphasizes that sudden angry feelings result from an identifiable sequence of events eliciting specific anger-engendering cognitions. Thus, treatment focuses on teaching clients to monitor cues associated with their anger and to employ specific skills for controlling their feelings and influencing others nonaggressively. Because feelings of anger are typically "justified" by external events, considerable effort is spent teaching clients to identify the way their interpretation of these events rather than the events themselves generate anger.

In a recent attempt to evaluate this treatment approach, individuals with chronic anger problems were instructed to monitor their responses to stressful situations and were taught either cognitive coping skills (reappraisal, self-instruction, etc.) or both cognitive and relaxation skills for controlling anger. On a variety of measures (daily recordings, response to role played, and unexpected provocations), both treatments proved superior to an attention-control procedure in reducing anger.

It is of particular interest that stress-coping procedures were effective in reducing blood pressure responses to provocations, since this finding suggests that these treatments may be effective in helping hypertensive individuals control pressor responses associated with the arousal of anger.

Depression. Depression has not only been associated with the onset of psychosomatic conditions (Luborsky *et al.*, 1973) but includes numerous somatic symptoms (Beck, 1967, 1976; Mendels, 1970). In fact, Mechanic (1974) has noted that the complaints that are most frequently presented to physicians are virtually indistinguishable from the somatic symptoms of depression.

The cognitive view of depression parallels the approach to stress that is presented here in that it emphasizes the depressed person's pessimistic appraisals of environmental demands and of his own ability to cope with these demands (Beck, 1967, 1976). Other somatic, affective, and behavioral symptoms of depression are assumed to follow from this distorted appraisal process. Similarly, the treatment approach that has evolved from this view of depression parallels the stress-coping procedures described above in that it is designed to

> help the patient learn to: (a) recognize the connections between cognition, affect, and behavior, (b) monitor his negative thoughts, (c) examine the evidence for and against his distorted cognitions, and (d) substitute more reality-oriented interpretations for his distorted negative cognitions. (Rush *et al.*, 1977, p. 19)

Since there is a serious motivational deficit associated with depression, structured activity schedules have been incorporated into the treatment procedures that are used with depression. Recent research suggests that such cognitively oriented self-control procedures are effective in reducing depression and may have advantages that other psychological and pharmacological treatments lack (Beck & Shaw, 1977; Rush *et al.*, 1977; Shaw, 1977; Taylor & Marshall, 1977).

Anxiety. At present, stress-coping procedures have most extensively been applied to the management of anxiety or fear that is aroused by relatively well-defined threatening situations. Thus, outcome studies have tended to focus on problems such as test and speech anxiety (Goldfried, Linehan, & Smith, 1978; Holroyd, 1976), interpersonal anxiety (DiLoretto, 1971; Kanter & Goldfried, 1976), and fears, such as fear of flying or small-animal fears (Girodo, 1979; Meichenbaum, 1971). Although the extent to which these findings will generalize to more insidious or traumatic stressors remains unclear, current evidence suggests that stress-coping procedures are effective in teaching individuals to manage a variety of situational stresses (see reviews by Goldfried, 1977, 1979).

Some of the most carefully controlled studies in the area of anxiety management have focused on the treatment of test anxiety, and they have thus benefited from research indicating that test anxiety is primarily characterized by deficits in cognitive coping skills rather than maladaptive levels of autonomic arousal (Holroyd & Appel, 1979; Holroyd, Westbrook, Wolf, & Badhorn, 1978; Wine, 1971). The fact that test anxiety is relatively well understood may account for the relatively clear-cut evidence of the effectiveness of stress-coping procedures obtained in these studies. Not only has stress-coping training proved more effective in reducing anxiety and improving academic performance than alternate anxiety reduction procedures, such as systematic desensitization (Goldfried, Linehan, & Smith, 1978; Holroyd, 1976; Meichenbaum, 1972), but there is relatively good evidence that these outcomes do not result from nonspecific treatment effects (Holroyd, 1976). In addition, laboratory research has demonstrated that the specific coping strategies taught during treatment are effective in modifying the symptoms of test anxiety (Sarason, 1973).

Treating Stress-Related Physical Disorders

In spite of recent interest in the cognitive–behavioral treatment of stress-related emotional problems, only a few studies have extended this treatment approach to stress-related physical disorders. However, results from the few existing studies suggest that this may be a promising approach to the treatment of at least some psychosomatic disorders.

Tension Headache. Tension headache is characterized by persistent sensations of bandlike pain or tightness located bilaterally in the occipital and/or forehead regions. It is gradual in onset and may last for hours, weeks, or even months. Of the 15 classes of headache identified by the Ad Hoc Committee on Classification of Headache (1962) of the American Medical Association, tension headache, also commonly termed *muscle contraction*, *psychogenic*, or *nervous headache*, is the most frequently occurring. The exact etiology of tension headache remains unclear (Bakal, 1975). However, there is a general consensus that tension headache (1) is an individual response to psychological stress (Ad Hoc Committee on the Classification of Headache, 1962; Wolff, 1963), and (2) may result from the sustained contraction of skeletal muscles about the face, scalp, neck, and shoulders (Bakal, 1975; Martin, 1972).

In a recent study, the effectiveness of stress-coping training and biofeedback have been compared in the treatment of chronic tension headache (Holroyd *et al.*, 1977). Clients receiving stress-coping training were taught to monitor subjective feelings of tension and to identify: (1) the cues triggering tension and anxiety; (2) the way they responded when anxious; (3) their thoughts prior to becoming aware of tension, while tense, and subsequently; and (4) the way these cognitions appeared to contribute to their tension and headache. As soon as they were fluent in verbalizing cognitions associated with distress, they were taught to deliberately interrupt the sequence of covert events preceding their emotional response at the earliest possible moment. In order to do this, clients were instructed to employ signs of impending distress as a signal to engage in cognitive strategies incompatible with the further occurrence of cognitive stress responses. The strategies provided were designed to enable clients to employ three types of cognitive coping responses that have been identified by Lazarus and his co-workers (Lazarus, Averill, & Opton, 1974): cognitive reappraisal, attention deployment, and fantasy. In addition, distress-eliciting cognitions were identified as emanating from unrealistic belief systems, and clients were encouraged to suppress such cognitions because they reflected unrealistic or irrational beliefs.

An index of headache activity obtained from daily headache recordings is presented for each of the treatment groups and a wait-list control group in Figure 1. It can be seen that the stress-coping treatment proved highly effective in reducing

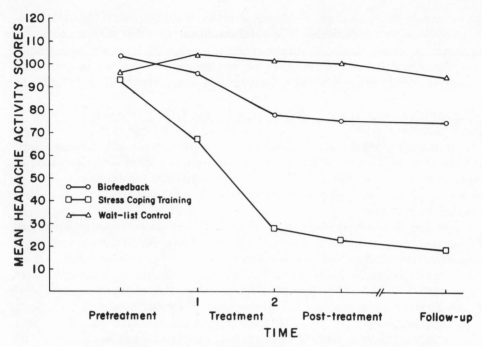

Figure 1.   Mean weekly headache activity scores in two-week blocks.

headaches at both the posttreatment and the 15-week follow-up evaluations. Significant reductions in other psychosomatic symptoms associated with headaches were
also reported. Although both the stress-coping and the biofeedback treatments were
accompanied by counterdemand instructions (Steinmark & Borkovec, 1974), only
the effectiveness of the biofeedback treatment seemed to be mitigated by these
instructions. Furthermore, reductions in resting levels of frontalis electromyographic
(EMG) activity were unrelated to headache improvement, suggesting that even for
clients receiving biofeedback, the ability to relax these muscles in the laboratory did
not necessarily enable the headache sufferer to employ these skills in actual stressful
situations (see also Epstein & Abel, 1977). Recently, the effectiveness of this stress-
coping treatment has been replicated in a study where the treatment was
administered in a group setting (Holroyd & Andrasik, 1978a).

   Migraine Headache. Migraine headaches are thought to be of vascular origin,
with pain resulting from the dilation of the cranial artery. The complete migraine
syndrome typically involves severe throbbing unilateral pain of sudden onset that
may be accompanied by nausea, irritability, photophobia, vomiting, constipation, or
diarrhea (Wolff, 1963). Attacks are frequently observed to follow periods of
psychological stress.

   In a series of studies, Mitchell and his colleagues (Mitchell, 1969, 1971a,b;
Mitchell & Mitchell,1971; Mitchell & White, 1977) have explored the use of a treatment that is designed to enable migraine sufferers to modify "both their environment and their reactions to their environment, and thus remain reasonably composed and better able to cope with those situations previously perceived as stressful"

(Mitchell & White, 1977, pp. 219–220). The rationale for this treatment emphasizes that migraines are precipitated by disruptive emotional responses to everyday stressful situations. Clients are taught to identify and recognize stressful transactions that precipitate migraine attacks, and a variety of cognitive–behavioral treatment procedures are employed to assist them in coping with these situations. This treatment thus follows the general stress-coping format outlined above.

In a recent evaluation of this treatment, Mitchell and White (1977) assigned 12 migraine sufferers either to one of two versions of this treatment or to one of two control conditions. Control subjects either recorded their headaches or recorded both headaches and stressful everyday situations. Clients in one treatment group were provided with audio cassettes describing a number of relaxation techniques for coping with stress. Clients in the second treatment group were provided a more systematic program for coping with stress, also by means of audio recordings. This program provided instructions in monitoring cognitive and behavioral responses to stressful situations and in employing a number of strategies for coping with stress (e.g., self-instruction, thought stopping, assertion training). It is this latter treatment that appears most similar to the stress-coping treatment approach described above.

Although subjects in the control conditions showed no reductions in migraine symptoms, both treatments produced significant improvements, with the more comprehensive treatment producing the greatest improvement (44.9% versus 73% improvement). Follow-up results indicated that these treatment gains were maintained for at least three months following treatment. These results suggest that treatments designed to alter the way clients cope with everyday stressful situations may be effective in the treatment of migraine headache.

Although the results that have been obtained in the treatment of tension and migraine headache are promising, additional information will be required before the utility of these treatments can be evaluated. Since a number of studies indicate that biofeedback procedures are also effective in treating these disorders (e.g., Blanchard, Theobald, Williamson, Silver, & Brown, 1978; Budzynski, Stoyva, Adler, & Mullaney, 1973), information concerning the relative effectiveness of these treatments is needed. The results of one study suggest that at least under some conditions, stress-coping training may be more effective than biofeedback in treating tension headache (Holroyd *et al.*, 1977). However, additional studies that include longer follow-up evaluations will be required before the relative effectiveness of these treatments can be evaluated. It is possible that each of these treatments may be more effective with certain individuals. Therefore, research is also needed to identify client characteristics that predict outcome with different treatments.

Since headache symptoms are readily perceptible, clients usually have little difficulty identifying stressful transactions that precipitate or aggravate symptoms. However, with other problems, the stressful interactions that aggravate or maintain symptoms may not be clear (e.g., peptic ulcers, essential hypertension). While it may be possible to monitor symptom-related physiological responses (e.g., stomach acid pH, blood pressure), this is often cumbersome and time-consuming. Therefore, it is important to determine if treatments that focus on helping clients cope with self-identified stresses are effective in modifying disorders where symptom-related physiological changes are not easily identified.

Peptic Ulcer. Ulcers are chronic lesions that extend into the wall of the stomach or the duodenum. When severe, these lesions may penetrate the stomach or duodenum wall allowing the contents of the gastrointestinal tract to leak into the peritoneum. Peptic ulcers cause about 10,000 deaths annually in the United States (Lachman, 1972).

Results from a study conducted over four decades ago suggest that treatments that are designed to modify cognitive and behavioral responses to daily stresses may prove useful in the treatment of peptic ulcer. In this study (Chappell, Stefano, Rogerson & Pike, 1936; Chappell & Stevenson, 1936), a newspaper announcement was employed to locate persons suffering from either gastric or duodenal ulcer. At the beginning of the experiment, each participant was prescribed antacids and a controlled diet. In addition, 32 participants attended small-group meetings that focused on teaching members to control cognitive and behavioral responses that were likely to unnecessarily elicit emotional arousal. Lectures focused on "the influence of thinking on bodily processes" (Chappell & Stevenson, 1936, p. 593). Participants were also taught to (1) disrupt worry and ruminative thinking by employing specific imaginal and self-instructional coping strategies; (2) cease discussing their symptoms with friends and relatives; and (3) avoid trying to demonstrate their independence by denying themselves relaxation or comfort.

At the end of six weeks, only one participant who received group treatment experienced a recurrence of symptoms when returning to a regular diet. Interestingly, the authors attributed this treatment failure to environmental stress, noting that this individual was "unemployed and about to lose his home on a foreclosure and his wife was about to have a baby" (Chappell et al., 1936, p. 816). However, within two weeks of the time participants in the control group expanded their diet, all but two had experienced a recurrence of symptoms, and both of these subjects experienced a recurrence of symptoms within two months. Furthermore, at an eight-month follow-up, only one of the 30 successfully treated participants who could be located reported a recurrence of symptoms. Of the treated subjects, 26 returned for laboratory tests and were "found to be in excellent health" Chappell et al., 1936, p. 816). Substantial treatment gains also appeared to be maintained at a three-year follow-up. It is unfortunate that these promising results have not stimulated further research, since only sketchy information is provided in the available reports of this study.

In a recent study, Beaty (1976) taught three patients with acute peptic ulcers to use relaxation as a coping skill for controlling their stress responses. Frontalis EMG biofeedback was employed to teach subjects to relax, and they were instructed in the use of relaxation as a coping skill. Results from this study suggest that both relaxation training and the active use of relaxation as a coping skill contributed to improvement.

Although results from these studies allow only tentative conclusions, the promising results reported by Chappell and his colleagues suggest that stress-coping training may be useful in the management of at least some peptic ulcers.

Essential Hypertension. Hypertension is not only common, occurring in 5–10% of the general population of the United States, but a serious health problem. Elevated levels of arterial blood pressure have been found to increase the risk of coronary heart disease, congestive heart failure, stroke, and arteriosclerosis, as well as other life-threatening disorders (Kannel & Dawber, 1974; Kannel, Gordon, & Schwartz, 1971). Mortality appears to be proportional to the severity of the hypertension, with the prognosis for severe cases of hypertension quite poor if they are left untreated (Farmer, Giffard, & Hines, 1963; Smirk, 1972). Even infrequent large increases in resting blood pressure may be associated with a shortening of the life span (Merrill, 1966).

Considerable recent attention has been paid to biofeedback procedures for reducing blood pressure as a treatment for essential hypertension (see reviews by Byassee, 1977; Blanchard & Young, 1974; Frumkin, Nathan, Prout, & Cohen, 1978; Shapiro & Surwit, 1976; Shapiro, Mainardi, & Surwit, 1977; Shapiro, Schwartz, Ferguson, Redmond, & Weiss, 1977). However, current evidence suggests that the initial hopes for this treatment are not being realized. Not only are the obtained blood pressure reductions small in magnitude, but therapeutic gains appear to be easily disrupted when stress is encountered outside the laboratory. Thus, Blanchard and Epstein (1978) have recently suggested that biofeedback "does not have much to offer the general treatment of hypertension" (p. 68).

Abundant evidence indicates that high levels of systemic arterial blood pressure are associated with environmental stress. For example, in an extensive review of both epidemiologic and experimental evidence, Gutmann and Benson (1971) concluded that high blood pressure levels were associated with environments requiring "continuous behavioral and physiologic adjustments" (p. 550) from the individual. More recently, Kaplan (1978) has concluded that "the literature increasingly incriminates psychogenic factors in human hypertension which presumably act through the sympathetic nerves" (p. 57).

There is some evidence that high levels of resting arterial blood pressure may be associated with specific behavioral responses to stress. For example, Harris and his colleagues have observed the behavior of "prehypertensive" women—whose casual readings exceeded 140/90 during college registration—in stressful laboratory situations (Harris, Sokolow, Carpenter, Freedman, & Hunt, 1953). When these women role-played situations involving interpersonal conflict (e.g., demanding proper service from an uncooperative proprietor, requesting the dean to postpone an exam), observers' ratings indicated that they were less able to respond with an appropriate level of assertiveness or to manage their feelings of anxiety and anger than were women whose readings were below 120/80 during registration. Q sorts of interview data collected over an 11-year period further suggested that these women exhibited similar patterns of behavior in important areas of their life outside the laboratory (Harris & Forsyth, 1973). In a final study in this series, ratings of the behavior of clinically hypertensive females in similar psychodramatic situations differentiated hypertensives from nonpatient controls (Kalis, Harris, Sokolow, & Carpenter, 1957). It may be that detailed analyses of these patterns of coping will enable us to identify those young people exhibiting labile hypertension who will later develop hypertensive disease. The successful identification of behavioral patterns associated with hypertension would also facilitate the development of rational preventive treatments for this disorder.

Support for a treatment approach directed at modifying patients' cognitive and behavioral response to stress has been provided by an important series of studies by Chandra Patel (1973, 1975a,b, 1976, 1977; Patel & North, 1975). According to Patel

(1977), her treatment approach is designed to teach hypertensive patients "to discriminate between realistic and unrealistic fear and between appropriate and inappropriate physiological responses to situations in daily life" and then to employ a "coping response" to control physiological stress responses (p. 12). Patients are taught to monitor their stress responses during the day by employing frequently occurring events as signals to assess their tension level. For example, a red dot is attached to the patient's wristwatch so that looking at the watch becomes a signal to self-monitor tension, rather than to hurry. Sounds of doorbells and telephones, or other stimuli such as traffic lights, are similarly utilized as cues to monitor tension, as is the occurrence of personally stressful events (e.g., meeting strangers and public speaking). When patients find themselves tense, they are instructed to relax themselves. Relaxation and meditation instructions, as well as galvanic skin response (GSR) and/or EMG biofeedback, have been employed during treatment sessions to teach clients techniques for relaxing both mentally and physically.

In a series of outcome studies, Patel has obtained impressive results with this treatment approach. For example, in a relatively well-controlled outcome study, hypertensive patients seen for 12 sessions showed substantial reductions in blood pressure (26.1/15.2 mm Hg) that were maintained over a six-month period. Controls who were also seen for 12 sessions but were simply told to relax during the sessions failed to show these gains (Patel & North, 1975). In other studies, similar gains have been obtained, even when antihypertensive medications have been reduced by as much as 40% (Patel, 1975a). In addition, treated patients have been found to exhibit smaller blood pressure responses to laboratory stressors (exercise and cold pressor tests) (Patel, 1975b). Taken as a whole, these findings suggest that hypertensive patients can alter their blood pressure by changing the way they cope with stress.

The effective elements of Patel's procedure remain to be determined. Undoubtedly, there are a variety of ways patients can modify their responses to stress that will have similar effects. In addition, the regular self-monitoring of tension levels may contribute substantially to the outcomes that are obtained by drawing stress-related behavior patterns to the patient's attention. Therefore, simpler self-control relaxation training or cognitive self-control procedures may prove equally effective (Bloom & Cantrell, 1978; Silver & Blanchard, 1979).

Other studies suggest that at least moderate reductions in blood pressure can be expected if any of a number of relaxation exercises are practiced regularly (see reviews by Blanchard & Miller, 1977; Jacob, Kraemer, & Agras, 1977; Shapiro *et al.*, 1977). For example, Taylor, Farquhor, Nelson, and Agras (1977) assigned 31 hypertensive patients to self-control relaxation, supportive psychotherapy, or medical treatment only. The self-control relaxation treatment involved five sessions of relaxation training and instruction in the use of relaxation as a coping skill. Coping-skills training was limited to the instruction "to take a deep breath, hold it momentarily, and to imagine they were in a peaceful place; then to think the word 'relax' as they exhaled" (p. 340), when in stressful situations.

The self-control relaxation group showed significantly larger reductions in blood pressure (13.6/4.9 mm Hg) than either of the other groups at the end of treatment. Although this improvement appeared to be maintained at six-month follow-up, attrition and improvements in the other groups prevented these differences from reaching significance at the follow-up.

The growing literature on relaxation exercises in the treatment of hypertension, and Patel's findings in particular, suggests that treatments that focus on altering the individual's response to daily stresses may prove useful in treating hypertension. Research to date has focused mainly on methods for teaching hypertensive patients to relax. However, it seems reasonable to expect that treatments that focus more comprehensively on altering patients' cognitive and behavioral responses to stress will prove move effective than relaxation treatments, which largely ignore the way cognitive and behavioral responses to environmental demands influence stress responses. Hopefully, future treatments studies will evaluate more comprehensive cognitive–behavioral approaches to stress management in the treatment of this disorder.

Coping with Illness: Examples

Illness itself may be stressful. Furthermore, the way the stress is handled may well influence the course of illness. In discussing this issue, Lipowski (1975) has suggested that there are six stages of illness: symptom perception, decision making (i.e., deciding what action to take), medical contact, acute illness, convalescence and rehabilitation, and chronic illness or disability. Each stage places somewhat different demands on the individual and requires somewhat different coping responses. Lipowski has attempted to impose some order on this complex process by discussing possible responses to illness and determinants of these responses at each of these stages. His formulation emphasizes the patient's appraisal of his condition and the resources available for coping.

Recent research on the coping responses of individuals with chronic asthma illustrates some of the ways coping behavior can influence the course of illness. High scorers on the panic–fear dimension respond to airway obstruction with helplessness and anxiety and, more generally, report being disinclined or unable to persist in the face of difficulty; low scorers on this measure appear to minimize or deny their symptoms (Dirks, Jones, & Kinsman, 1977). Although these coping styles appear to be independent of pulmonary function measures of the severity of asthma, they affect the length of time patients are hospitalized, the amount of steroid medication prescribed, and rehospitalization rates (e.g., Dirks *et al.*, 1977; Dirks, Kinsman, Horton, Fross, & Jones, 1978; Kinsman *et al.*, 1977). These results suggest that the way the patient copes with the chronic threat of airway obstruction may be as important as the actual severity of symptoms in determining the course of illness. As Dirks *et al.* (1978) have noted, effective treatment of a chronic disorder such as asthma must be directed at the patients' attempts to regulate and cope with their symptoms and not just the primary symptoms themselves.

Coronary heart disease provides a good example of the way stress-related behavior may influence the course of illness at a number of different points. It was noted above that the coronary-prone behavior pattern has been implicated in the pathogenesis of this disorder. In addition, the way individuals cope with the stress of acute cardiovascular incidents, attendant medical care, and recovery influences their chance of surviving.

To illustrate, more than 50% of deaths from myocardial infarction may result from unnecessary delays in receiving medical care. In a review of literature in this area, Gentry (1975) has emphasized the role of faulty symptom appraisals and maladaptive coping behavior in understanding this delay. According to Gentry, as many as 70% of the individuals suffering a myocardial infarct misinterpret or deny the source of their symptoms. If faulty symptom appraisals are influenced by some of the same variables that influence the appraisal of other threatening events, more effective strategies for appraising and coping with this threat can probably be systematically taught. Similarly, delay that results from maladaptive attempts to cope with symptoms (e.g., use of patent medications) might be prevented if individuals at risk were taught how to appraise and cope with their symptoms appropriately.

Reviews by Pranulis (1975) and Klein (1975) indicate that the way patients cope with hospitalization and coronary care may influence their chance of survival. Pranulis has suggested that disruptive anxiety and extreme helplessness are the most common outcomes of faulty coping, and Klein has outlined the way these responses might induce a cardiovascular incident. In an attempt to minimize this problem, Hackett and Cassem (1975) have developed a program to assist patients to cope with the stress involved in coronary care. Patients are provided information about their condition and the medical interventions to which they are exposed and are taught relaxation skills for reducing anxiety. Although this treatment has yet to be evaluated, Langer, Janis, and Wolfer (1975) found that a similar intervention, consisting of information and cognitive strategies for coping with the stress of surgery, significantly reduced the need for postoperative pain medication. In the latter study, only the cognitive coping strategies contributed to the treatment outcome; preoperative information was of little use.

There is a large literature on the period of recovery following myocardial infarction (see Croog & Levine, 1977). However, there are few controlled studies of interventions that are designed to assist patients in coping with the stresses that are encountered during this period. As a number of investigators have noted, it is the psychological, rather than the physical, aspects of recovery that are likely to be most trying (e.g., Garrity, 1975). Gulledge (1975) has reviewed evidence indicating that many postinfarction patients are highly anxious, fearful, and depressed for months following their release from the hospital. For example, Wishnie, Hackett, and Cassem (1971) reported that six months to one year after leaving the hospital, 88% of their patients were anxious or depressed, and almost 40% had failed to return to work for psychological reasons.

Patients who show signs of ineffective coping in the hospital (inability to manage their emotional responses) have been found to have a higher mortality rate during the subsequent six-month period than patients who cope more effectively with hospitalization (Garrity, 1975; Pancheri, Bellaterra, Matteoli, Cristofari, Polizzi, & Puletti, 1978). Garrity (1975) has also noted that following hospitalization, patients develop idiosyncratic, and frequently maladaptive, strategies for coping with the threat of a myocardial infarction, suggesting that interventions that help patients "to acquire more effective coping skills" (p. 131) could have a major impact on rehabilitative outcome.

A comprehensive behavioral approach to the postinfarction patient has yet to be developed. Such a treatment program should not only provide the patient with skills for coping with the predictable stresses of recovery but help the patient alter chronic stress-related behavior patterns and relevant behavioral risk factors, such as smoking, diet, and exercise.

The Cardiac Stress Management Program developed by Suinn (1977) is an initial step in this direction (see also Chesney, 1978, and Roskies, 1978). Patients are taught to monitor signs of stress and to identify maladaptive coping behaviors associated with the coronary-prone behavior pattern. Cognitive modeling procedures are employed to rehearse new ways of responding in stressful situations and to develop skill in the use of relaxation to manage stress responses. Suinn (1974, 1975; Suinn & Bloom, 1978; Suinn, Brock, & Edie, 1975) has presented preliminary data indicating that significant reductions in serum cholesterol and triglycerides, as well as behavioral change, follow only five hours of stress management training. Although this treatment approach requires further evaluation, the preliminary results suggest that stress management training may prove a useful component of treatment programs for the postinfarction patient.

SUMMARY

In this chapter, the implications of recent developments in stress research for behavioral medicine were discussed. In an attempt to clarify conceptual difficulties that have plagued the study of stress and disease, convergent trends in epidemiology, psychosomatic medicine, and psychophysiology were examined. It was argued that formulations of stress solely in terms of environmental events or solely in terms of the organism's response have tended to obscure important relationships between coping activity, pathophysiology, and disease outcome. Therefore, research is needed that focuses on the self-regulatory or coping activity that is called into play in managing stressful transactions. The potential advantages of such a transactional perspective were illustrated with research that has begun to elucidate relationships between stressful transactions, characteristic coping responses, and the pathogenesis of coronary heart disease.

Behavioral approaches to the treatment of stress-related illness have also tended to ignore the coping activity that mediates between environmental demands and symptom-related physiological activity. In fact, the behavioral literature has been dominated by research on biofeedback. When stress-related illness is viewed from a transactional perspective, however, biofeedback often appears to be an illogical and inefficient treatment. Since stress reactions are dependent on cognitive and behavioral responses to environmental demands, patients are frequently unable to alter specific physiological stress responses outside the laboratory without also altering their interactions with the environment. Therefore, effective treatment strategies must focus not only on specific stress responses but on functionally related cognitive and behavioral activity. A review of emerging research employing cognitive–behavioral interventions in the treatment of stress-related illness suggested that this treatment strategy deserves the increased attention of researchers in behavioral medicine.

ACKNOWLEDGMENTS

Appreciation is expressed to Margret Appel and Michael Wolf for comments on an earlier draft of this chapter.

REFERENCES

Ad Hoc Committee on Classification of Headache. Classification of Headache. *Journal of the American Medical Association*, 1962, *179*, 717–718.

Alexander, F. *Psychosomatic medicine: Its principles and applications.* New York: Norton, 1950.

Alexander, F. Discussion of a paper by Mahl and Karpe. *Psychosomatic Medicine*, 1953, *15*, 327.

Andrasik, F., & Holroyd, K. A test of the specific effects in the biofeedback treatment of tension headache. Paper presented at the Association for the Advancement of Behavior Therapy Convention, Chicago, Nov. 1978.

Antonovsky, A. Conceptual and methodological problems in the study of resistance resources and stressful life events. In B. S. Dohrenwend & B. P. Dohrenwend (Eds.), *Stressful life events: Their nature and effects.* New York: Wiley, 1974.

Bakal, D. Headache: A biopsychological perspective. *Psychological Bulletin*, 1975, *82*, 369–382.

Bandura, A. *Social learning theory.* Englewood Cliffs, N.J.: Prentice-Hall, 1977.

Beaty, E. T. Feedback-assisted relaxation training as a treatment for gastric ulcers. Paper presented at Seventh Annual Meeting of Biofeedback Research Society, Colorado Springs, Co., 1976.

Beck, A. T. *Depression: Clinical, experimental, and theoretical aspects.* New York: Hoeber, 1967.

Beck, A. T. *Cognitive therapy and the emotional disorders.* New York: International Universities Press, 1976.

Beck, A. T., & Shaw, B. F. Cognitive approaches to depression. In A. Ellis & R. Grieger (Eds.), *Handbook of rational emotive theory and practice.* New York: Springer, 1977.

Birk, L. (Ed.). *Biofeedback: Behavioral medicine.* New York: Grune & Stratton, 1973.

Birnbaum, F., Coplon, J., & Scharff, I. Crisis intervention after a natural disaster. In R. H. Moos (Ed.), *Human adaptation, coping with life crises.* Lexington, Mass.: D. C. Heath, 1976.

Blanchard, E. B., & Epstein, L. H. *A biofeedback primer.* Reading, Mass.: Addison-Wesley, 1978.

Blanchard, E. B., & Miller, S. T. Psychological treatment of cardiovascular disease. *Archives of General Psychiatry*, 1977, *34*, 1402–1413.

Blanchard, E. B., & Young, L. D. Clinical applications of biofeedback training: A review of the evidence. *Archives of General Psychiatry*, 1974, *30*, 530–589.

Blanchard, E. B., Theobald, D. E., Williamson, D. A., Silver, B. V., & Brown, D. A. A controlled comparison of temperature biofeedback in the treatment of migraine headaches. *Archives of General Psychiatry*, 1978, *35*, 581–588.

Bloom, L. J., & Cantrell, D. Anxiety management training for essential hypertension in pregnancy. *Behavior Therapy*, 1978, *9*, 377–382.

Bourne, P. G. (Ed.). *The psychology and physiology of stress.* New York: Academic, 1969.

Budzynski, T. H., Stoyva, J. M., Adler, C. S., & Mullaney, D. J. EMG biofeedback and tension headache: A controlled outcome study. *Psychosomatic Medicine*, 1973, *35*, 484–496.

Burnam, M. A., Pennebaker, J. W., & Glass, D. C. Time consciousness, achievement striving, and the Type A coronary-prone behavior pattern. *Journal of Abnormal Psychology*, 1973, *84*, 76–79.

Byassee, J. E. Essential hypertension. In R. B. Williams & W. D. Gentry (Eds.), *Behavioral approaches to medical treatment.* Cambridge, Mass.: Ballinger, 1977.

Caffrey, B. Reliability and validity of personality and behavioral measures in a study of coronary heart disease. *Journal of Chronic Diseases*, 1968, *21*, 191–204.

Cannon, W. B. *The wisdom of the body.* New York: Norton, 1932.

Cannon, W. B. The role of emotion in disease. *Annals of Internal Medicine*, 1936, *9*, 1453–1456.

Carver, C. S., Coleman, A. E., & Glass, D. C. The coronary-prone behavior pattern and the suppression of fatigue on a treadmill test. *Journal of Personality and Social Psychology*, 1976, *33*, 460–466.

Cassel, J. Social science in epidemiology: Psychosocial processes and "stress" theoretical formulation. In E. L. Struening & M. Guttentag (Eds.), *Handbook of evaluation research*. Beverly Hills, Calif.: Sage, 1975.

Cassel, J. The contribution of the social environment to host resistance. *American Journal of Epidemiology*, 1976, *104*, 107–123.

Chappell, M. N., & Stevenson, T. I. Group psychological training in some organic conditions. *Mental Hygiene*, 1936, *20*, 588–597.

Chappell, M. N., Stefano, J. J., Rogerson, J. S., & Pike, F. H. The value of group psychological procedures in the treatment of peptic ulcer. *American Journal of Digestive Diseases*, 1936, *3*, 813–817.

Chesney, M. A. Coronary-prone behavior and coronary heart disease: Intervention strategies. Paper presented at the annual meeting of the American Psychological Association, Toronto, Canada, Aug. 1978.

Cobb, S., & Rose, R. M. Hypertension, peptic ulcer and diabetes in air traffic controllers. *Journal of the American Medical Association*, 1973, *224*, 489–492.

Cohen, S. I., Silverman, A. J., Waddell, W., & Zuidema, G. D. Urinary catecholamine levels, gastric secretion and specific psychological factors in ulcer and nonulcer patients. *Journal of Psychosomatic Research*, 1961, *5*, 90–115.

Croog, S. H., & Levine, S. *The heart patient recovers*. New York: Human Sciences, 1977.

Davies, M. H. Is high blood pressure a psychosomatic disorder. *Journal of Chronic Diseases*, 1971, *24*, 239–258.

Dembroski, T. M., & MacDougall, J. M. Stress effects on affiliation preferences among subjects possessing the Type A coronary prone behavior pattern. *Journal of Personality and Social Psychology*, 1978, *36*, 23–33.

Dembroski, T. M., MacDougall, J. M., & Shields, J. L. Physiologic reactions to social challenge in persons evidencing the Type A coronary-prone behavior pattern. *Journal of Human Stress*, 1977, *3*, 2–9.

DiGuseppe, R. A., & Miller, N. J. A review of outcome studies on rational-emotive therapy. In A. Ellis & R. Grieger (Eds.), *Handbook of rational emotive therapy*. New York: Springer, 1977.

DiLoretto, A. O. *Comparative psychotherapy: An experimental analysis*. Chicago: Aldine-Atherton, 1971.

Dirks, J. F., Jones, N. F., & Kinsman, R. A. Panic-fear: A personality dimension related to untractability in asthma. *Psychosomatic Medicine*, 1977, *39*, 120–126.

Dirks, J. F., Kinsman, R. H., Horton, D. J., Fross, K. H., & Jones, N. F. Panic-fear in asthma: Rehospitalization following intensive long-term treatment. *Psychosomatic Medicine*, 1978, *40*, 5–13.

Dohrenwend, B. S., & Dohrenwend, B. P. Overview and prospects for research on stressful life events. In B. S. Dohrenwend & B. P. Dohrenwend (Eds.), *Stressful life events: Their nature and effects*. New York: Wiley, 1974.

Dubos, R. *The mirage of health: Utopias, progress and biological change*. New York: Doubleday, 1961.

Dunbar, H. F. *Emotions and bodily changes: A survey of literature on psychosomatic interrelationships, 1910–1933*. New York: Columbia University Press, 1935.

Dyer, E. D. Parenthood as crisis: A re-study. In R. H. Moos (Ed.), *Human adaptation: Coping with life crises*. Lexington, Mass.: D. C. Heath, 1976.

Eitinger, L., & Strom, A. *Mortality and morbidity after excessive stress*. New York: Humanities, 1973.

Ellis, H., & Grieger, R. (Eds.). *Handbook of rational emotive therapy*. New York: Springer, 1977.

Epstein, L. H., & Abel, G. G. Analysis of biofeedback training effects for tension headache patients. *Behavior Therapy*, 1977, *8*, 37–47.

Erhardt, C., & Berlin, J. E. *Mortality and morbidity in the United States*. Boston, Mass.: Harvard University Press, 1974.

Estes, W. K. (Ed.). *Handbook of learning and cognitive processes:* Vol. 1. *Introduction to concepts and issues*. New York: Halsted, 1975.

Faire, U., & Theorell, T. Life changes and myocardial infarction. *Preventive Medicine*, 1977, *6*, 302–311.

Farmer, R. G., Giffard, R. W., & Hines, E. A. Effect of medical treatment of severe hypertension: A follow-up study of 161 patients with group 3 and group 4 hypertension. *Archives of Internal Medicine*, 1963, *112*, 161–174.

Folkins, C. H. Temporal factors and the cognitive mediators of stress reaction. *Journal of Personality and Social Psychology*, 1970, *14*, 173–184.

Foreyt, J. P., & Rathjen, G. J. (Eds.). *Cognitive-behavior therapy: Research and application*. New York: Plenum, 1978.

Frankenhaeuser, M. Behavior and circulating catecholamines. *Brain Research*, 1971, *31*, 241–262.

Frankenhaeuser, M. The role of peripheral catecholamines in adaptation to understimulation and over-stimulation. In G. Serban (Ed.), *Psychopathology of human adaptation*. New York: Plenum, 1976.

Frankenhaeuser, M., & Rissler, A. Effects of punishment on catecholamine release and efficiency of performance. *Psychopharmacologia*, 1970, *17*, 378–390.

Friedman, M. *Pathogenesis of coronary artery disease*. New York: McGraw-Hill, 1969.

Friedman, M. Modification of Type A behavior to reduce risk of heart disease. Paper presented at the 85th annual convention of the American Psychological Association, San Francisco, 1977.

Friedman, M., Byers, S. O., Diamant, J., & Rosenman, R. H. Plasma catecholamine response of coronary-prone subjects (Type A) to a specific challenge. *Metabolism*, 1975, *24*, 205–210.

Frumkin, K., Nathan, K. J., Prout, M. F., & Cohen, B. A. Nonpharmacologic control of essential hypertension in man: A critical review of the experimental literature. *Psychosomatic Medicine*, 1978, *40*, 294–320.

Garma, A. On pathogenesis of peptic ulcer. *International Journal of Psychoanalysis*, 1950, *31*, 53–72.

Garrity, T. F. Morbidity, mortality, and rehabilitation. In W. D. Gentry & R. B. Williams, Jr. (Eds.), *Psychological aspects of myocardial infarction and coronary care*. St. Louis: Mosby, 1975.

Garrity, T. F., Marx, M. B., & Somes, G. W. Langner's 22-item measure of psychophysiological strain as an intervening variable between life changes and health outcome. *Journal of Psychosomatic Research*, 1977, *21*, 195–199.

Gentry, W. D. Preadmission behavior. In W. D. Gentry & R. B. Williams, Jr. (Eds.), *Psychological aspects of myocardial infarction and coronary care*. St. Louis: Mosby, 1975.

Gerard, M. W. Genesis of psychosomatic symptoms in infancy. In F. Deutsch (Ed.), *The psychosomatic concept in psychoanalysis*. New York: International Universities Press, 1953.

Gersten, J. C., Langner, T. S., Eisenberg, J. G., & Orzek, L. Child behavior and life events: Undesirable change or change per se? In B. S. Dohrenwend & B. P. Dohrenwend (Eds.), *Stressful life events: Their nature and effects*. New York: Wiley, 1974.

Girodo, M. Self-talk: Mechanisms in anxiety and stress management. In I. G. Sarason & C. Spielberger (Eds.), *Stress and anxiety*, Vol. 4. Washington, D.C.: Hemisphere/Wiley, 1979.

Glass, D. C. *Behavior patterns, stress, and coronary disease*. New York: Lawrence Erlbaum, 1977.

Glass, D. C., Snyder, M. L., & Hollis, J. F. Time urgency and the Type A coronary-prone behavior pattern. *Journal of Applied Social Psychology*, 1974, *4*, 125–140.

Glazier, W. H. The task of medicine. *Scientific American*, 1973, *228*, 13–17.

Goldfried, M. R. The use of relaxation and cognitive relabeling as coping skills. In R. B. Stuart (Ed.), *Behavioral self-management: Strategies and outcomes*. New York: Brunner/Mazel, 1977.

Goldfried, M. R. Anxiety reduction through cognitive-behavioral intervention. In P. C. Kendall & S. D. Hollon (Eds.), *Cognitive-behavioral interventions: Theory, research and procedures*. New York: Academic, 1979.

Goldfried, M. R., & Davison, G. C. *Clinical behavior therapy*. New York: Holt, Rinehart, & Winston, 1976.

Goldfried, M. R., Linehan, M. M., & Smith, J. L. The reduction of test anxiety through rational restructuring. *Journal of Consulting and Clinical Psychology*, 1978, *46*, 32–39.

Grace, W. J., & Graham, D. T. Relationship of specific attitudes and emotions to certain bodily diseases. *Psychosomatic Medicine*, 1952, *14*, 243–251.

Grace, W. J., Wolf, S., & Wolff, H. G. *The human colon*. New York: Hoeber, 1951.

Graham, D. T. Psychosomatic medicine. In N. S. Greenfield & R. A. Sternbach (Eds.), *Handbook of psychophysiology*. New York: Holt, Rinehart, & Winston, 1972.

Green, R. A., & Murray, E. J. Expression of feeling and cognitive reinterpretation in the reduction of hostile aggression. *Journal of Consulting and Clinical Psychology*, 1975, *43*, 375–383.

Gulledge, A. D. The psychological aftermath of a myocardial infarction. In W. D. Gentry & R. B. Williams, Jr. (Eds.), *Psychological aspects of myocardial infarction and coronary care*. St. Louis: Mosby, 1975.

Gutmann, M. C., & Benson, H. Interaction of environmental factors and systemic arterial blood pressure: A reveiw. *Medicine*, 1971, *50*, 543–553.

Haan, N. *Coping and defending*. New York: Academic, 1977.

Hackett, T. P., & Cassem, N. H. Psychological intervention in myocardial infarction. In W. D. Gentry & R. B. Williams, Jr. (Eds.), *Psychological aspects of myocardial infarction and coronary care*. St. Louis: Mosby, 1975.

Haggerty, K. J. Changing lifestyles to improve health. *Preventive Medicine*, 1977, *6*, 276–289.

Hamburg, D. A., Hamburg, B., & DeGoza, S. Adaptive problems and mechanisms in severely burned patients. *Psychiatry*, 1953, *16*, 1–20.

Hamilton, M. *Psychosomatics*. New York: Wiley, 1955.

Harris, R. E., Sokolow, M., Carpenter, L. G., Freedman, M., & Hunt, S. P. Response to psychologic stress in persons who are potentially hypertensive. *Circulation*, 1953, *7*, 874–879.

Harris, R. E., & Forsyth, R. P. Personality and emotional stress in essential hypertension in man. In G. Onesti, K. W. Kim, & J. H. Moyer (Eds.), *Hypertension: Mechanisms and management*. New York: Grune & Stratton, 1973.

Hinkle, L. E. The concept of "stress" in the biological and social sciences. *International Journal of Psychiatry in Medicine*, 1974, *5*, 355–357.

Holmes, T. H., & Masuda, M. Life change and illness susceptibility. In B. S. Dohrenwend & B. P. Dohrenwend (Eds.), *Stressful life events: Their nature and effects*. New York: Wiley, 1974.

Holmes, T. H., & Rahe, R. H. The social readjustment rating scale. *Journal of Psychosomatic Research*, 1967, *11*, 213.

Holroyd, K. Cognition and desensitization in the group treatment of test anxiety. *Journal of Consulting and Clinical Psychology*, 1976, *44*, 991–1001.

Holroyd, K., & Andrasik, F. Coping and the self-control of chronic tension headache. *Journal of Consulting and Clinical Psychology*, 1978, *46*, 1036–1045. (a)

Holroyd, K., & Andrasik, F. Treating tension headache: New data, new problems. Paper presented in symposium on Biofeedback and the Behavioral Treatment of Stress Related Disorders at the 50th Annual Convention of the Midwestern Psychological Association, Chicago, 1978. (b)

Holroyd, K., & Appel, M. Test anxiety and physiological responding. In I. Sarason (Ed.), *Test anxiety: Theory, research and applications*. Hillsdale, N.J.: Lawrence Erlbaum, 1979.

Holroyd, K., Andrasik, F., & Westbrook, K. Cognitive control of tension headache. *Cognitive Therapy and Research*, 1977, *1*, 121–133.

Holroyd, K., Westbrook, T., Wolf, M., & Badhorn, E. Performance, cognition and physiological responding in test anxiety. *Journal of Abnormal Psychology*, 1978, *87*, 442–451.

Howard, J., Cunningham, D., & Rechnitzer, P. Health patterns associated with Type A behavior: A managerial population. *Journal of Human Stress*, 1976, *2*, 24–33.

Hudgens, R. W. Personal castastrophe and depression: A consideration of the subject with respect to medically ill adolescents, and a requeuem for retrospective life-event studies. In B. S. Dohrenwend & B. P. Dohrenwend (Eds.), *Stressful life events: Their nature and effects*. New York: Wiley, 1974.

Jacob, R. G., Kraemer, H. C., & Agras, W. S. Relaxation therapy in the treatment of hypertension. *Archives of General Psychiatry*, 1977, *34*, 1417–1427.

Jenkins, C. D. Recent evidence supporting psychological and social risk factors for coronary disease. *New England Journal of Medicine*, 1976, *294*, 987, 994, 1066, 1088.

Jenkins, C. D., Zyzanski, S. J., & Rosenman, R. H. Coronary-prone behavior: One pattern or several. *Psychosomatic Medicine*, 1978, *40*, 25–43.

Kalis, B. L., Harris, R. E., Sokolow, M., & Carpenter, L. G. Response to psychological stress in patients with hypertension. *American Heart Journal*, 1957, *53*, 572–578.

Kannel, W. B., & Dawber, T. R. Hypertension as an ingredient of a cardiovascular risk profile. *British Journal of Hospital Medicine*, 1974, *11*, 508–528.

Kannel, W. B., Gordon, T., & Schwartz, M. J. Systolic versus diastolic blood pressure and risk of coronary heart disease. *American Journal of Cardiology*, 1971, *27*, 335–343.

Kanter, N. J., & Goldfried, M. R. Relative effectiveness of rational restructuring and self-control desensitization for the reduction of interpersonal anxiety. Unpublished manuscript, State University of New York at Stony Brook, 1976.

Kaplan, N. M. *Clinical hypertension* (2nd ed.). Baltimore: Williams & Wilkins, 1978.

Katz, J., Weiner, H., Gallagher, T., & Hellman, L. Stress, distress and ego defenses. *Archives of General Psychiatry*, 1970, *23*, 131–142.

Kellam, S. G. Stressful life events and illness: A research area in need of conceptual development. In B. S. Dohrenwend & B. P. Dohrenwend (Eds.), *Stressful life events: Their nature and effects*. New York: Wiley, 1974.

Kendall, P. C., & Hollon, S. D. (Eds.). *Cognitive-behavioral interventions: Theory, research, and procedures*. New York: Academic, 1979.

Kenigsberg, D., Zyzanski, S. J., Jenkins, C. D., Wardwell, W. I., & Licciardello, A. T. The coronary-prone behavior pattern in hospitalized patients with and without coronary heart disease. *Psychosomatic Medicine*, 1974, *36*, 344–351.

Kilpatrik, D. G. Differential responsiveness of two electrodermal indices to psychological stress and performance of a complex cognitive task. *Psychophysiology*, 1972, *9*, 218–226.

Kinsman, R. A., Dahlem, N. W., Spector, S., & Staudenmayer, H. Observations on subjective symptomatology coping behavior, and medical decisions in asthma. *Psychosomatic Medicine*, 1977, *39*, 102–119.

Klein, R. F. Relationship between psychological and physiological stress in the coronary care unit. In W. D. Gentry & R. B. Williams, Jr. (Eds.), *Psychological aspects of myocardial infarction and coronary care*. St. Louis: Mosby, 1975.

Krantz, D. S., Glass, D. C., & Snyder, M. L. Helplessness, stress level, and the coronary-prone behavior pattern. *Journal of Experimental Social Psychology*, 1974, *10*, 284–300.

Lacey, B. C., & Lacey, J. J. Two-way communication between the heart and the brain. *American Psychologist*, 1978, *33*, 99–113.

Lacey, J. I. Somatic response patterning and stress: Some revisions of activation theory. In M. H. Appley & R. Trumbull (Eds.), *Psychological stress*. New York: Appleton-Century-Crofts, 1967.

Lacey, J. I., Kagan, J., Lacey, B. C., & Moss, H. A. The visceral level: Situational determinants and behavioral correlates of autonomic response patterns. In P. H. Knapp (Ed.), *Expression of the emotions in man*. New York: International Universities Press, 1963.

Lachman, S. J. *Psychosomatic disorders: A behavioristic interpretation*. New York: Wiley, 1972.

Langer, E. J., Janis, I. L., & Wolfer, J. A. Reduction of psychological stress in surgical patients. *Journal of Experimental Social Psychology*, 1975, *11*, 155–165.

Lazarus, R. S. *Psychological stress and the coping process*. New York: McGraw-Hill, 1966.

Lazarus, R. S. Discussion. In G. Serban (Ed.), *Psychopathology of human adaptation*. New York: Plenum, 1976.

Lazarus, R. S. Psychological stress and coping in adaptation and illness. In Z. J. Lipowski, D. R. Lipsitt, & P. C. Whybrow (Eds.), *Psychosomatic medicine: Current trends and clinical applications*. New York: Oxford University Press, 1977.

Lazarus, R. S., & Launier, R. Stress-related transactions between person and environment. In L. A. Pervin & M. Lewis (Eds.), *Internal and external determinants of behavior*. New York: Plenum, 1978.

Lazarus, R., Averill, J., & Opton, E. The psychology of coping: Issues of research and assessment. In G. Coelho, D. Hamburg, & J. Adams (Eds.), *Coping and adaptation*. New York: Basic, 1974.

Levine, S. V. Draft dodgers: Coping with stress, adapting to exile. In R. H. Moos (Ed.), *Human adaptation: Coping with life crises*. Lexington, Mass.: D. C. Heath, 1976.

Lipowski, Z. J. Physical illness, the patient and his environment: Psychosocial foundations of medicine. In S. Arieti (Ed.), *American handbook of psychiatry*, Vol. 4. New York: Basic, 1975.

Lipowski, Z. J. Psychosomatic medicine in the seventies: An overview. *American Journal of Psychiatry*, 1977, *134*, 233–244.

Luborsky, L., Docherty, J. P., & Penick, S. Onset conditions for psychosomatic symptoms: A comparative review of immediate observation with retrospective research. *Psychosomatic Medicine*, 1973, *35*, 187–204.

Lynn, S. J., & Freedman, R. R. Transfer and evaluation of biofeedback treatment. In A. P. Goldstein & F. Kanfer (Eds.), *Maximizing treatment gains: Transfer enhancement in psychotherapy*. New York: Academic, 1979.

Mahl, G. F. Anxiety, HCl secretion and peptic ulcer etiology. *Psychosomatic Medicine*, 1950, *12*, 158–169.

Mahoney, M. *Cognition and behavior modification*. Cambridge, Mass.: Ballinger, 1974.

Mahoney, M. J., & Arnkoff, D. E. Cognitive and self-control therapies. In S. L. Garfield & A. E. Bergin (Eds.), *Handbook of psychotherapy and behavior change*, Vol. 2. New York: Wiley, 1978.

Margolin, S. G. Genetic and dynamic psychophysiological determinants of pathophysiological processes. In F. Deutsch (Ed.), *The psychosomatic concept in psychoanalysis*. New York: International Universities Press, 1953.

Martin, M. J. Muscle-contractions headache. *Psychosomatics*. 1972, *13*, 16–19.

Mason, J. W. Organization of psychoendocrine mechanisms. *Psychosomatic Medicine*, 1968, *30*, 565–808.

Mason, J. W. Strategy in psychosomatic research. *Psychosomatic Medicine*, 1970, *32*, 427–439.

Mason, J. W. A re-evaluation of the concept of "nonspecificity" in stress theory. *Journal of Psychiatric Research*, 1971, *8*, 323–333.

Mason, J. W. Specificity in the organization of neuroendocrine response profiles. In P. Seeman, & G. Brown (Eds.), *Frontiers in neurology and neuroscience research*. Toronto: University of Toronto, 1974.

Mason, J. W. Clinical psychophysiology. In M. F. Reiser (Ed.), *American handbook of psychiatry*, Vol. 4. New York: Basic, 1975.

Mason, J. W., Maher, J. T., Hartley, L. H., Mougey, E., Perlow, M. J., & Jones, L. G. Selectivity of corticosteroid and catecholamine responses to natural stimuli. In G. Serban (Ed.), *Psychopathology of human adaptation*. New York: Plenum, 1976.

Mattila, V. J., & Solokangas, R. K. Life changes and social group in relation to illness onset. *Journal of Psychosomatic Research*, 1977, *21*, 167–174.

Mechanic, D. Social psychologic factors affecting the presentation of bodily complaints. *New England Journal of Medicine*, 1972, *286*, 1132–1139.

Mechanic, D. Discussion of research programs on relations between stressful life events and episodes of physical illness. In B. S. Dohrenwend & B. P. Dohrenwend (Eds.), *Stressful life events: Their nature and effects*. New York: Wiley, 1974.

Meichenbaum, D. Examination of model characteristics in reducing avoidance behavior. *Journal of Personality and Social Psychology*, 1971, *17*, 298–307.

Meichenbaum, D. Cognitive modification of test anxious college students. *Journal of Consulting and Clinical Psychology*, 1972, *39*, 370–380.

Meichenbaum, D. A self-instructional approach to stress management: A proposal for stress-inoculation training. In C. Spielberger & I. Sarason (Eds.), *Stress and anxiety in modern life*. New York: Winston and Sons, 1976.

Meichenbaum, D. *Cognitive-behavior modification*. New York: Plenum, 1977.

Meichenbaum, D., Turk, D., & Burnstein, S. The nature of coping with stress. In I. Sarason & C. Spielberger (Eds.), *Stress and anxiety*, Vol. 2. New York: Wiley, 1975.

Mendels, J. *Concepts of depression*. New York: Wiley, 1970.

Merrill, J. P. Hypertensive vascular disease. In J. V. Harrison, R. D. Adams, I. J. Bennett, W. H. Resnik, G. W. Thorn, & M. M. Wintrobe (Eds.), *Principles of internal medicine*. New York: McGraw-Hill, 1966.

Miller, N. E. Learning of visceral and glandular responses. *Science*, 1969, *163*, 434–445.

Miller, N. E. The role of learning in physiological response to stress. In G. Serban (Ed.), *Psychopathology of human adaptation*. New York: Plenum, 1976.

Miller, N. E. Biofeedback and visceral learning. In *Annual Review of Psychology*, Vol. 29. Palo Alto, Calif.: Annual Reviews, 1978.

Miller, N. E., & Dworkin, B. R. Critical issues in therapeutic applications of biofeedback. In G. E. Schwartz & J. Beatty (Eds.), *Biofeedback*. New York: Academic, 1977.

Mischel, W. Toward a cognitive social learning reconceptualization of personality. *Psychological Review*, 1973, *80*, 252–283.

Mitchell, K. R. The treatment of migraine. An exploratory application of time-limited behavior therapy. *Technology*, 1969, *14*, 50–55.

Mitchell, K. R. A note on the treatment of migraine using behavior therapy techniques. *Psychological Reports*, 1971, *28*, 191–192. (a)

Mitchell, K. R. A psychological approach to the treatment of migraine with behavior therapy techniques. *British Journal of Psychiatry*, 1971, *119*, 533-534. (b)

Mitchell, K. R., & Mitchell, D. M. Migraine: An exploratory treatment application of programmed behavior therapy techniques. *Journal of Psychosomatic Research*, 1971, *15*, 137-157.

Mitchell, K., & White, R. Behavioral self-management: An application to the problem of migraine headache. *Behavior Therapy*, 1977, *8*, 213-221.

Mordkoff, A. M., & Parsons, O. A. The coronary personality: A critique. *International Journal of Psychiatry*, 1968, *5*, 413-426.

Mostofsky, D. I., & Balaschak, B. A. Psychobiological control of seizures. *Psychological Bulletin*, 1977, *84*, 723-750.

Murphy, L. B., & Moriarty, A. E. *Vulnerability, coping, and growth*. New Haven, Conn.: Yale University Press, 1976.

Murray, E. J., & Jacobson, L. I. Cognition and learning in traditional and behavioral therapy. In S. L. Garfield & A. E. Bergin (Eds.), *Handbook of psychotherapy and behavior change* (2nd ed.). New York: Wiley, 1979.

National Center for Health Statistics, 1977, Series 10, Nos. 62 and 119.

Novaco, R. W. *Anger control: The development and evaluation of an experimental treatment*. Lexington, Mass.: D.C. Heath, 1975.

Nuckolls, C. B., Cassel, J., & Kaplan, B. H. Psycho-social assets, life crises and the prognosis of pregnancy. *American Journal of Epidemiology*, 1972, *95*, 431-441.

Obrist, P. The cardiovascular-behavioral-interaction—As it appears today. *Psychophysiology*, 1976, *13*, 95-107.

Oken, D. The psychophysiology and psychoendocrinology of stress and emotion. In M. H. Appley & R. Trumbull (Eds.), *Psychological stress*. New York: Appleton-Century-Crofts, 1967.

Pancheri, P., Bellaterra, M., Matteoli, S., Cristofari, M., Polizzi, C., & Puletti, M. Infarct as a stress agent: Life history and personality characteristics in improved versus not-improved patients after severe heart attack. *Journal of Human Stress*, 1978, *4*, 16-22, 41-42.

Parkes, C. M. *Bereavement*. New York: International Universities Press, 1972.

Patel, C. A 12-month follow-up of yoga and biofeedback in the management of hypertension. *Lancet*, 1975, *1*, 62-65. (a)

Patel, C. Yoga and biofeedback in the management of "stress" in hypertensive patients. *Clinical Science and Molecular Medicine*, 1975, *48*, Suppl., 171-174. (b)

Patel, C. Reduction of serum cholesterol and blood pressure in hypertensive patients by behavior modification. *Journal of the Royal College of General Practitioners: British Journal of General Practice*, 1976, *26*, 211-215.

Patel, C. H. Yoga and biofeedback in the management of hypertension. *Lancet*, 1973, *2*, 1053-1055.

Patel, C. H. Biofeedback-aided relaxation and meditation in the management of hypertension. *Biofeedback and Self-Regulation*, 1977, *2*, 1-41.

Patel, C. H., & North, W. R. S. Randomized controlled trial of yoga and biofeedback in the management of hypertension. *Lancet*, 1975, *2*, 93-95.

Pranulis, M. Coping with acute myocardial infarction. In W. D. Gentry & R. B. Williams, Jr. (Eds.), *Psychological aspects of myocardial infarction and coronary care*. St. Louis: Mosby, 1975.

Price, K. P. The application of behavior therapy to the treatment of psychosomatic disorders: Retrospect and prospect. *Psychotherapy: Theory, Research and Practice*, 1974, *11*, 138-155.

Price, K. P., Gaas-Abrams, E., & Browder, S. Research developments in behavioral interventions with psychophysiological disorders. A paper presented at the American Psychological Association Meeting, San Francisco, 1977.

Rabkin, J. G., & Struening, E. L. Life events, stress, and illness. *Science*, 1976, *194*, 1013-1020.

Rahe, R. H. The pathway between subject's recent life changes and their near-future illness reports: Representative results and methodological issues. In B. S. Dohrenwend & B. P. Dohrenwend (Eds.), *Stressful life events: Their nature and effects*. New York: Wiley, 1974.

Rahe, R. H. & Ransom, R. J. Life change and illness studies: Past history and future directions. *Journal of Human Stress*, 1978, *4*, 3-15.

Robinson, J. O. A possible effect of selection on the test scores of a group of hypertensives. *Journal of Psychosomatic Research*, 1964, *8*, 239.

Rosenman, R. H., Rahe, R. H., Borhani, N. O., & Feinleib, M. Heritability of personality and behavior pattern. Proceedings of the First International Congress on Twins, Rome, Italy, Nov. 1974.

Roskies, E. Considerations in developing a treatment program for the coronary-prone (Type A) behavior pattern. In P. Davidson (Ed.), *Behavioral medicine: Changing health life styles*. New York: Brunner/Mazel, 1978.

Rowland, K. F., & Sokol, B. A review of research examining the coronary-prone behavior pattern. *Journal of Human Stress*, 1977, *3*, 26-33.

Rush, A. J., Beck, A. T., Kovacs, M., & Hollon, S. Comparative efficacy of cognitive therapy and pharmacotherapy in the treatment of depressed outpatients. *Cognitive Therapy and Research*, 1977, *1*, 17-37.

Sarason, I. G. Test anxiety and cognitive modeling. *Journal of Personality and Social Psychology*, 1973, *28*, 58-61.

Sarason, I. G. Methodological issues in the assessment of life stress. In L. Levi (Ed.), *Emotions: Their parameters and measurement*. New York: Raven, 1975.

Scherwitz, L., Berton, K., & Leventhal, H. Type A assessment and interaction in the behavior pattern interview. *Psychosomatic Medicine*, 1977, *39*, 229-240.

Schucker, B., & Jacobs, D. K. Assessment of behavioral risk for coronary disease by voice characteristics. *Psychosomatic Medicine*, 1977, *39*, 219-227.

Schwartz, G. E. Biofeedback as therapy: Some theoretical and practical issues. *American Psychologist*, 1973, *28*, 666-673.

Schwartz, G. E. Psychosomatic disorders and biofeedback: A psychobiological model of disregulation. In J. D. Maser & M. E. P. Seligman (Eds.), *Psychopathology: Experimental models*. San Francisco: W. H. Freeman, 1977.

Selye, H. *The stress of life*. New York: McGraw-Hill, 1956.

Selye, H. *Stress without distress*. Philadelphia: Lippincott, 1974.

Selye, H. *The stress of life* (rev. ed.). New York: McGraw-Hill, 1976.

Selye, H. On the real benefits of eustress. *Psychology Today*, March 1978, 60-63, 69-70.

Shapiro, A. P., Schwartz, G., Ferguson, D., Redmond, D., & Weiss, S. M. Behavioral approachs to the treatment of hypertension: Clinical status. *Annals of Internal Medicine*, 1977, *86*, 626-636.

Shapiro, D., & Surwit, R. Learned control of physiological function and disease. In H. Leitenberg (Ed.), *Handbook of behavior modification and behavior therapy*. Englewood Cliffs, N.J.: Prentice-Hall, 1976.

Shapiro, D., Mainardi, J. A., & Surwit, R. S. Biofeedback and self-regulation in essential hypertension. In G. E. Schwartz & J. Beatty (Eds.), *Biofeedback*. New York: Academic, 1977.

Shaw, B. F. A comparison of cognitive therapy and behavior therapy in the treatment of depression. *Journal of Consulting and Clinical Psychology*, 1977, *45*, 543-551.

Silver, B. V., & Blanchard, E. B. Biofeedback and relaxation training in the treatment of psychophysiologic disorders: Or, are the machines really necessary? *Journal of Behavioral Medicine*. 1979, *1*, 217-239.

Smirk, F. H. The prognosis of untreated and treated hypertension and advantages of early treatment. *American Heart Journal*, 1972, *83*, 825-840.

Spaulding, R. C., & Ford, C. V. The *Pueblo* incident: Psychological reactions to the stresses of imprisonment and repatriation. In R. H. Moos (Ed.), *Human adaptation: Coping with life crises*. Lexington, Mass.: D. C. Heath, 1976.

Spitz, R. A. The psychogenic diseases in infancy: An attempt at their etiologic classification. *The Psychoanalytic Study of the Child*, 1951, *6*, 255-275.

Steinmark, S., & Borkovec, T. Active and placebo treatment effects on moderate insomnia under counterdemand and positive demand instruction. *Journal of Abnormal Psychology*, 1974, *83*, 157-163.

Sterman, M. B. Neurophysiological and clinical studies of sensorimotor EEG biofeedback training: Some effects on epilepsy. In L. Birk (Ed.), *Biofeedback: Behavioral medicine*. New York: Grune & Stratton, 1974.

Suinn, R. M. Behavior therapy for cardiac patients. *Behavior Therapy*, 1974, *5*, 569-571.

Suinn, R. M. The cardiac stress management program for Type A patients. *Cardiac Rehabilitation*, 1975, *15*, 13-15.

Suinn, R. M. Type A behavior pattern. In R. B. Williams & W. D. Gentry (Eds.), *Behavioral approaches to medical treatment*. Cambridge, Mass.: Ballinger, 1977.

Suinn, R. M., & Bloom, L. J. Anxiety management training for pattern A behavior. *Journal of Behavioral Medicine*, 1978, *1*, 25–35.

Suinn, R. M., Brock, L., & Edie, C. A. Behavior therapy for Type A patients. *American Journal of Cardiology*, 1975, *36*, 269.

Taylor, C. B., Farquhor, J. W., Nelson, E., & Agras, W. S. Relaxation therapy and high blood pressure. *Archives of General Psychiatry*, 1977, *34*, 339–342.

Taylor, F. G., & Marshall, W. J. A cognitive-behavioral therapy for depression. *Cognitive Therapy and Research*, 1977, *1*, 59–72.

Turk, D. C. Cognitive-behavioral techniques in the management of pain. In J. P. Foreyt & D. J. Rathjen (Eds.), *Cognitive-behavior therapy: Research and application*. New York: Plenum, 1978.

Turk, D. C. Application of coping-skills training to the treatment of pain. In C. D. Spielberger & I. G. Sarason (Eds.), *Stress and anxiety*, Vol. 5. New York: Brunner/Mazel, 1979.

Weiner, H., Thaler, M., Reiser, M. F., & Mirsky, I. A. Etiology of duodenal ulcer. *Psychosomatic Medicine*, 1957, *19*, 1–10.

Weisman, A. D., & Worden, J. W. The existential plight in cancer: Significance of the first 100 days. *International Journal of Psychiatry in Medicine*, 1976, *7*, 1–15.

Weiss, J. H. The current state of the concept of a psychosomatic disorder. In Z. J. Lipowski, D. R. Lipsitt, & P. C. Whybrow (Eds.), *Psychosomatic medicine*. New York: Oxford University Press, 1977.

Weiss, J. M. Psychological factors in stress and disease. *Scientific American*, June 1972, 104–113.

Weiss, J. M. Ulcers. In J. D. Maser & M. E. P. Seligman (Eds.), *Psychopathology: Experimental models*. San Francisco: W. H. Freeman, 1977.

Weiss, J. M., Stone, E. A., & Harrell, N. Coping behavior and brain norepinephrine level in rats. *Journal of Comparative and Physiological Psychology*, 1970, *72*, 153–160.

Weiss, J. M., Glazer, H. I., & Pohorecky, L. A. Coping behavior and neurochemical changes: An alternative explanation for the original "learned helplessness" experiments. In G. Serban & A. Kling (Eds.), *Animal models of human psychobiology*. New York: Plenum, 1976.

Wine, J. Test anxiety and direction of attention. *Psychological Bulletin*, 1971, *76*, 92–104.

Wishnie, H. A., Hackett, T. P., & Cassem, N. H. Psychological hazards of convalescence following myocardial infarction. *Journal of the American Medical Association*, 1971, *215*, 1292–1296.

Wittkower, E. D. Historical perspective of contemporary psychosomatic medicine. In Z. J. Lipowski, D. R. Lipsitt, & P. C. Whybrow (Eds.), *Psychosomatic medicine*, New York: Oxford University Press, 1977.

Wolf, S. *The stomach*. New York: Oxford University Press, 1965.

Wolf, S., & Goodell, H. *Harold G. Wolff's stress and disease* (2nd ed.). Springfield, Ill.: Charles C Thomas, 1968.

Wolf, S., Cardon, P. V., Shepard, E. M., & Wolff, H. G. *Life stresses and essential hypertension*. Baltimore: Williams & Wilkins, 1950.

Wolff, C. T., Friedman, S. B., Hofer, M. A., & Mason, J. W. Relationship between psychological defenses and mean urinary 17-hydroxycorticosteroid excretion rates: I & II. *Psychosomatic medicine*, 1964, *26*, 576–609.

Wolff, H. G. Life stress and bodily disease—A formulation. In H. G. Wolff, S. Wolf, & C. C. Hare (Eds.), *Life stress and bodily disease*. Baltimore: Williams & Wilkins, 1950.

Wolff, H. G. *Headache and other head pain*. New York: Oxford University Press, 1963.

Wolff, H. G., Wolf, S., & Hare, C. C. *Life stresses and bodily disease*. Baltimore: Williams & Wilkins, 1950.

Yager, J., & Weiner, H. Observations in man with remarks on pathogenesis. In H. Weiner (Ed.), *Duodenal ulcer*. New York: Karger, 1971.

9

Behavioral Intervention in a Pediatric Setting

C. EUGENE WALKER

INTRODUCTION

While psychologists have worked with children for many years, recognition of pediatric psychology as a distinct area, having some relationship to child psychology but differing in many ways, is a relatively recent phenomenon. The term *pediatric psychology* appears originally to have been proposed by Wright in an article in the *American Psychologist* in 1967. The Society of Pediatric Psychology was founded in 1968, and publication of the *Pediatric Psychology* newsletter began in 1969. In 1976, the name of the newsletter was changed to the *Journal of Pediatric Psychology*.

Starting with a relatively small group of psychologists scattered around the country, who began to realize that what they were doing was different from traditional child psychology, pediatric psychology in the last decade has grown from an infant to a rather healthy toddler. The types of settings that employ pediatric psychologists have similarly expanded. These range from most major medical schools and many hospitals to private clinics and private settings throughout the country. In a recent survey of clinical training centers, 63 of 153 centers reported that they offered training in pediatric psychology at some level (Tuma, 1977). Since this was strictly a voluntary survey, there are many other centers offering such training that are not included in the report. Thus, there is little doubt that pediatric psychology is an area of specialization that is being seen as an interesting, challenging, and growing field by more and more psychologists.

Pediatric psychology differs from traditional child psychology in terms of (1) conceptualization; (2) point of intervention; and (3) manner of intervention. In terms of conceptualization, pediatric psychology is best regarded as a specialty within

C. EUGENE WALKER • Division of Pediatric Psychology, University of Oklahoma Medical School, Oklahoma City, Oklahoma 73190.

medical psychology dealing with children and their behavioral-developmental problems. Traditional child psychology is more closely aligned with mental health and psychiatric models and conceptualizations.

In terms of the point of intervention, the pediatric psychologist generally becomes involved in a case via consultation with the pediatrician. The typical psychologist becomes involved after the patient has had a number of contacts with various professionals that have led to a referral to a mental health practitioner. However, the pediatric psychologist frequently sees patients who originally came in for a routine checkup or as a result of some minor problem such as a runny nose or a sore throat. In the course of the examination, the physician may have noted something of concern, or the mother may have asked a question having to do with the psychological and emotional development of the child. At this point, the pediatric psychologist is called upon. As a result of this point of entry, the pediatric psychologist typically sees an extremely wide range of psychopathology of childhood and sees the problems when they are still fresh and in their formative stages, rather than after the patient has been through a number of shaping procedures in developing an appropriate repertoire of "mental health patient" behaviors. In addition, the pediatric psychologist is frequently called upon to deal with emotional and behavioral problems related to medical disorders. Thus, the pediatric psychologist may see a child who will not comply with a regimen to control diabetes; he/she may deal with the emotional and family problems surrounding a chronic illness or the imminent death of a child; he/she may deal with a child who is experiencing excessive anxiety over upcoming surgery or, as in a recent case seen in our hospital, assist a family in coping with the stress attendant in a situation in which the father accidentally ran over a young child with a tractor lawn mower, severing three limbs and causing considerable damage to the child.

The type of intervention offered by pediatric psychologists also varies from traditional child clinical psychology. The pediatric psychologist serves as a consultant to the pediatrician and the family with respect to all manner of children's medical and psychological problems. In this role, he/she is able to provide guidance and training in effective parenting skills, thus preventing the development of problems before they have an opportunity to become serious. The pediatric psychologist also serves a very useful evaluation and screening function in enabling the pediatrician and the family to know when a child should be referred to another specialist and what specialist would be of the most help. The pediatric psychologist is also frequently called upon when management of behavior is crucial to the successful treatment of medical disorders. Serving in this role, the pediatric psychologist's therapeutic intervention usually takes the form of crisis management and short-term treatment.

Perhaps the nature of pediatric psychology can be made more clear by reference to the referrals typically made to a pediatric psychology service. Table 1 indicates the frequency of referral for various problems in 1975–1978 in the Pediatric Psychology Service of Oklahoma Childrens Memorial Hospital. It should be noted that these were the main reasons given for referral. In many cases, multiple problems were discovered on examination. These are not reflected in the table but would considerably increase the frequency in some of the categories were they included.

Studies in other pediatric settings reveal very similar patterns of referral (e.g., Mesibov, Schroeder, & Wesson, 1977; Monnelly, Ianzito, & Stewart, 1973). Examination of this table reveals a wide range of problems, including all of the normal or typical problems that are referred to child psychologists as well as some relatively unusual problems. The basic nature and philosophy of pediatric psychology would

Table 1.   Referral Frequency

Category	Definition	Frequency of referral	Percentage of total
Death	Understanding the concept, adjusting to death of someone who was close	18	1.19
Developmental delays	Perceptual motor problems, slow development, school readiness, speech problems	98	6.49
Divorce, separation	Adoption, guardianship, advice on proper placement, what to tell the child, court referral for testing	24	1.59
Family problems	Parents disagree on discipline, mother feels isolated, parents argue a lot, child abuse	143	9.47
Food/eating problems			
Obesity	Overweight	29	1.92
Anorexic	Underweight	7	.46
Guidance of talented child	Need for special programs, appropriate stimulation	3	.19
Hyperactivity	Active to the extent that child is considered unmanageable	73	4.83
Infant management	Feeding, nursing, postpartum depression, cries all the time (colicky), failure to thrive	4	.26
Miscellaneous			
Depression		117	7.75
Hallucinations		10	.66
Suicide		37	2.45
Instability—difficulty in making decisions		8	.53
Moving	Preparation for a new home, problems of adjustment after moving	2	.13
Negative behaviors	(Toward parents) won't listen to parents, doesn't obey, is bossy, demanding, cries and whines	155	10.27
Mental retardation		75	4.97
Parents' negative feelings toward child	Generally don't like child, no enjoyment from child	2	.13
Personality problems	Emotional, lacks self-control, no motivation, won't assume responsibility, lies, steals, dependent, etc.	63	4.17

(*Continued*)

Table 1.   (Continued)

Category	Definition	Frequency of referral	Percentage of total
Physical complaints			
Headaches		22	1.45
Stomachaches		25	1.65
Asthma		18	1.19
Diabetes		16	1.06
Meningomyocele		11	.72
Spinal cord injury		8	.53
Cerebral palsy		7	.46
Overdose (drugs, alcohol, etc.)		43	2.84
General		190	12.59
School problems	Hates school, not doing well in school, reading or math problems, aggression by child toward teacher. Is the child getting what is needed?	134	8.88
Sex-related problems	Trying on opposite-sexed parent's clothes, no same-sexed friends, lack of sex-appropriate interests, sex abuse of child	30	1.98
Sibling–peer problems	Won't share, has no friends, aggressive toward peers and siblings, fights a lot, sibling rivalry	10	.66
Sleeping problems	Won't go to bed, wakes up at night, nightmares	20	1.32
Specific bad habits	Nail biting, tics, thumb sucking	23	1.52
Specific fears	Dogs, the dark, trucks, etc.	13	.86
Toileting			
Enuresis		25	1.65
Encopresis		42	2.78
Encopresis and enuresis		4	.13
	Total	1509	

seem to invite a behavioral orientation, though many other approaches are taken by practitioners in the area.

The remainder of this chapter deals with the philosophy and structure of the clinic procedures, assessment procedures, and treatment procedures used in handling cases referred to a pediatric psychologist.

CLINIC PROCEDURES

Since the philosophy of intervention employed in pediatric psychology dictates clinical procedures and office management to a considerable extent, a brief description of the manner in which these issues are handled in a typical pediatric psychology service is presented here. Since the pediatric psychologist must be available for consultation and must be able to intervene in crises, it is imperative that he/she guard against filling his/her schedule with relatively long-term treatment cases. It would be very easy for the pediatric psychologist to have a full schedule of relatively long-term treatment cases. However, the pediatric psychologist spends a good deal of time "on call" and is available to consult with pediatricians and others on relatively short notice. In our service, this has been accomplished in a variety of ways. On occasion, we have arranged with clinics in our hospital to have a psychology intern or staff member be present at the clinic during the treatment hours to be available to consult with medical personnel and patients. Since there are many more clinics and ongoing activities within the hospital than can be handled in this manner, most of the consulting has to be by request. Thus, on any given day, we attempt to have in the pediatric psychology office at least one person, and, if possible, more than one, who can go to any clinic or ward in the hospital for consultation. Sometimes, the consultation requires one session only and can be handled on the spot. Some reassurance, information, or advice may be given to the physician or the family that will handle the problem under consideration. However, in many cases, it is obvious that longer-term treatment and additional follow-up will be needed. When this occurs, the pediatric psychologist generally makes contact with the family and arranges to see them later in the office if it is a problem that the psychologist wishes to deal with personally. Or an appropriate referral to other resources in the community may be made if the pediatric psychologist does not wish to handle the case personally. In any event, he/she serves as a gate keeper and ensures that the patient gets prompt and efficient attention for the presenting problems.

In making referrals to community agencies and practitioners, it is essential that the pediatric psychologist not simply say to the patient that they should go to a certain mental health center or see a certain professional in the community. Under such circumstances, the likelihood that the person will actually find his/her way to that source of help is relatively low. A much better course of action is to call the place and make an appointment for the patient. Then, the psychologist contacts the patient and lets him/her know what arrangements have been made. Or if the agency or professional in question prefers to contact the patient, the information can be given to the agency, and the patient is informed that the agency will be contacting her/him in the near future.

For consultations that are not urgent and do not need to be made on the spot, a card requesting consultation services is used. When the psychologist sees the case, brief notes on the back of the card are made as to where the case stands. Our service has also found it helpful to keep a chronological log of the incoming consultation requests. When new cases are picked up, the logbook is scanned for cases of high priority or for the next case in line. These are then scheduled for visits.

On the first occasion that a patient in seen in pediatric psychology, a number of forms, including a release-of-information form, are completed by the patient or the family of the patient. The standardized release-of-information form is extremely valuable in permitting the pediatric psychologist to converse with other professionals who may be involved with the child. We have found that it is extremely helpful if the receptionist or the psychologist explains to the family the purpose of this release.

The family can then be guided to list those with whom they wish us to be in contact and to omit any that they do not. Some families choose to leave the form blank. This is quite acceptable. Names can be filled in later, if necessary. However, by having most patients fill in the forms on the first visit, unnecessary delays and inconveniences are avoided.

PSYCHOLOGICAL ASSESSMENT IN A PEDIATRIC PSYCHOLOGY CENTER

Because of the historical development of the field of clinical psychology and the fact that psychologists for many years marketed their skills as psychological testers and examiners, many of the referrals received by psychologists have to do with psychological evaluation and testing. This is particularly true for child patients because such areas as developmental progress and school achievement require careful measurement. However, even behavioral problems in the child are much more difficult to assess than in the adult, largely because the age and the developmental level of the child are major considerations in determining whether or not a behavior is appropriate and acceptable. Psychology as a profession has matured to the point where most psychologists prefer not to present knowledge and experience derived from psychological testing as the psychologist's most important contribution. They prefer rather to emphasize the high degree of skill and expertise needed to conduct psychotherapy, consultation, research, and other scientific or professional activities.

Behavioral psychologists have been particularly vocal regarding the need to emphasize other aspects of the clinical psychologist's role. There are several reasons for this. First, behavior therapy developed historically at a time when psychologists began to emphasize skills other than testing. In addition, many of the commonly used psychological tests are based on theoretical notions of psychodynamics and traits connected with internal states and conditions that do not fit very well with behavioral theory and its emphasis on environmental determinants. Finally, many of the tests are interpreted on the basis of normative data, while behavioral approaches frequently emphasize careful examination of the individual case.

Initially, many behavioral therapists completely rejected psychological testing and assessment, substituting direct observations of patient behavior, either in the natural setting or in simulated conditions in the office, for test scores and protocols. However, over the years, it became increasingly evident that additional techniques were needed for assessment and evaluation. Thus, behavior therapists began to develop questionnaires and checklists to assist them in their work. More psychometrically sophisticated critics were quick to point out that these types of instruments were discarded by other psychologists decades ago in favor of more rigorously developed instruments (Evans & Nelson, 1974). Behavioral psychologists generally countered this argument with comments to the effect that their instruments had content validity, which was the most appropriate form of validity for their purposes. Their instruments, they pointed out, were used primarily to save time and to serve as a guide when interviewing the patient. Some behavioral psychologists began to use direct observation of peers of the identified patient as a type of control or normative group and found that this observation helped combine the "best of two worlds" in that the result was direct observation with norms (Nelson & Bowles, 1975). Other behavioral psychologists began to refine their paper-and-pencil assessment techniques in an attempt to improve them in terms of more traditional approaches to reliability and validity. This is where the field currently stands. Direct observations are much preferred and used by behaviorists, though they tend to be time-consuming and costly. Some of the paper-and-pencil instruments in use have the beginnings of research data that make them useful and interpretable in the therapeutic setting. Others are still in such embryonic stages that they represent little more than the author's ideas about what are good questions to ask.

For the behaviorally oriented pediatric psychologist, the controversy regarding assessment procedures is particularly important. Schoolteachers, parents, and other professionals still view the psychologist as a major resource for psychological testing. Therefore, many of the referrals made to the pediatric psychologist request psychological evaluation. It is also true that on many occasions, a careful assessment of the developmental progress of the child in various areas is most advantageous and helpful. Therefore, the pediatric psychologist, even if he/she is behaviorally inclined, finds himself/herself doing considerably more psychological testing than other behaviorally oriented psychologists. An additional practical consideration is that since many professionals request psychological testing and are more accepting of recommendations that are based on testing, it is often politically wise for the pediatric psychologist to do a certain amount of psychological testing before making comments or recommendations regarding the handling of the child. It may well be true that the same general recommendations could be made without the testing, but the likelihood of their being accepted and implemented may be greatly enhanced by buttressing them with testing results. This is not to say that the behavioral psychologist should not attempt to educate other professionals and wean them away from excessive or unnecessary testing. However, this takes time, and if one wishes to accomplish a purpose, often one will have to do it by means of a vehicle that may not be the vehicle of choice.

Another reason for testing occurs if the pediatric psychologist is in a training setting. For example, in our service, we frequently require interns to evaluate a case through selected psychological testing instruments. Following this, the intern formulates a treatment program and sees the patient in treatment. Thus, the intern is able, with prolonged observation of the case, to evaluate test interpretations critically. As a result, the intern learns what kinds of statements it is possible to make on the basis of such data and what kinds of statement are not possible. It is often a rather sobering experience.

A brief review of the particular psychological tests and instruments that we find helpful in the Pediatric Psychology Service at Oklahoma Childrens Memorial Hospital may further illustrate our philosophy of assessment. In a large majority of the cases referred to our clinic, school and behavioral problems are closely intertwined. That is, the child is frequently having a variety of behavioral difficulties both at home and at school. Many times, determining which came first is a chicken-and-egg problem. However, it is often possible to make a judgment in this area. Thus, a child may be experiencing emotional problems that are causing school performance to deteriorate. Or the child may be having unusual difficulty in school, which is causing emotional upset. If the problem is obviously in one area or the other, we generally proceed with an assessment of the problem area. However, in the majority of cases, we perform some type of assessment in both areas. Our general procedure is to begin with an initial interview of an hour, or more if needed. In this interview, we attempt to get a clear statement of the problems about which the patient or the family is concerned. We obtain a brief picture of the child's functioning in a variety of areas and attempt to get some idea of the family situation. We do not attempt an exhaustive social and developmental history; rather, we interview specifically with respect to the presenting symptoms. In general, the interview is structured to gather information from the following five areas in order to clarify the problem at hand: presenting complaint, habits, attitudes and emotional behavior, interpersonal social behavior, and development.

Following the initial interview phase of the assessment process, some evaluation of intellectual ability and school performance is generally made. If the problems in the school situation or the behavioral problems appear to be due to intellectual factors and are relatively severe, we use the standard instruments, such as the Wechsler tests (Wechsler, 1967, 1974) or the Stanford–Binet (Terman & Merrill, 1960). If the intellectual or cognitive factors involved in the child's problem do not appear to be particularly prominent, we frequently use a relatively brief screening device, such as the Peabody Picture Vocabulary Test (Dunn, 1965), to determine whether or not further evaluation in this area is required. If the child has a particular handicap, we use the intelligence tests designed for children with such handicaps, for example, the Leiter (Leiter, 1969) for children with language deficits or the Hiskey–Nebraska Test of Learning Aptitude (Hiskey, 1966) for a child with significant hearing impairment. If a child has a relatively short attention span or is uncooperative, we frequently give a simple test like the Peabody to capitalize on what little involvement and cooperation is present. In other cases where the child is essentially untestable, we use the Vineland Social Maturity Scale (Doll, 1965) and various other scales based on developmental milestones. Through these types of instruments, we are able to roughly determine the intellectual ability of the child relative to his/her peers. This approach often yields very useful information in determining the nature of the problem and in selecting a behavioral strategy to deal with it. It also enables us to counsel effectively with the parents and the schoolteachers. As suggested earlier, the scores tend to buttress our recommendations and ensure greater cooperation than if we made the same recommendations without the scores.

Second, we attempt to make an assessment of academic progress, if this appears to be an issue. School reports and telephone conversations with the teachers are very helpful. The testing instruments in this area are much less reliable and valid, but there are several that are commonly employed, such as the Bender–Gestalt test (Bender, 1946) to evaluate perceptual–motor functioning and the Wide Range Achievement Test (Jastak, Bijou, & Jastak, 1965) for a crude index of academic achievement. Various diagnostic tests, such as the Illinois Test of Psycholinguistic

Abilities (Kirk, McCarthy, & Kirk, 1968) and the Spache Reading Diagnostic Test (Spache, 1963), provide some indication of the nature of the learning problems that the child may be experiencing.

Emotional problems and behavioral disorders of children seen in pediatric psychology are evaluated by a wide range of techniques. Much useful information is obtained from the interviews conducted. In addition, observations are frequently made of the child's behavior. These may be made in our office or playroom as well as at the school or at home. Numerous checklists completed by the parents are also often helpful. The Cassel Child Behavior Rating Scale (Cassel, 1962) provides information on the child's functioning in several different areas, including self-adjustment, home adjustment, social adjustment, school adjustment, physical adjustment, and overall adjustment rated by the parents. The scales developed by the Devereaux Foundation (Spivack & Spotts, 1966; Spivack & Swift, 1967) also provide useful information regarding the child's behavior in a variety of areas. In addition, there are scales that can be completed by the schoolteachers and others (e.g., Burks, 1969).

Scales are available that assess the parents' attitudes toward their child and child rearing (Hereford, 1963; Schaefer & Bell, 1958). These forms are frequently filled out by the parents in the waiting room while interviews or observations are being made of the child. This procedure yields much useful information without requiring any additional time. Errors in parenting skills or attitudes of the parents that serve essentially as "expectancies" and elicit unacceptable behavior may be uncovered. A variety of questionnaires and scales are also available that are completed by the child. Table 2 presents a fear survey developed for use with child patients, and Table 3 presents a reinforcement survey. Both instruments are used to better understand the problem(s) and assist in therapeutic planning with the child. Both of these instruments are currently used as checklists and are followed up with interview and discussion. No normative or research data are available on them at present. However, such data have been gathered and are in the process of being analyzed.

A variety of standardized personality instruments are also available for assessment. Most instruments available for children suffer greatly from the difficulty of developing a reliable and valid instrument that is suitable for use with children at all educational and developmental levels. However, we have made good use of the series of tests developed at the Institute for Personality and Ability Testing (IPAT). These instruments begin at the first grade and run through adulthood. The tests included in the series are the Early School Personality Questionnaire for children from 6 to 8, the Children's Personality Questionnaire for ages 8-12, the Junior–Senior High School Personality Questionnaire for adolescents, and the Sixteen P–F test for adults (Cattell, 1972; Cattell, Coan, & Beloff, 1969; Coan & Cattell, 1972; Porter & Cattell, 1968). While the psychometric properties of these instruments leave much to be desired, they are the most suitable instruments available. All forms of the IPAT tests have been evaluated for their reliability and validity and have available norms that are helpful in interpreting the results. Each produces essentially the same factors from one age group to another, though the factors vary

Table 2. Student's Attitude Survey

The things below are things that sometimes make people scared or afraid. Mark the box that tells if they do that to you or not. If you have any questions or don't know some of the words, ask the person who gave you this paper. You should be sure to tell the truth in your answers. What you say will help us know how to help you.

Fears	Doesn't scare me at all	Scares me a little	Scares me very much
1. Being alone			
2. Being in a strange or funny place			
3. Loud talking			
4. Dead people			
5. People who seem crazy			
6. Cars and trucks on the road			
7. Being teased			
8. Thunder			
9. Failure			
10. Being in a high place and looking down			
11. Imaginary creatures (monsters, animals, etc.)			
12. Strangers			
13. Riding in a car or bus			
14. Old people			
15. Bugs, spiders, or worms			
16. Sudden noises			
17. Crowds of people			
18. Large open spaces			
19. Cats or dogs			
20. Somebody hitting or being mean to someone else			
21. Tough-looking people			
22. Being watched when I'm doing something			
23. Guns			
24. Sick people			
25. People telling me I'm wrong			
26. People who are mad			
27. Knives			
28. Being kidnapped			
29. Blood			
30. Someone in the family dying			
31. Things that are messy			
32. When people don't like me			
33. When somebody tells me to stop doing something			
34. When people won't listen to me			
35. Being in the dark			
36. Lightning			
37. Doctors			
38. Doing things wrong			
39. When people say I'm silly			
40. Getting sick			
41. Going crazy			
42. Taking tests			
43. Feeling different from other people			
44. Arguing with people			
45. When my heart beats funny			
46. Growing up and getting older			
47. Boys			
48. Girls			
49. Talking to my teacher			
50. Talking in front of class			
51. Homework			
52. Taking a shower with other kids at school or someplace			

Table 2. (*Continued*)

Fears	Doesn't scare me at all	Scares me a little	Scares me very much
53. Going on dates			
54. People without their clothes on			
55. Going to the bathroom when other people are around			
56. Getting good grades at school			
57. Not being chosen for a team or being chosen near the end			
58. If people don't like me			
59. Dreams or nightmares			
60. Wetting the bed			
61. Finding spots on my underwear			
62. Getting clothes dirty			
63. Spankings			
64. Breaking things			
65. People swearing			
66. Getting married someday			
67. Mornings			
68. Going to bed			
69. Being lost			
70. Mom and Dad arguing			
71. Mom or Dad shouting			
72. Hurting myself			
73. Not having any friends			
74. Getting into fights			
75. School			
76. Teachers			
77. The future			
78. Drugs			
79. Drinking			
80. Forgetting things			
81. Being late			
82. People laughing at me			
83. Not doing what I am told			
84. People who show off			
85. Older kids			
86. Not being invited to parties			
87. Going to parties			
88. Staying overnight with a friend			
89. Riding the school bus			
90. Looking funny in my clothes			
91. Not telling the truth			
92. Getting caught doing something			
93. Water			
94. Not having a home			
95. Losing my breath			
96. Being ugly			
97. Not being smart enough			
98. Not understanding things			
99. Parents getting divorced			
100. Hospitals			
101. Falling			
102. Elevators			
103. Dying			
104. People who are drunk			
105. Being poisoned			
106. End of the world			
107. People from outer space			

Table 3. Student's Attitude Survey

The things below are things that make some people happy because they like them. Mark the box that tells if they make you happy or not. If you have any questions or don't know some of the words, ask the person who gave you this paper.

Reinforcements	Doesn't make me happy at all	Makes me a little happy	Makes me very happy
1. Watching TV			
2. Money			
3. Reading			
4. Friends			
5. Parents			
6. Clothes			
7. Dancing			
8. Music			
9. Eating			
10. Playing games			
11. Going to movies			
12. Playing sports			
13. Making things			
14. Playing pinball machines			
15. Going on trips			
16. Going to amusement parks			
17. Horseback riding			
18. Swimming			
19. Drawing and painting pictures			
20. Solving puzzles			

slightly from one age group to another. The advantages of the tests are that they are short and relatively easy to administer even to young children. Also, work is currently being conducted on a preschool version of these tests (Cattell & Dreger, 1976).

Occasional use is also made of projective instruments. Instruments such as the Rorschach (Rorschach, 1954), the Thematic Apperception Test (Murray, 1943), the Children's Apperception Test (Bellak & Bellak, 1965), the Education Apperception Test (Thompson & Sones, 1973), the Pain Apperception Test (Petrovich, 1973), and the Michigan Pictures Test (Michigan Pictures Test, 1953) are used as a means of observing children's behavior under unique but standardized conditions. In addition, interviewing the child regarding the responses given to the test stimuli often elicits much valuable information that can be used in developing a treatment program.

Frequent use of drawings and paintings is made in working with children. On occasion, the child may simply be given some crayons or paints and asked to produce something. Or the child may be asked to draw a specific picture, such as a "family" or "yourself doing what you like to do best." Interpretation of these materials is not based on psychodynamic principles or related to details of the drawings produced. Rather, the drawings or productions serve as a vehicle through which the examiner can ask questions and elicit further responses from the patient. Many times, children who will not answer questions or respond in an interview produce drawings and may then be encouraged to discuss the drawings. Thus, the drawing serves as a vehicle for relating to the child and eliciting conversation.

Structured doll play is used in a similar manner in the evaluation process. Most of the original doll play techniques (e.g., Lynn, 1959) were developed for the use of psychoanalytic principles for interpretation. However, we keep a set of dolls and furniture available to use in interviewing the child and simply attempt to elicit information regarding the child's behavior and reactions in various situations through doll play. For example, in a case of suspected child abuse, we might say, "This is the little boy who has just spilled some milk on the floor. This is the mommy. Here, you take the boy and the mommy and show us what happens." By structuring situations that are of interest and letting the child act out in doll play what he/she perceives to be happening, it is possible to uncover valuable information regarding the child's perception of his/her behavior and the behavior of others around him/her. This technique is particularly helpful with younger children.

It is perhaps appropriate to comment here on the interpretations generally given to psychological tests. The research literature of the last several decades clearly leads to the conclusion that psychological tests must be interpreted conservatively and very cautiously. The most generous interpretation of the evidence suggests that accurate statements may be made about broad categories and general trends. However, once one gets into more refined and esoteric interpretations, the evidence regarding validity indicates that such interpretations are more often wrong than right. Therefore, throughout our interpretation of results, we tend to be conservative, dealing with general categories and basic interpretations that then lead to action-oriented recommendations for correction, rather than dwelling on elaborate descriptions and refined interpretations, most of which are likely to be wrong. For example, in dealing with a school problem, we do not attempt to specify the exact nature of the problem and tell the teacher the exact page of a particular workbook to begin with. We find more often than not that when the teacher begins with the page recommended by some tester, he/she finds that the tests were in error and that the child either cannot handle this material or can handle it with ease. The teacher then proceeds with a trial-and-error process until the right materials and the right approach are found. However, knowing that the child does have a problem and that it is in a particular area usually serves to help the teacher get started in the right direction. We therefore make an effort to serve this function but shy away from overly elaborate and specific interpretations and recommendations based on testing. Likewise, in personality testing, we do not attempt to present any elaborate descriptions of, or details about, behaviors that we have not observed. Rather, we discuss what was observed and make certain inferences from the test results about the general directions that therapy should take, recognizing that more precise behavioral analyses will be performed as each problem area is dealt with in treatment.

Report Writing

Following completion of the psychological assessment, a report is generally prepared. The type of report prepared by a behavioral pediatric psychologist differs from that usually prepared following psychological testing. Historically, psychologists earned their way into clinical practice through psychological testing. In the early days, little psychotherapy was done by psychologists, and what was done was with selected cases under the supervision of psychiatrists. Having highly capable, intelligent, and verbal psychologists funneling most of their energies into psychological testing and report writing resulted in a unique situation. Under these circumstances, the psychological testing process came to involve anywhere from five to six hours with the patient, followed by another three to five hours of report preparation. Each response on each test was carefully studied and weighed. In the report, elaborate discussions were presented dealing with all of the results, and a highly involved description of the patient's "psychodynamics" emerged. This procedure generally resulted in a long, relatively pedantic, and esoteric report. Many of these reports were never read because of their length or, if they were read, proved incomprehensible to the reader. The recommendations made on the basis of the evaluation frequently were either absent or extremely weak because the psychologist was aware that a newcomer should not be too forceful in making recommendations. The treatment of the case was the responsibility of the psychiatrist.

However, with the movement of psychologists into a more active treatment role, spending that amount of time in psychological testing and report writing has become highly suspect. In terms of cost efficiency, it would appear to be far better to spend a much briefer period of time in evaluation and to increase the amount of time spent in therapy. If a psychologist is to spend 12 hours on a case, it would be much better to spend 2 or 3 hours in assessment, followed by 8 or 10 in treatment rather than to spend all of that time in assessment. Thus, in pediatric psychology, we typically spend a relatively short period of time in psychological assessment and attempt to get on with the treatment as quickly as possible. Testing is not done if it is not needed. The report that is prepared by the behavioral pediatric psychologist is not a lengthy one that reads like a textbook but a brief, crisp communication regarding the patient's problem and what should be done about it. At Oklahoma Childrens Memorial Hospital, we label our reports "Narrative Consultation Summary." The report typically takes the form of a sentence or two regarding the reason for referral, followed by a list of the procedures used and the results section, in which the general findings are discussed. Behavioral observations and items from the history are worked into this section where appropriate rather than being included in separate sections. In a couple of paragraphs, an attempt is made to describe the nature of the problem and the information pertinent to the problem. Following this is a section regarding recommendations. The recommendations section is regarded as the most important part of the report. An attempt is made to indicate exactly what kind of treatment or help should be given to this patient. This report is generally prepared prior to feedback with the patient. Following the feedback session, an addendum is added to the bottom indicating the patient's response to the recommendations and a note about what plans are being implemented to follow up the recommendations. All of this is accomplished in approximately a page and a half to two pages. It has been our experience that this style of report communicates well and facilitates treatment.

TREATMENT

In this section, the treatment approaches that have been found to be helpful with the problems represented in Table 1 are briefly reviewed. In cases where adequate literature exists, the procedures are briefly discussed, with references to pertinent sources provided for details. In cases where ideas or approaches have developed out of the clinical application of behavioral principles, more detail is given. Because of the wide variety of topics covered in this chapter, literature citation is selective—in terms of approaches and presentations that have been found to be most helpful—rather than exhaustive.

Tension-Related Disorders

Examination of Table 1 indicates several categories of disorders in which anxiety and tension play a major role. Such factors are believed to be important in the physical complaint of chronic recurrent abdominal pain. The general treatment principles outlined in connection with the treatment of abdominal pain would apply to any of the categories in Table 1 where tension or anxiety either is the source of the problem or contributes to it.

A typical case history for abdominal pain might be a young child between the ages of 3 and 12, more commonly female than male, who reports severe stomach pain to her parents and is obviously in such great distress that she is rushed to the emergency room of a local hospital. On examination, the physician is unable to determine any physiological reason for the pain. The pain frequently persists for many hours but often is relieved by reassurance or prescription of a placebo. In our hospital, the child is generally sent home following the emergency treatment and is referred for psychological assessment and treatment. Frequently, the parents do not follow up on the psychological referral. They tend to feel that there is no significant psychological problem and that the physicians have not property diagnosed the physical condition. The first attack is usually followed by several similar incidents over a period of weeks, months, or years. Eventually, the family decides to follow up on the psychological referral. Psychological examination generally reveals a normal, well-functioning but tense child. Investigation of the family frequently reveals family situations that place great pressure on the child. For example, the child is being pressured for outstanding school performance that he/she feels unable to deliver; or there may be an impending divorce, with both parents attempting to win the loyalty of the child; or there may be significant rivalries among the children; or a host of similar problems. At any rate, the result is that the child becomes aware of intestinal reactions while under pressure. These frighten the child and a pain reaction develops. The child then learns that this pain reaction significantly alters the environment. The parents generally become very concerned about the child and reduce the pressure because he/she is "sick." This reaction serves to reinforce the pain behavior and makes it very likely that the pain will recur in the future. Many physicians who treat these patients refer to this malady as the chronic recurrent abdominal pain syndrome (CRAP)—and the abbreviation for the syndrome is not an accident. In traditional nomenclature, this symptom represents a rather shadowy area between psychophysiological reactions and hysterical reactions. Hysterical reactions, while thought to be rare in adult behavior, are surprisingly common in pediatric settings (Laybourne & Churchill, 1972). Interruption of the reinforcers along with training in relaxation and more effective ways of coping with problems is generally helpful in treating these problems.

Behavioral treatment of recurrent abdominal pain requires intervention in several areas. First, the physician involved is consulted to be sure that all probable organic causes have been ruled out. The physician counsels the parents regarding his findings in a positive rather than negative manner. That is, he/she explains that there is no organic illness that is threatening the child and thus no immediate physical danger. The physician, however, points out that the pain is real, not imaginary, and that it is the result of tension. The phychologist in the case then explains to the family that the child is not "mentally ill" but points out that just as tension can produce ulcers and other physical symptoms, it can result in abdominal pain in children. Relaxation training is then explained and recommended to reduce tension. Following this, muscle relaxation is taught. EMG biofeedback is employed, if needed. Details of relaxation therapy are discussed elsewhere (Bernstein & Borkovec, 1973; Goldfried & Davison, 1976; Walker, Hedberg, Clement, & Wright, in press). Numerous tape recordings are available, but we have found the Peace, Harmony, and Awareness series (Lupin, 1974) most useful. Other behavioral procedures, such as assertive training, behavioral contracting among the family members, social training, and environmental restructuring to reduce sources of tension, are also used as needed.

While the above example describes a physical symptom, the basic procedures in relaxation training may be employed with a wide variety of problem behaviors and symptoms as long as anxiety and tension are prominent features. Thus, this treatment is useful with such problems as nightmares, fears, and anxiety reactions. Relaxation training has also been found to be effective with hyperactive children (Lupin, Braud, & Deur, 1974) and is very useful in cases where school performance deteriorates because of excessive tension. Relaxation training may be the only form of treatment offered in some cases. However, more commonly, it is used as part of a treatment package involving other forms of therapy.

Phobias

When a specific stimulus is identifiable as a source of conditioned anxiety, systematic desensitization is employed. Children may be desensitized to relatively common fear-evoking stimuli, such as dogs, elevators, water, and separation from parents. In addition, numerous occasions for systematic desensitization occur in a pediatric clinic that are relatively unique to the setting. For example, we recently desensitized a young male patient to a phobia regarding needles. The patient was to be a kidney donor for his sister and was quite willing to donate a kidney. However, he was extremely phobic about needles and was terrified at the prospect of the various medical procedures involving needles. Systematic desensitization enabled him to cooperate with the medical procedures with comfort. Similarly, when the local school district began to enforce its rules regarding immunization prior to enrolling in school, several referrals for desensitization of needle phobias were received.

Since many patients seen by the pediatric psychologist are involved in learning disabilities or academic performance problems of one sort or another, systematic desensitization may be employed in these cases also. Frequently, what began as a difficulty in learning (possibly as a result of some sort of developmental delay or lack of readiness on the part of the child) over time becomes a source of conditioned anxiety. That is, the child originally may have been called upon to perform tasks that he/she was not capable of handling. Continued pressure and stress resulting from attempts to accomplish the tasks produce a conditioned anxiety reaction. Then, the child becomes unable to do the work because of the severe anxiety reaction experienced when confronted with the material. Thus, some children would be able to read, except that they become extremely tense and block mentally when they are presented with a printed page. We begin treatment of such children with desensitization for the reading phobia. Generally, the child is able to make rapid progress with remedial training following the desensitization.

Systematic desensitization with children is often accomplished by use of the standard imaginal procedures. However, with young children, it is often necessary to use variations in the procedures because they are not able to cooperate with the procedures generally used with adults. Thus, *in vivo* desensitization is often used if the child is unable to cooperate with imaginal procedures (Tasto, 1969). Similarly, Croghan and Musante (1975) used playing games in the presence of the feared object, and Kissel (1972) used pictures, reading, and storytelling to desensitize a child's phobia to dogs. In addition, emotive imagery has been used (Lazarus & Abramovitz, 1962). In emotive imagery, the visualization encourages the child to see himself/herself as an agent of Superman or some other fictitious character and to confront the feared stimulus with help from the hero character. Modeling has also been effective in helping children overcome fears (Adelson & Goldfried, 1970; Clement, 1976).

School Refusal

School refusal is a common problem that the pediatric psychologist is called upon to deal with. While it seems like a relatively simple problem and most psychologists would agree that it is necessary to get the child to school (Lassers, Nordon, & Bladholm, 1973) as soon as possible, the situation is often more complex than it first appears. The first issue that must be dealt with is to determine the nature of the problem more precisely. School refusal may be due to a phobic reaction to something in the school situation, but it may also be a symptom of some other problem, such as depression, delinquency, or even psychosis (Marine, 1968–1969; Smith, 1970). If one of the latter is involved, it is generally a mistake to focus on the school refusal until later. Assuming, however, that the problem can be defined as a phobic reaction, a careful behavioral analysis should be done. Of particular importance is the length of time the child has been out of school, whether the onset was acute or occurred over a period of time, the age of the child, the general adjustment of the child, and the degree of cooperation that can be expected from the school (Weinberger, Leventhal, & Beckman, 1973). Additional considerations are discussed by Kennedy (1965) and Berecz (1968). Two general patterns typically emerge from the behavioral analysis (Coolidge, Hahn, & Peck, 1957). One is the younger child, under 12, who appears to be functioning well but suddenly begins to refuse to go to school. The second is the older, teenage child, who has numerous signs of emotional problems and who gradually, over a period of months or even years, begins to refuse more and more often to go to school until he/she is not attending at all.

With the first type, simply seeing that the child is taken to school and required to remain there is the major treatment (Kennedy, 1965). It is helpful to have someone who is able to be firm with the child and whom the child will cooperate with to take the child to school. This may be mother, father, grandparents, uncle, or neighbor. The child will be met at the door by a counselor or teacher who escorts him/her to classes throughout the day. The teachers and counselors are instructed to physically retain the child in the building until he/she is picked up at the end of the day. If the child is able to identify a specific source of the fear (e.g., a certain teacher or another student who has threatened him/her), this problem is discussed with the child prior to taking him/her to school. Then, any environmental manipulation possible is made (e.g., conference with the teacher or assurance of protection from the other child). However, in many cases, the child is unable or unwilling to identify any specific source contributing to the refusal. If such is the case, it is nevertheless necessary to proceed with treatment. The psychologist can be helpful to the child by agreeing to see him/her immediately after school for support during the first few days. Generally, with such a program, the child is quite resistant, cries, attempts to run away, etc., for the first few days. This behavior diminishes rapidly, and within a few weeks the child is completely over the phobia.

In the second pattern, a more gradual approach appears justified (Kelly, 1973). It is generally best to begin treatment by establishing a good relationship with the patient and helping with general problems of coping. Following this, the problem of reentry in school is approached. Imaginal or *in vivo* desensitization may be employed before reentry is attempted. In addition, successive approximations may be employed by having the child begin by going to the school each moring to pick up assignments to take home and complete. After doing this for a period of time, the child is required to stay for the first period of the day before leaving. Later, the second period is added, and so on until the child is in school all day. Similar approaches have been described by Berryman (1959), as well as Ayllon, Smith, and Rogers (1970).

Discipline and Tantrums

As is evident from the table, one of the most frequent reasons for referral is negative behavior and related discipline problems. Such problems generally require a behavioral analysis of family interactions and the way in which discipline is applied. Eliminating sources of reinforcement for inappropriate behavior and providing sufficient reinforcement for appropriate behavior, along with opening channels of communication and understanding between family members, generally resolve these problems. Improving communication and understanding is often crucial in these cases. Frequently, inappropriate use of reinforcement and punishment is based on misunderstandings and lack of accurate perception. Thus, the parent may have expectations regarding the child's behavior that are inappropriate for a child of that age. Or the child may not be aware of principles that the parents take into account in determining appropriate or inappropriate behavior. Having discussions and providing information in these areas are often very important. With older children, behavioral contracting is frequently useful. For example, if a teenager wants to stay out later than the parents will permit, it is often helpful to review such points as (1) the parents sincere concern for the teenager's safety; (2) the legal responsibility that parents have for things that the teenager may get involved in late at night; and (3) the anxiety experienced by the parents when the teenager is out late. It can then be pointed out that parents probably try to be overly conservative and that teenagers tend to be overly liberal in determining the time they should be in at night. Within this framework, a behavioral contract may be negotiated in which hours to be home are specified and the conditions for staying out are clearly stated (e.g., the parents should know where the teenager will be in case they need to contact him).

The typical behavioral prescription for tantrum behavior is to ignore the tantrums. However, careful behavioral analysis of tantrum behavior would suggest a slightly different approach. Clinical observation suggests that tantrums generally occur for two reasons. First, the tantrum is an attempt by the child to communicate with the parents. The message of the tantrum is that the child is unhappy with the way things are proceeding and that he/she feels that it will be impossible to have any input into the system without completely disrupting the ongoing process. Thus, a tantrum is initiated. The second reason that tantrums occur (and the reason they persist over time) is that they frequently are reinforced. Thus, when children throw tantrums, they frequently get what they want. Thus the tantrum behavior is reinforced and increased.

In dealing with tantrums, we generally discuss these two points with parents and then explain to them how to deal with the behavior. We encourage them first to recognize the tantrum as an attempt to communicate. The parents are generally instructed to face the child when a tantrum is about to occur and to say "No! We will not have that behavior! If you have a problem, tell us about it. We will try to help, but we will not have that behavior!" If the child ceases the behavior, the parents discuss the problem and resolve it in a suitable manner. For example, if the child were to request a soft drink, the parents might respond by simply saying, "No, you cannot have any soda pop before supper." This statement would be met by a tantrum from the child. However, if the parents attempt to communicate with the child, they might find that the child is thirsty and had merely selected soda pop to quench the thirst. If this is the case, the parent might reply, "You may have a drink of water and have some soda pop following supper, but you cannot have soda pop now." Thus, the main problem, which is that the child is thirsty, is dealt with in an effective way, and useful communication has taken place between the parents and the child. To simply deny a thirsty child something to quench thirst produces understandable frustration. The tantrum is the child's attempt to communicate this frustration.

If the child refuses to communicate or refuses to accept the offered solution, the parent is instructed to observe the rule that the tantrum will *never* produce the desired result. Whatever the child was after will absolutely not be given if he/she engages in a tantrum. In addition, the parent is instructed to place the child in a chair and require that he/she remain there until the tantrum ceases (parents occasionally have had to stand behind the chair and hold the child in the chair to enforce this rule).

With the use of this basic procedure, the child quickly learns that if there is a problem, the parents will be willing to discuss it and seek a reasonable solution. However, if he/she chooses to engage in tantrum behavior, the result will be that the desired outcome will absolutely not be possible and the effect of the tantrum itself will merely be that the child will sit in a chair until it ceases. Structuring the situation in this manner encourages communication and compromise on solutions rather than tantruming.

One further instruction given to parents is that they should attempt to anticipate tantrum behavior and to communicate with the child in advance. Thus, if the child is playing with the toys in a department store, the parent may try simply to remove the child and leave the store. However, it is unpleasant for the child to be interrupted in the midst of an activity that is very enjoyable. Therefore, the parent might anticipate this and say to the child, "You're having a good time playing with the toys, aren't you?" When the child replies, "Yes," the parent can say "We are going to have to leave in five minutes, so look at anything you want to and do what you want to, but we will be leaving in five minutes." At the appointed time, the parent can take the child and leave. Communicating with the child in this manner enables the child to prepare for departure. In addition, if the parent can indicate to the child that he/she understands the child's wishes, this will often make a tantrum unnecessary as a means of communication. Thus, when the appointed time to depart from the store comes, the parent might say, "You would like to stay here and play longer, wouldn't you?" The child will generally respond in the affirmative. The parent can then say, "I understand that and I wish we could stay longer too, but we really must leave. We will try to come back again sometime later. It's a lot of fun to play with the toys here. Isn't it?"

Other useful approaches to dealing with tantrums have been reported by Coe (1972), Kaufmann and Wagner (1972), Williams (1959), and Webster and Azrin (1973). While the approaches suggested by these authors differ somewhat from the approach described above, they represent creative approaches to the problem and merit further use.

Compliance with Commands

A problem somewhat related to tantruming that is very commonly brought to the pediatric psychologist is the problem of the child who refuses to perform functions at the request of the parent. Many times this results because the child has mastered a discrimination learning task with respect to the parents' behavior. That is, many parents tend to repeat a command numerous times, not really expecting the child to complete the act on the first request. The child generally becomes very adept at knowing exactly how many times a parent will repeat a command, noting changes in the tone and volume of the voice of the command in order to comply only when the last minute approaches. Occasional miscalculations on the part of the child result, and the parent physically punishes the child for failure to complete the activity.

Behavioral counseling for this problem generally takes the following form. The parents are first told to expect philosophically that children will not do everything the first time they are commanded to. They need to be reminded and instructions need to be repeated. However, a definite pattern needs to be established for commands. The parent is instructed to give a command twice in a calm voice. If the child fails to respond, the parent is instructed to get up and walk the child through the activity with physical prompts. These should be given in a supportive and gentle rather than aggressive manner, and the child should be complimented for completing the task. The prompts can be faded later as compliance becomes more habitual. The child is praised and given occasional rewards for prompt compliance. If this is done, the child generally learns that an instruction will be given followed by a reminder and finally physical prompting. Therefore, he/she learns that compliance is the best course.

While this program requires a great deal of effort initially, in the long run it requires less effort than other methods that are less efficient. The general principle should be clear to the child that appropriate compliance with commands meets with approval and reinforcement. Ignoring commands results in mild disapproval and behavioral enforcement of the command. This kind of process shapes the child into appropriate behavior without undue physical or psychological assault.

When severe stubbornness becomes a problem, an additional feature that may be added to the above approach is mild punishment. A procedure that we recommend is that commands be presented with clearly defined consequences for compliance and noncompliance. For example, the parent might say, "It is time for you to take your bath and get ready for bed. If you would like to, you can go take your bath, have a snack, watch TV for a half hour, and go to bed. However, if you are unwilling to take a bath on your own and get ready for bed, I will give you a bath and put you to bed immediately. Which do you want to do?" Physical punishment in the form of one or two swats on the buttocks may be a useful consequence for noncompliance. However, if used, it should be mild, controlled, and used only occasionally for emphasis and enforcement. It should never be used frequently or as a means of venting parental anger. In practice, use of physical punishment is rarely needed, especially after other means of behavior management have been employed for a period of time. Excessive or frequent physical punishment generally ceases to be effective because such measures only temporarily suppress selected behaviors. They do not teach or reinforce more appropriate behavior. Also, the emotional reactions resulting from such measures generally predispose the child to future disruptive behavior.

In their classic review of the punishment literature, Azrin and Holz (1966) noted that punishment should be intense to suppress behavior. They were also not much impressed with the negative consequences that generally result. It should be noted that the principles discussed by Azrin and Holz are appropriate for selective use to handle specific symptoms. They are, however, not advised for daily use in child rearing. Frequent application of intense punishment may have very devastating effects on the child (e.g., Bandura, 1973; Welsh, 1976; Williams, 1978). The basic principle that behavior is best shaped and trained by reinforcement, modeling, and other positive means is as applicable to child rearing as it is to other situations. A major part of dealing with noncompliance, stubbornness, hostility, and related behaviors in children involves counseling the parents on more positive behaviors for themselves.

The present author favors these more general programs of reinforcement and punishment over the more rigorus programs that involve charts, record keeping, specific rewards, etc., because they are more intrinsic to the situation. Problems of extrinsic systems have recently been discussed by Levine and Fasnacht (1974). However, the literature abounds with such programs and they are useful in selected cases.

Teaching Values

An additional discipline problem frequently reported by parents has to do with the general problem of teaching values to the developing child. This is a particularly difficult task and results in much stress for parents and children. A good example is lying. Behaviorally, this is a very difficult situation to deal with. If one punishes a child following telling the truth, this tends to discourage telling the truth. However, if the child learns that he/she can do most anything as long as it is confessed immediately, this is an unfortunate situation also. Some principles that we have clinically found useful in dealing with this situation are the following. Child-rearing procedures should be discussed with the parents, and they should be encouraged to provide the child with a generally reinforcing and supportive environment. The child should feel sufficiently rewarded and reinforced to wish to be cooperative and to desire to model the parents' behavior. The parents may then provide instruction in values by modeling the values that they wish the child to have. Parents should be encouraged to verbalize the principle involved in a given situation. For example, if the child is observed to tell a distorted version of a story, the parent may stop the child and say, "Wait, we tell the truth around here. One should be truthful in what one says. Now, let's discuss what happened again." The child can then be encouraged step by step to tell the story in an undistorted fashion. When the truthful version of the story is completed, the parent can praise the child and tell him/her that that is what is expected. Verbalizing the principle of truthfulness and reinforcing truthful accounts, on as many occasions as present themselves, teach the child appropriate behavior. When the parent is unaware of the facts of the situation, which is a common occurrence, the manner in which the child is approached is crucial. It is best not to ask questions in such a way that lying is encouraged. Thus, direct questions such as "Did you do such and such?" should be avoided. Rather, the first approach to the child might be to ask the child to describe from the start exactly what occurred and caution him/her beforehand that the truth is desired and that the matter will be thoroughly investigated. After the child has given an account of the story, the parent may question the others involved and arrive at the closest version of the truth possible. If the child has been truthful, he/she should be praised, and a satisfactory resolution of the problem should be worked out. However, if the child has not been completely truthful, this should be pointed out and some degree of consequence should be given. The consequence should fit the crime as nearly as possible, and the child should be encouraged to be truthful on the next occasion.

Sometimes, it is impossible to determine the truth in a given situation. It often boils down to one person's word against another's. In these cases, the parent will have to decide which version of the story seems more likely. The parent may then inform the child of the version of the story that he/she believes to be true and mete out consequences based on that. It can be made clear in an honest and straightforward manner that the parent is simply attempting to ascertain the facts and act on the facts as he/she sees them. It is not necessary for the parent to be right in every case, as long as the basis on which the consequences are meted out are explained to the child and the parent is acting in good faith in terms of his/her understanding of the facts. In cases where the facts are really difficult to ascertain, the parent may acknowledge that it is difficult to know exactly what happened on this occasion and indicate that no consequences will be forthcoming. However, the child should be reminded that truthfulness and honesty are important and will be rewarded in the household. Consequences, when employed, should rectify the misdeed, if this is possible. For example, if the child makes an unkind statement intended to hurt another child's feelings, the child may be cautioned not to say that and the reason explained. The child may also be instructed to apologize for the statement and be rewarded for showing more positive behaviors toward the other child.

If children are having difficulties sharing a toy, the principle that toys must be shared can be expressed to the children. The parent can then help them work out a system of taking turns and permit them to play with the toy under those circumstances. They can be cautioned that if they are unable to play with the toy in that manner, the toy will be removed and they will not be permitted to play with it. As they take turns and play successfully with the toy, the parent can express approval and point out to them that this is a much better way to handle the situation.

If children have a tendency to fight, as they often do, the parent may interrupt the fight and insist that they discuss the situation and resolve it in some manner other than fighting. If they are unable to solve their difficulty in a manner other than physical violence, they may be required to submit to a mild punishment, such as sitting in a chair for a period of time. When they are ready to discuss the problem and solve it in a more appropriate manner, they may be permitted to leave their seats. Throughout the process, the principle is repeated that problems are resolved by discussing them and finding an appropriate solution rather than fighting about them.

Explicitly stating the principles involving family interactions makes behavior control and the contingencies regarding reinforcement and punishment clear to the child, resulting in more effective child-rearing and discipline. For example, if children are involved in rivalry and competitiveness, the parent may need to state the principle that everything around the household will be handled in a fair manner, with everyone getting his or her share and no one getting more than his or her share. The parent can then explain to the children why given situations are fair and equitable. Usually, the child will see the fairness of the situation when it is delineated by the parent. However, on some occasions, the child may actually point out to the parent that there is an inequitable situation that the parent has not been aware of. In these cases, the parent needs to be faithful to the principle and take steps to rectify the situation.

The above examples constitute rather simple applications of behavioral principles to common child-rearing situations. Although not described in detail, the principles of reinforcement, punishment, prompting, shaping, stimulus control, modeling, time out, and overcorrection in the above examples are critical to the success of an intervention. The pediatric psychologist devotes considerable time to tailoring behavioral principles to child-rearing problems presented by parents. Extended discussions of these techniques and of the use of parents as therapists may be found in McIntire (1975), Mash, Handy, and Hamerlynck (1976), and Mash, Hamerlynck, and Handy (1975).

Child Custody

Several categories in Table 1 have to do with custody or placement of the child following a divorce, removal from the home, adoption, or some other related circumstance. In such cases, an assessment of the child's behavior is made by means of observation, psychological testing, and interviews with the significant people in the child's life. Then, an operational definition of the kind of environment that would be most beneficial to the child for his/her future development is derived. To the extent possible, the various alternatives available for placement of the child are considered with respect to the goodness of fit with this operational definition. The alternatives and their suitability are then discussed with the person or persons responsible for making the placement. Once the placement is made, consultation is offered to assist those responsible for the child in carrying out the program felt to be most beneficial to the child. These are often very sensitive and delicate situations involving the feelings of parents and others involved in the life of the child. The pediatric psychologist is careful to be aware of and respond to the feelings and problems of those involved in an honest and helpful way. While the main consideration is the welfare of the child, the welfare of the significant others in the child's life can by no means be ignored.

Child Abuse

Closely related to the above discussion of custody is the area of child abuse. The pediatric psychologist may be the first to discover and report abuse; he/she may be called upon to evaluate and testify to the effects of abuse and/or neglect; and finally, the pediatric psychologist may be involved in the treatment of the child and/or the parents. It is an interesting commentary on our attitudes regarding children to learn that the first child abuse case on record in the United States occurred in 1874 and involved a young girl who was severely beaten every day by her parents (Fontana, 1964). A church worker discovered this and attempted to intervene, but no way could be found to do so. In desperation, the worker sought and received help from the Society for the Prevention of Cruelty to Animals. One year later, the New York Society for the Prevention of Cruelty to Children was founded.

Extensive reviews of the literature are available concerning the characteristics of abusing parents, recognition of abuse in children, and the psychologist's role in handling these cases ("Abused and Neglected Children," 1976; Paulson & Blake, 1967; "Violence against Children," 1973). Leake and Smith (1977) have presented information for the professional called upon to testify in child abuse cases, and Jensen (1976) developed a behavioral treatment program for training personnel who have direct contact with abusing parents. The treatment personnel were trained in behavioral management procedures that they in turn taught to the abusing parent. The program consisted of two phases: an implementation phase and a follow-up data collection phase. During the initial implementation phase, the participants received a series of instructional sessions on behavior management. These sessions were then followed by an equal number of consultation and follow-up sessions in which the treatment personnel discussed current cases in terms of the earlier material presented.

Developmental Problems

Another major group of referrals have to do with developmental delay and infant management problems, including such things as failure to thrive, slow development, and possible retardation. These problems are handled by assessing the developmental status of the child. From this, the most suitable environment and stimulation program for the child may be determined. Provision is then made for counseling the parents or responsible adults in carrying out the needed program. Often, instruction and training of the parents is accomplished by private sessions with them. Frequently, they observe the therapist working with the child as he/she demonstrates the recommended procedures. The therapist then has the parents attempt the procedures and gives them additional guidance and instruction. Parent groups are also conducted in which group discussion, lectures, and training are given in child care and rearing relevant to the problems encountered. Use is also frequently made of social workers, public health nurses, and others who make home visits to enhance the program. Consultation with school officials frequently results in a revision of the child's program and handling at the school. Various clubs, such as Scouts and Indian Guides, as well as various civic groups such as the Big Brother and Big Sister organizations, provide additional input. College student volunteers have also been involved in such programs.

A number of developmental programs have been devised and targeted for special groups. For example, various programs are available for infant and child stimulation (e.g., Meier, Segner, & Grueter, 1970), and Mahrer, Levinson, and Fine (1976) have recently discussed the theory and practice of infant psychotherapy. Guidelines for counseling parents of retarded children are presented in Campanelle (1965), and numerous programs for training retarded children are available (e.g., Bensberg, 1965; Bijou, Birnbrauer, Kidder, & Tague, 1966).

Hyperactivity

Frequently, children referred for pediatric psychology consultation are described as hyperactive. As is well known, hyperactivity is a wastebasket label in child psychopathology. *Hyperactivity* and related terms have been applied relatively indiscriminately to a wide number of behavioral problems. The term is also overburdened with numerous theoretical notions regarding etiology and treatment, few of which have substantial data to back them up. Thus, some children seen for hyperactive behavior are found to be children who have simply been subjected to very poor child management techniques. Others are found to be extremely anxious and tense, with their hyperactivity reflecting their general unease. Others are found to have mild to moderate symptoms of brain dysfunction, which are frequently considered the hallmark of such disorders. Still others are found to be the victims of unrealistic expectations regarding their behavior on the part of the adults around them. Fortunately, regardless of the exact etiology of the problem, the therapeutic approach that has been found to be successful is highly similar in all these cases. Parents and other responsible adults may be instructed in behavioral management techniques to patiently reinforce appropriate behavior while ignoring or mildly punishing inappropriate behavior. Consistent application of reinforcement principles has a dramatic effect upon hyperactive behavior (e.g., Ayllon, Laymon, & Kandel, 1975; Rosenbaum, O'Leary, & Jacob, 1975).

Ray, Shaw, and Cobb (1970) have described an ingenious approach to reducing hyperactivity in the school classroom. The child sits with a "workbox" in view. A light on the workbox lights up if the child has been working attentively for a specified period of time. The child and the class receive rewards contingent on the number of times the light flashes.

Relaxation training and electromyograph (EMG) feedback have also proved helpful in reducing hyperactive behavior (Lupin, 1974; Nall, 1973). This approach appears to be one of the most promising for future development. Breathing control (Simpson & Nelson, 1974) and even massage have been reported as effective in reducing hyperactivity, possibly because of the relaxing effect of such procedures.

Meichenbaum and Goodman (1971) have presented a treatment approach that involves teaching the child to talk to himself/herself, thus bringing behavior under stimulus control. A similar procedure proposed by Douglas (1972) suggests that the child be taught to stop, look, and listen before acting.

Tics and Mannerisms

A variety of specific habits, mannerisms, and tics are the occasion for referral to the pediatric psychologist. Reviews of the literature in these areas (e.g., Hersen & Eisler, 1973; Yates, 1970) have indicated that behavioral treatment, or any treatment, of these disorders is difficult and has been only minimally successful. Among the most successful treatments are massed practice and negative practice. However, a recent treatment that appears to be very promising has been proposed by Azrin and Nunn (1973). This approach involves providing the patient with feedback regarding when the tic is occurring and training the patient to make a muscle movement that is in direct opposition to the muscle movement involved in the tic. The result is that the tic or mannerism is neutralized and the habit is broken.

Fire Setting

A problem that occurs with relative frequency is fire setting, which generally causes great concern. In contrast to the numerous theoretical notions regarding the psychodynamics and the psychoanalytic significance of fire setting, massed practice has been found to be effective in the treatment of this problem (Welsh, 1968). The general procedure is to have several sessions with the child in which he/she is to be permitted to light matches, candles, small fires, etc., resulting in a certain amount of satiation. In addition, the child is trained in the appropriate and safe use of fire, and the family is encouraged to give him/her frequent opportunities to light matches, candles, etc., under supervision. It is easier to partially satiate the behavior and teach proper control of the behavior than to suppress it completely.

Toilet Training, Enuresis, and Encopresis

Numerous cases involving toilet training, enuresis, and encopresis are referred for pediatric psychological treatment. Many questions of parents presented to the pediatric psychologist have to do with the toilet training of the normally developing child. A basic principle in dealing with this problem is to reassure the parents that 2 years of age is not a magical number by which every child must be trained. Many children are not trained until 3, 4, or 5 years of age or even older (Walker, 1978). Simply encouraging the parents to be patient; to instruct the child in proper toilet habits; to model the behavior for him/her; and to show considerable pleasure when proper toileting occurs is sufficient in general to accomplish the task.

If the child reaches school age and is still having difficulty, the principles outlined in *Toilet Training in Less Than a Day* by Azrin and Foxx (1976) may be employed. Studies of this method have indicated that the procedures often are not successful when carried out by parents on their own (Butler, 1976; Matson & Ollendick, 1977). However, the techniques are highly successful if completed with professional consultation and guidance. Extensive reviews of the literature (e.g., Yates, 1970) reveal that serious psychopathology is seldom related to the symptoms of enuresis and encopresis. There is some evidence that mild tension or family conflict may be involved in a fair number of cases. A careful review of the literature in this area may be found in Walker (1978). Effective behavioral treatments of enuresis include random awakening at night (Creer & Davis, 1975; Young, 1964), bladder retention training (Kimmel & Kimmel, 1970; Muellner, 1960; Starfield & Mellits, 1968), and conditioning by means of the pad and bell apparatus (Costello, 1970; Yates, 1970). A rigorous behavioral treatment of encopresis that involves careful use of reinforcement, punishment, and selected cathartics has been described by Wright and Walker (1977). This treatment program has been used extensively in pediatric psychology settings for several years and has been found to be virtually 100% effective.

Academic Underachievement

School problems are common reasons for referral. One of the most common problems presented is the child who hates school and refuses to perform any of the required tasks. Working with these situations requires first that the parents be helped to understand the situation as the child perceives it. Care is taken to point out to the parents that for a child, doing well in school is not very high on the list of priorities and often does not seem to be very important. The child has many other things in his/her life that are much more rewarding and enjoyable. The immediate reinforcement from these activities tends to govern behavior much more than any long-range consequences of failure to achieve in school. Valuing school and the lessons learned from it are things that will come with maturity and adulthood. It is often helpful to point out that this is true of many more children than is realized. However, many children continue to perform school tasks not because they are intrinsically interested or impressed with the importance of learning the material but because they are rewarded by approval from parents and teachers. Walker (in press) has described a behavioral program for promoting educational achievement. In brief, the program divides the school day into periods and assigns points to each period, so that if a child does adequate schoolwork all day, he/she receives 100 points. The points are assigned according to the length of the time spent on each lesson and the difficulty of the material studied. Thus, math may be worth 30 points, while art is worth 5 points and reading 20. A reinforcement menu is prepared. Items on the menu are then assigned points roughly in the ratio of one point being worth one cent. The child can also request money for the points rather than purchasing items from the menu. The teacher initials a card or makes a record that is sent home each day indicating to the parent how many points have been earned. Work not completed at school is sent home to be completed. No points are earned for work completed at home. This program has been found to be highly successful with children in need of extrinsic motivation for schoolwork.

Eating Problems

Eating-related problems are frequently presented to the pediatric psychologist. For the normal child who is simply a "picky" eater and will not eat certain foods, the principle may be established that the child should take at least one mouthful of each item of food on the table. Then, the child may self-select more items to eat. The parents make an effort to provide food at each meal that the child does like, and the child may be encouraged to take part in planning the menus from day to day. Over a period of time, tasting a variety of foods while eating more of those that the child likes results in a broadening of food preferences. A variety of reinforcers and punishers may be used to ensure that the principle of tasting each food is carried out. For example, allowing the child to help prepare the food sometimes makes him/her more willing to taste it. In addition, such techniques as permitting the child to light a candle and blow the candle out when finished eating reinforces eating behavior. This effect can be enhanced if there is more than one child by having extra candles that the first child finished eating can blow out. Playing games with the child following supper or allowing him/her to stay up a little bit later can also be used as reinforcers. Punishers may involve loss of privileges, time out from pleasurable activities following dinner such as playing games and watching TV, etc. Palmer, Thompson, and Linsheid (1975) and Bernal (1972) have discussed behavioral treatment of the child who refuses solid food as he/she grows out of infancy. A similar problem, psychogenic vomiting, has been treated by aversive procedures (Komechak, 1972; Wright & Thalassinos, 1973) and positive reinforcement. Behavioral treatment of pica has also been discussed, using positive and aversive procedures (e.g., Ausman, Ball, & Alexander, 1974; Magness & Ball, 1972).

Anorexia Nervosa

An eating disorder that is becoming considerably more prevalent than in the past is anorexia nervosa. Relatively mild cases can be treated on an outpatient basis (e.g., Scrignar, 1971). However, severe cases require hospitalization. Numerous studies have employed reinforcement techniques to induce eating and weight gain (e.g., Azerrad & Stafford, 1969; Garfinkel, Kline, & Stancer, 1973). These have been quite successful in producing the desired weight gain (Bhanji & Thompson, 1974). However, this is only a partial treatment. The original development of the symptom results from disturbed family relationships and interpersonal difficulties (Liebman, Minuchin, & Baker, 1974a,b). Thus, anorexic patients frequently need training in assertion, decision making, desensitization, and other forms of treatment in order for the condition to be completely resolved (e.g., Agras, Barlow, Chapin, Abel, & Leitenberg, 1974; Halsten, 1965; Schnurer, Rubin, & Roy, 1973).

Obesity

A very common referral for pediatric psychology is the opposite of the above two problems, that is, the problem of obesity or overeating. The overweight child and teenager are an increasing problem. Reviews of the literature in this area (Abramson, 1973; Brightwell & Sloan, 1977; Stunkard & Mahoney, 1976) indicate generally modest treatment effects for most programs. However, behavior programs appear to show considerable promise. As is well known, the basic therapeutic principle involved in weight loss is a matter of input versus output (Stuart & Davis, 1972). In order to lose weight, the person must reduce the intake of food, particularly fattening foods, and increase the amount of energy output, or in other words become more active and involved in exercise. In our treatment of such children, this basic principle is explained to the parent and the child. The child may then be asked to commit himself/herself to a rigorous program based on this principle (Wright, 1976). To encourage cooperation, a variety of reinforcers, such as gifts, money, and privileges, are offered for remaining on the program. The therapist meets with the child and the family at regular intervals to suggest ways of reducing weight, such as chewing food slowly, keeping snack foods out of sight, substituting less fattening foods for more fattening ones, and watching calories. The therapist is the ally of the child in losing weight so that the reinforcers may be obtained. Numerous discussions of such techniques are available in the literature (e.g., Christensen, Jeffrey, & Pappas, 1973; Stuart & Davis, 1972).

Other approaches to the problem have been discussed, but none is outstandingly successful. Recent reviews of this literature appear in Abramson (1973) and Bornstein (1972). It appears that for the child who works on a behavioral program and for whom significant reinforcers can be found, success is relatively high. With children, some success is assured if caloric intake can merely be stabilized rather than decreased, because as the child grows, he/she will be less obese if the same weight is maintained. However, a significant number of teenagers are unwilling to commit themselves to such a program, and sufficiently potent reinforcers are not available to produce the desired results. This remains an unsolved problem in the treatment of such behaviors. An interesting development in this area is the work of Haber (1978), which suggests that a fear of thinness may develop in patients who lose large amounts of weight. This fear may then hinder further efforts at weight control.

Sexual Problems

A fairly common sexual problem of children is compulsive masturbation. On examination, this problem generally is found to be highly similar, in principle, to thumb sucking and other tension-reducing habits. The child has simply discovered that manipulating the genitals is pleasurable and tends to reduce tension. Thus, the child engages in this behavior when tense or bored or otherwise upset (Levine, 1951). Working with the family to reduce pressures and tensions in the environment as well as to reinforce periods that are free of masturbation is one simple element in the treatment of this problem. The parents, of course, must be reassured that this behavior does not signal sexual perversion or future pathology. Training the child in relaxation has been found clinically effective.

Many parents become concerned about the child who appears to be developing inappropriate sex interests in terms of being unusually precocious in interest, or not developing the right sex-role identity, or desiring to behave as a member of the opposite sex. Generally, counseling the parents regarding reinforcement of appropriate behavior and mild discouragement of inappropriate behavior is a central part of this treatment. In addition, reassurance, factual information, and therapeutic sex education are often required. For the older child, modeling and discussion of appropriate sexual behavior is helpful. Rekers and Lovaas (1974) and Rekers, Lovaas, and Low (1974) have discussed treatment of children with sexual identity problems, and Money (1968) has provided much useful information about the child with genetic sexual anomalies.

A recent case treated in our clinic (Shaw & Walker, in press) was that of an 8-year-old, moderately retarded child who had developed a sexual attraction to feet. When possible (at home when visitors were there, in church, etc.), the patient would get on the floor, fondle the feet of females present, and masturbate. This behavior was causing him and his family serious problems in the rural Oklahoma town in which they lived. The history revealed that when the child was younger, the mother frequently stroked the child's stomach with her foot while he played on the floor. She also nibbled and played with his feet while changing his diapers, etc. The child was trained in the use of relaxation procedures as a form of self-control. Following training, his parents, his teachers, and significant others, simply said, "Relax, G." when they saw him becoming aroused. The training was effective in eliminating the symptom, and it has not returned for two years.

Drug Abuse

A large number of teenagers are referred for a variety of substance abuse problems involving everything from teenage alcoholism to use of hard drugs, glue sniffing, etc. Parents who present these young people for treatment generally are relatively hostile and negative toward the child. They frequently bring the child to treatment and make it clear that they expect the therapist to see that the drug use stops. If this is not accomplished in relatively short order, they tend to become upset and feel that the treatment is not working. In view of this attitude, it is essential to point out to parents when such children are brought for treatment that the therapist will make an effort to help the young person resolve whatever problems he/she has and to examine his/her use of drugs, but no promise can be made regarding cessation of the drug usage. By the time chidren become teenagers, there is no way, short of locking them up, to prevent them from involving themselves in substance abuse if they so desire.

Treatment of the problems generally revolves around enabling the young person to reduce anxiety by means of relaxation training, systematic desensitization, and related means, as well as developing better coping and problem solving skills by means of assertiveness training, behavior rehearsal, and other modalities. Factual information is presented regarding drug abuse and use when the time is appropriate. As a result of this effort, the young person may either cease to use drugs or become highly selective and responsible in his/her use of them as other problems are brought under control. Training in the techniques of self-reinforcement prove invaluable in developing self-confidence and self-control in young people who are abusing drugs. When the young person learns to monitor his/her own behavior, reinforcing desirable behavior and mildly punishing undesirable behavior, a degree of self-control and self-confidence is achieved that results in effective coping and less need for drugs. For a more extensive review of the literature on the behavioral treatment of drug abuse, see Callner (1975).

Delinquency

Dealing with the delinquent child and teenager is a formidable challenge. Training in social skills and effective problem-solving makes antisocial behavior less necessary. Exploration of values and interpersonal behavior may be accomplished by use of the techniques developed by Schwitzgebel (1964) in which the young person is rewarded for filling a tape with conversation. Discussing and developing values are rewarded with bonuses. Rational–emotive therapy brings behavior under more appropriate cognitive control (Ellis & Grieger, 1977). Behavioral contracting is useful in setting limits on behaviors and reconciling family differences (e.g., Malouf & Alexander, 1974; Parsons & Alexander, 1973). Token economies (Tyler, 1967) have also been used with success. Fixsen, Phillips, and Wolf (1973) described a program called "Achievement Place," where principles of democratic self-government were taught to delinquents through a type of token economy. Davidson and Seidman (1974) have recently carefully reviewed behavioral therapy approaches to juvenile delinquency.

Psychoses

Interestingly, psychotic children and young people are relatively infrequently referred to pediatric psychologists. These symptoms are more commonly referred to psychologists in other settings, particularly inpatient settings and mental health clinics. However, successful treatment of psychoses has been accomplished by means of selective use of reinforcement and punishment to shape normal behavior (Nordquist & Wahler, 1973). Likewise, extensive environmental manipulation and family reorganization are often necessary. Rigorous and highly structured programs, such as token economies, have proved highly effective in the treatment of these behaviors on an inpatient basis (Ayllon & Azrin, 1968; Knepler, Sewall, & Boor, 1972; Lovaas, 1977; Lovaas, Koegel, Simmons, & Long, 1973). Often a family-operated token economy can be developed for outpatient care.

Depression and Suicide

Depression and suicidal behavior are common referrals to pediatric psychologists. If the child is depressed but not suicidal, a variety of treatment approaches are found to be worthwhile. It is interesting to note that in the very young child, depression frequently is expressed in a variety of other symptoms. Thus, a child may be hyperactive, overly aggressive, or cruel; may refuse to eat; or may display other behaviors when depressed. As a child gets older, sadness and the more typical signs of depression become more prominent and common. Behavioral analyses of depression generally stress the loss or lack of reinforcement for behavior (Miller, 1975). Thus, in treating the young child, environmental manipulation is necessary to provide the child with sufficient material and social reinforcement. In the older child, such as the teenager, similar procedures are used along with self-reinforcement and basic principles of rational–emotive psychotherapy (Ellis & Harper, 1961) to promote realistic thinking and evaluation of situations, as well as to prevent catastrophizing ideation. The cognitive–behavioral approach of Rush and Beck (1978) has also been employed with success. This approach uses individual and group training sessions to change cognitions that are producing depression. The approach draws heavily on rational–emotive principles of therapy.

Suicidal threats and behaviors in children and adolescents must be carefully handled. The basic principles of Schneidman and Farberow (1957) may be employed to determine the seriousness of the suicidal threat. In addition, the child's age must be taken into account. The youngest suicidal attempt reported in the literature (Bakwin & Bakwin, 1973) involved a 3-year-old child who was found along with his 18-month-old sibling in a room with the gas jet turned on. The child reported that he was angry with his parents for not taking him for a walk that day and had therefore attempted to kill himself. The father had discussed in front of the child the manner in which an acquaintance committed suicide by turning on the gas. However, for all practical purposes, suicide is very rare and unlikely up to the age of 10. From age 10 to puberty, suicide is still a relatively small risk. However, with the advent of the teenage years, suicide becomes a significant threat and is one of the major causes of death in this age group (Wright, in press).

Principles for handling such cases are well known and have been discussed extensively in the literature (Resnik, 1968). They will not be further discussed here. Needless to say, distinguishing between real suicidal attempts and suicidal gestures is crucial. Failure to do this may result in inadvertent reinforcement of suicidal behavior, which is extremely unfortunate, especially when it occurs at a young age. A very common occurrence is for a young person, particularly female, to take a large dose of pills following a family conflict or argument (often regarding a boyfriend) in an effort to dramatize her unhappiness and manipulate the family situation. If this situation is not handled carefully, the young person will be encouraged to attempt suicide in the future as a problem-solving technique. Suicidal gestures and attempts may be interpreted as cries for help (Farberow & Schneidman, 1961), and the basic problems involved should be dealt with in a way that promotes more effective functioning and coping.

Handicapped Children

Referrals are not infrequently made to pediatric psychologists for handicapped children who have a disfiguring or limiting handicap. Therapy in these cases revolves around dealing with the expectancies of the child and the parents regarding what the child is capable of and what he/she is not capable of in a positive manner so that the effects of the handicap are minimized rather than exaggerated (Moos, 1976).

Rational–emotive and the cognitive–behavioral therapies are helpful in enabling the child to realistically assess the situation and to effectively achieve realistic goals. Bibliotherapy, in which the child is guided in reading about other handicapped people and their accomplishments, is frequently used, and modeling may also be very helpful.

Chronic Illness

Dealing with the feeelings of depression, helplessness, guilt, anger, and related emotions of the child and the family when the child is chronically ill often falls to the pediatric psychologist. Support, environmental manipulation to reduce stress, education and straight thinking about the illness, and life planning for the child are important principles of handling such cases (Battle, 1975). Dealing with the child's development of adequate social skills, peer relationships, education, and self-concept are crucial. For children who are hospitalized for long periods of time, the pediatric psychologist works with ward personnel in providing an enriching and rewarding environment. Studies of children who have been seriously ill indicate some difficulties in later adjustment that have been labeled the *vulnerable child syndrome* (e.g., Sigal, Chagoya, Villeneuve, & Mayerovitch, 1978). However, others have stressed the strengths and the more positive coping skills of such children (e.g., Gayton, Friedman, Tavormina, & Tucker, 1977; Tavormina, Boll, Gayton, & Mattsson, in press).

Death

Death and dying in the life of a child are dealt with by pediatric psychologists. In the case of the child who has lost a parent or a loved one or is in danger of losing one because of illness, assuring the child that he/she is not responsible for the death is important. Likewise, offering support and understanding regarding the child's loss of reinforcement and fears about his/her own safety and well-being are also important considerations. Discussions regarding the meaning of life, death, and values are important. In the case of the child with a terminal illness, counseling for the family and the child are needed to reduce conflicts, guilt, and pressures. Parents and child can be encouraged to make the most of the remaining time of life, rather than becoming depressed and adopting a futile attitude that precludes any further development of the child. Extended discussions of this area may be found in the special issue of the *Journal of Clinical Child Psychology* devoted to this topic (1974) and in Schaefer's section on death and dying in Wright, Schaefer, and Solomans (in press).

Unusual Problems

Unique medical problems are frequently brought to the attention of the pediatric psychologist. Behavioral methods are often successful in dealing with these.

For example, Walker (in press) and Sackett and Haynes (1976) discuss procedures for children who will not comply with important medical regimens, such as insulin intake for the control of diabetes. Behavioral programs can be elaborated to deal with these compliance problems. For instance, children who refuse to take oral medication have been treated by Wright (1969b). Behavioral treatment of tracheostomy addiction in the infant has also been reported (Wright, 1969a). Other medically related problems are frequently encountered that lend themselves to a behavioral treatment approach. Treatment of these disorders represents an exciting and interesting challenge for the fields of psychology and medicine.

SUMMARY

Pediatric psychology is a relatively new specialty in child clinical psychology. The pediatric psychologist must deal with a wide variety of behavioral and medical problems. Careful assessment and behavior analysis are often required in order to make appropriate referrals and to plan treatment. Pediatric psychologists emphasize short-term therapy, crisis intervention, consultation, and educational intervention methods. A broad-spectrum, multimodal approach has proved most useful. Frequently, unique behavioral problems related to medical care of the child are presented to the pediatric psychologist for solution. Creative application of the basic principles of behavioral therapy is required in such situations.

REFERENCES

Abramson, E. A review of behavioral approaches to weight control. *Behaviour Research and Therapy*, 1973, *11*, 547–556.

Abused and neglected children. *Pediatric Psychology*, 1976, *2*, entire issue.

Adelson, R., & Goldfried, M. Modeling and the fearful child patient. *Journal of Dentistry for Children*, 1970, *37*, 34–37.

Agras, S., Barlow, D., Chapin, H., Abel, G., & Leitenberg, H. Behavior modification of anorexia nervosa. *Archives of General Psychiatry*, 1974, *30*, 279–286.

Ausman, J., Ball, T., & Alexander, D. Behavior therapy of pica with a profoundly retarded adolescent. *Mental Retardation*, 1974, *12*, 16–18.

Ayllon, T., & Azrin, N. *The token economy: A motivational system for therapy and rehabilitation*. New York: Appleton-Century-Crofts, 1968.

Ayllon, T., Smith, D., & Rogers, M. Behavioral management of school phobia. *Journal of Behavior Therapy and Experimental Psychiatry*, 1970, *1*, 125–138.

Ayllon, T., Laymon, D., & Kandel, H. A behavioral, educational alternative to drug control of hyperactive children. *Journal of Applied Behavioral Analysis*, 1975, *8*, 137–146.

Azerrad, J., & Stafford, R. Restoration of eating behavior in anorexia nervosa through operant conditioning and environmental manipulation. *Behaviour Research and Therapy*, 1969, *7*, 165–171.

Azrin, N., & Foxx, R. *Toilet training in less than a day*. New York: Pocket, 1976.

Azrin, N., & Holz, W. Punishment. In W. K. Honig (Ed.), *Operant behavior: Areas of research and application*. New York: Appleton-Century-Crofts, 1966.

Azrin, N., & Nunn, R. Habit reversal: A method of eliminating nervous habits and tics. *Behaviour Research and Therapy*, 1973, *11*, 619–628.

Bakwin, H., & Bakwin, R. *Behavior disorders in children*. Philadelphia, Pa.: Saunders, 1973.

Bandura, A. *Aggression: A social learning analysis*. Englewood Cliffs, N.J.: Prentice-Hall, 1973.

Battle, C. Chronic physical disease. *Pediatric Clinics of North America*, 1975, *22*, 525–531.

Bellak, L., & Bellak, S. *Children's Apperception Test*. New York: CPS, 1965.

Bender, L. *The Visual Motor Gestalt Test*. New York: American Orthopsychiatric Association, 1946.

Bensberg, G. *Teaching the mentally retarded*. Atlanta, Ga.: Southern Regional Educational Board, 1965.

Berecz, J. Phobias of childhood: Etiology and treatment. *Psychological Bulletin*, 1968, *70*, 694–720.

Bernal, M. Behavioral treatment of a child's eating problem. *Journal of Behavior Therapy and Experimental Psychiatry*, 1972, *3*, 43–50.

Bernstein, D., & Borkovec, T. *Progressive relaxation training: A manual for the helping professions*. Champaign, Ill.: Research, 1973.

Berryman, E. School phobia: Management problems in private practice. *Psychological Reports*, 1959, *5*, 19–25.

Bhanji, S. & Thompson, J. Operant conditioning in the treatment of anorexia nervosa: A review and retrospective study of 11 cases. *British Journal of Psychiatry*, 1974, *124*, 166–172.

Bijou, S., Birnbrauer, J., Kidder, J., & Tague, C. Programmed instruction as an approach to teaching reading, writing, and arithmetic to retarded children. *The Psychological Record*, 1966, *16*, 505–522.

Bornstein, P. Obesity: A review of the literature. *JSAS Catalog of Selected Documents in Psychology*, 1972, *2*, 70.

Brightwell, D., & Sloan, C. Long-term results of behavior therapy for obesity. *Behavior Therapy*, 1977, *8*, 898–905.

Burks, H. *Burks Behavior Rating Scales*. Huntington Beach, Calif.: Arden Press, 1969.

Butler, J. F. The toilet training success of parents after reading "Toilet training in less than a day." *Behavior Therapy*, 1976, *7*, 185–191.

Callner, D. Behavioral treatment approaches to drug abuse: A critical view of the research. *Psychological Bulletin*, 1975, *82*, 143–164.

Campanelle, T. C. *Counseling parents of mentally retarded children*. Milwaukee: Bruce, 1965.

Cassell, R. *Child Behavior Rating Scale:* Los Angeles, Calif.: Western Psychological Services, 1962.

Cattell, R. *Sixteen P-F*. Champaign, Ill.: IPAT, 1972.

Cattell, R., & Dreger, R. Alignment and identification of factors in the early and preschool personality questionnaires. *Multivariant Experimental and Clinical Research*, 1976, *2*, 155–165.

Catell, R. B., Coan, R. W., & Beloff, H. *Jr.-Sr. High School Personality Questionnaire*. Champaign, Ill.: IPAT, 1969.

Christensen, E., Jeffrey, B., & Pappas, J. A therapist manual for a behavior modification weight reduction program. Research and development reprint #37, Counseling and Psychology Services, University of Utah, 1973.

Clement, P. Tailor made peer therapy for groups for children. In B. Lubin (Chairman), *Parents and Psychologists: The New Team*. Symposium presented at the American Psychological Association Convention, Washington, D.C., Sept. 1976.

Coan, R. & Cattell, R. *Early School Personality Questionnaire*. Champaign, Ill.: IPAT, 1972.

Coe, W. A behavioral approach to disrupted family interactions. *Psychotherapy: Theory, Research, and Practice*, 1972, *9*, 80–85.

Coolidge, J., Hahn, P., & Peck, A. School phobia: Workshop, 1955: School Phobia: Neurotic crisis or way of life? *American Journal of Orthopsychiatry*, 1957, *27*, 296–309.

Costello, C. *Symptoms of psychopathology: A handbook*. New York: Wiley, 1970.

Creer, T., & Davis, M. Using a staggered wakening procedure with enuretic children in an institutional setting. *Journal of Behavior Therapy and Experimental Psychiatry*, 1975, *6*, 23–25.

Croghan, L. & Musante, G. The elimination of a boy's high building phobia by in vivo desensitization and game playing. *Journal of Behavior Therapy and Experimental Psychiatry*, 1975, *6*, 87–88.

Davidson, W. & Seidman, E. Studies of behavior modification and juvenile delinquency: A review, methodological critique, and social perspective. *Psychological Bulletin*, 1974, *81*, 988–1011.

Death and children. *Journal of Clinical Child Psychology*, 1974, *3*, entire issue.

Doll, E. *Vineland Social Maturity Scale*. Circle Pines, Minn.: American Guidance Service, 1965.

Douglas, V. Stop, look, listen: The problem of sustained attention and impulse control in hyperactive and normal children. *Canadian Journal of Behavioral Science*, 1972, *4*, 259–282.

Dunn, L. *Peabody Picture Vocabulary Test*. Minneapolis: American Guidance Service, 1965.

Ellis, A., & Grieger, R. *Handbook of rational emotive therapy*. New York: Springer, 1977.

Ellis, A., & Harper, R. *A new guide to rational living*. Englewood Cliffs, N.J.: Prentice-Hall, 1961.

Evans, I., & Nelson, R. A curriculum for the teaching of behavior assessment. *American Psychologist*, 1974, *29*, 598–606.

Farberow, N., & Schneidman, E. *The cry for help*. New York: McGraw-Hill, 1961.

Fixsen, D., Phillips, E., & Wolf, M. Achievement place: Experiments in self-government with pre-delinquents. *Journal of Applied Behavior Analysis*, 1973, *6*, 31–47.

Fontana, J. *The maltreated child: The maltreatment syndrome in children*. Springfield, Ill.: Charles C Thomas, 1964.

Garfinkel, P., Kline, S., & Stancer, H. Treatment of anorexia nervosa using operant conditioning techniques. *Journal of Nervous and Mental Disease*, 1973, *6*, 428–433.

Gayton, W., Friedman, S., Tavormina, J., & Tucker, F. Children with cystic fibrosis: I. Psychological test findings of patients, siblings, and parents. *Pediatrics*, 1977, *59*, 888–894.

Goldfried, M., & Davison, G. *Clinical behavior therapy*. New York: Holt, Rinehart, & Winston, 1976.

Haber, S. Fear of thinness: An alternative approach to the treatment of obesity. Paper presented at the American Psychological Association, Toronto, Aug. 1978.

Halsten, E. Adolescent anorexia nervosa treated by desensitization. *Behaviour Research and Therapy*, 1965, *3*, 87–91.

Hereford, C. *Changing parental attitudes through group discussions*. Austin: University of Texas Press, 1963.

Hersen, M., & Eisler, R. Behavioral approaches to study and treatment of psychogenic tics. *Genetic Psychology Monographs*, 1973, *87*, 289–312.

Hiskey, M. *Hiskey-Nebraska Test of Learning Aptitude*. Lincoln, Neb.: Union College Press, 1966.

Jastak, J., Bijou, S., & Jastak, S. *Wide Range Achievement Test*. Wilmington, Dela.: Guidance Associates, 1965.

Jensen, R. A behavior modification program to remediate child abuse. *Journal of Clinical Child Psychology*, 1976, *5*, 30–32.

Kaufmann, L., & Wagner, B. BARB: A systematic treatment technology for temper control disorders. *Behavior Therapy*, 1972, *3*, 84–90.

Kelly, E. School phobia: A review of theory and treatment. *Psychology in the Schools*, 1973, *10*, 33–42.

Kennedy, W. School phobia—rapid treatment of fifty cases. *Journal of Abnormal Psychology*, 1965, *70*, 285–289.

Kimmel, H., & Kimmel, E. An instrumental conditioning method for the treatment of enuresis. *Journal of Behavior Therapy and Experimental Psychiatry*, 1970, *1*, 121–123.

Kirk, S., McCarthy, J., & Kirk, W. *Illinois Test of Pscyholinguistics*. Urbana: University of Illinois Press, 1968.

Kissel, S. Systematic desensitization therapy with children: A case study and some suggested modifications. *Professional Psychology*, 1972, *3*, 164–168.

Knepler, K., Sewall, S. & Boor, M. Token economy as a ward management approach in a psychiatric inpatient service for children. *Journal of Behavior Therapy and Experimental Psychiatry*, 1972, *3*, 289–295.

Komechak, M. Extinction of vomiting behavior in a retarded child. *JSAS Catalog of Selected Documents in Psychology*, 1972, *2*.

Lassers, E., Nordon, R., & Bladholm, S. Steps in the return to school of children with school phobia. *American Journal of Psychiatry*, 1973, *130*, 265–268.

Laybourne, P., & Churchill, S. Symptom discouragement in treating hysterical reactions of childhood. *International Journal of Child Psychotherapy*, 1972, *1*, 111–123.

Lazarus, A., & Abramovitz, A. The use of emotive imagery in the treatment of children's phobias. *Journal of Mental Science*, 1962, *108*, 191–195.

Leake, H., & Smith, D. Preparing for and testifying in a child abuse hearing. *Clinical Pediatrics*, 1977, *16*, 1057–1063.

Leiter, R. *Leiter International Performance Scale*. Chicago: Stoelting, 1969.

Levine, F. Pediatric observations on masturbation in children. Paper presented at Interval Meeting of the New York Psychoanalytic Society, Feb. 13, 1951.

Levine, F., & Fasnacht, G. Token economies may lead to token learning. *American Psychologist*, 1974, *29*, 816–820.

Liebman, R., Minuchin, S., & Baker, L. An integrated program for anorexia nervosa. *American Journal of Psychiatry*, 1974, *131*, 432–435. (a)

Liebman, R., Minuchin, S., & Baker, L. The role of the family in the treatment of anorexia nervosa. *Journal of the American Academy of Child Psychiatry*, 1974, *3*, 264–274. (b)

Lovaas, O. *The autistic child*. New York: Irvington Publishing, 1977.

Lovaas, O., Koegel, R., Simmons, J., & Long, J. Some generalizations and follow up measures on autistic children in behavior therapy. *Journal of Applied Behavior Analysis*, 1973, *6*, 131–166.

Lupin, M. *Peace, harmony, and awareness*. Houston, Texas: Self-Management Tapes, 1974.

Lupin, M., Braud, W., & Deur, W. Effects of relaxation upon hyperactivity using relaxation tapes for children and parents. Unpublished paper, 1974.

Lynn, B. *Structured Doll Play Test*. Denver: Test Developments, 1959.

Magness, R., & Ball, T. Behavior therapy with a profoundly retarded adult coprophagic. Pomona, Calif.: Pacific State Hospital, 1972.

Mahrer, A., Levinson, J., & Fine, S. Infant psychotherapy: Theory, research, and practice. *Psychotherapy: Theory, Research, & Practice*, 1976, *13*, 131–139.

Malouf, R., & Alexander, J. Family crisis intervention: A model and technique of training. In R. E. Hardy & J. G. Cull (Eds.), *Therapeutic needs of the family*. Springfield, Ill.: Charles C Thomas, 1974.

Marine, E. School refusal—who should intervene? (Diagnostic and treatment categories) *Journal of School Psychologists*, 1968–1969, *1*, 63–70.

Mash, E. Hamerlynck, L., & Handy, L. *Behavior modification and families*. New York: Brunner/Mazel, 1975.

Mash, E., Handy, L., & Hamerlynck, L. *Behavior modification approaches to parenting*. New York: Brunner/Mazel, 1976.

Matson, J. L., & Ollendick, T. Issues in toilet training normal children. *Behavior Therapy*, 1977, *8*, 549–553.

McIntire, R. W. *Child psychology: A behavioral approach to everyday problems*. Kalamazoo, Mich.: Behaviordelia, 1975.

Meichenbaum, D., & Goodman, J. Training impulsive children to talk to themselves: A means of developing self-control. *Journal of Abnormal Psychology*, 1971, *77*, 115–126.

Meier, J., Segner, L., & Grueter, B. An education system for high risk infants: A preventive approach to developmental learning disabilities. In J. Helmuth (Ed.), *Disadvantaged child*, Vol. 3. New York: Brunner/Mazel, 1970.

Mesibov, G., Schroeder, C., & Wesson, L. Parental concerns about their children. *Journal of Pediatric Psychology*, 1977, *2*, 13–17.

Michigan Pictures Test. Michigan State Department of Mental Health. Chicago: Science Research, 1953.

Miller, W. Psychological deficits in depression. *Psychological Bulletin*, 1975, *82*, 238–260.

Money, J. *Sex errors of the body*. Baltimore: Johns Hopkins University Press, 1968.

Monnelly, E., Ianzito, B., & Stewart, M. Psychiatric consultations in a children's hospital. *American Journal of Psychiatry*, 1973, *130*, 789.

Moos, R. *Coping with physical illness*. New York: Plenum, 1976.

Muellner, S. Development of urinary control in children: A new concept in cause, prevention, and treatment of primary enuresis. *Journal of Urology*, 1960, *84*, 714–716.

Murray, H. *Thematic Apperception Test*. Cambridge, Mass.: Harvard University Press, 1943.

Nall, A. Alpha training and the hyperkinetic child: Is it effective? *Academic Therapy*, 1973, *9*, 5–19.

Nelson, R., & Bowles, P. E., Jr. The best of two worlds—Observations with norms. *Journal of School Psychology*, 1975, *13*, 3–9.

Nordquist, M., & Wahler, R. Naturalistic treatment of an autistic child. *Journal of Applied Behavioral Analysis*, 1973, *6*, 79–87.

Palmer, S., Thompson, R., & Linsheid, T. Applied behavioral analysis in the treatment of childhood feeding problems. *Developmental Medicine and Child Neurology*, 1975, *17*, 333–339.

Parsons, B., & Alexander, J. Short term family intervention: A therapy outcome study. *Journal of Counseling and Clinical Psychology*, 1973, *41*, 195–201.

Paulson, M., & Blake, P. The abused, battered, and maltreated child: A review. *Trauma*, 1967, *9*, 3–134.

Petrovich, D. *Pain Apperception Test*. Los Angeles: Western Psychological Services, 1973.

Porter, R., & Cattell, R. *Children's Personality Questionnaire.* Champaign, Ill.: IPAT, 1968.

Ray, R., Shaw, D., & Cobb, J. The work box: An innovation in teaching attentional behavior. *The School Counselor*, 1970, *18*, 15–35.

Rekers, G., & Lovaas, O. Behavioral treatment of deviant sex-role behaviors in a male child. *Journal of Applied Behavior Analysis*, 1974, *7*, 173–190.

Rekers, G., Lovaas, O., & Low, B. The behavioral treatment of a "transsexual" pre-adolescent boy. *Journal of Abnormal Child Psychology*, 1974, *2*, 99–116.

Resnik, H. *Suicidal behavior: Diagnosis and management*, Boston: Little, Brown, 1968.

Rorschach, H. *Rorschach.* New York: Grune & Stratton, 1954.

Rosenbaum, A., O'Leary, D., & Jacob, R. Behavioral intervention with hyperactive children: Group consequences as a supplement to individual contingencies. *Behavior Therapy*, 1975, *6*, 315–323.

Rush, A., & Beck, A. Adults with affective disorders. In M. Hersen & A. Bellack (Eds.), *Behavior therapy in the psychiatric setting.* Baltimore: Williams & Wilkins, 1978.

Sackett, D., & Haynes, R. *Compliance with therapeutic regimes.* Baltimore: Johns Hopkins University Press, 1976.

Schaefer, A. Death and dying. In L. Wright, A. Schaefer, & G. Solomans (Eds.), *Encyclopedia of pediatric psychology.* Baltimore: University Park Press, in press.

Schaefer, E., & Bell, R. Development of a parental attitude research instrument (PARI). *Child Development*, 1958, *29*, 339–361.

Schneidman, E., & Farberow, N. *Clues to suicide.* New York: McGraw-Hill, 1957.

Schnurer, A., Rubin, R., & Roy, A. Systematic desensitization of anorexia nervosa seen as a weight phobia. *Journal of Behavior Therapy and Experimental Psychiatry*, 1973, *4*, 149–153.

Schwitzgebel, R. *Streetcorner research.* Cambridge: Harvard University Press, 1964.

Scrignar, C. Food as the reinforcer in the outpatient treatment of anorexia nervosa. *Journal of Behavior Therapy and Experimental Psychiatry*, 1971, *2*, 31–36.

Shaw, W., & Walker, C. Relaxation treatment of sexual foot fetish and hyperactivity in an eight year old patient with phenylketonuria. *Journal of Pediatric Psychology*, in press.

Sigal, J., Chagoya, L., Villeneuve, C., & Mayerovitch, J. Later psychosocial sequelae of early childhood illness (severe group). *American Journal of Psychiatry*, 1973, *130*, 786–788.

Simpson, D., & Nelson, A. Attention training through breathing control to modify hyperactivity. *Journal of Learning Disabilities*, 1974, *7*, 274–283.

Smith, S. School refusal with anxiety: A review of sixty-three cases. *Canadian Psychiatric Association Journal*, 1970, *15*, 257–264.

Spache, G. *Diagnostic Reading Scales.* Monterey, Calif.: McGraw-Hill, 1963.

Spivack, G., & Spotts, J. *Deveraux Child Behavior Rating Scale.* Devon, Pa.: Devereaux, 1966.

Spivack, G., & Swift, M. *Elementary School Behavior Rating Scale.* Devon, Pa.: Devereaux, 1967.

Starfield, B., & Mellits, E. Increase in functional bladder capacity and improvements in enuresis. *Journal of Pediatrics*, 1968, *72*, 483–487.

Stuart, R., & Davis, B. *Slim chance in a fat world: Behavioral control of obesity.* Champaign, Ill.: Research, 1972.

Stunkard, A., & Mahoney, M. Behavior treatment of the eating disorders. In H. Leitenberg (Ed.), *Handbook of behavior modification and behavior therapy.* Englewood Cliffs, N.J.: Prentice-Hall, 1976.

Tasto, D. Systematic desensitization, muscle relaxation, and visual imagery in the counter conditioning of a 4-year-old phobic child. *Behaviour Research and Therapy*, 1969, *7*, 409–411.

Tavormina, J., Boll, T., Gayton, W., & Mattsson, A. Psychosocial effects of physical illness on child and family functioning. *Pediatrics*, in press.

Terman, L., & Merrill, M. *Stanford–Binet Intelligence Scale.* Cambridge, Mass.: Houghton-Mifflin, 1960.

Thompson, J., & Sones, R. *Education Apperception Test.* Los Angeles: Western Psychological Services, 1973.

Tuma, J. Practicum, internship, and postdoctoral training in pediatric psychology: A survey. *Journal of Pediatric Psychology*, 1977, *2*, 9–12.

Tyler, V. Application of operant token reinforcement to academic performance of an institutionalized delinquent. *Psychological Reports*, 1967, *21*, 249–260.

Violence against children. *Journal of Clinical Child*, Fall 1973, entire issue.

Walker, C. Enuresis and encopresis. In P. Magrab (Ed.), *Psychological management of pediatric problems*. Baltimore: University Park Press, 1978.

Walker, C. Behavior therapy for medical/psychological problems. In L. Wright, A. Schaefer, & G. Solomans (Eds.), *Encyclopedia of pediatric psychology*. Baltimore: University Park Press, in press.

Walker, C., Hedberg, A., Clement, P., & Wright, L. *Clinical procedures for behavior therapy*. Englewood Cliffs, N.J.: Prentice-Hall, in press.

Webster, D., & Azrin, N. Required relaxation: A method of inhibiting agitative disruptive behavior of retardates. *Behaviour Research and Therapy*, 1973, *11*, 67–78.

Wechsler, D. *Wechsler PreSchool and Primary Scale of Intelligence*. New York: Psychological Corporation, 1967.

Wechsler, D. *Wechsler Intelligence Scale for Children—Revised*. New York: Psychological Corporation, 1974.

Weinberger, G., Leventhal, T., & Beckman, G. The management of a chronic school phobic through the use of consultation with school personnel. *Psychology in the Schools*, 1973, *10*, 83–87.

Welsh, R. Stimulus satiation as a technique for the elimination of juvenile fire setting behavior. Paper presented at Eastern Psychological Association Convention, Washington, D.C., Apr. 1968.

Welsh, R. Severe parental punishment and delinquency: A developmental approach. *Journal of Clinical Child Psychology*, 1976, *5*, 17–23.

Williams, C. The elimination of tantrum behavior by extinction procedures. *Journal of Abnormal and Social Psychology*, 1959, *59*, 269.

Williams, G. Child abuse. In P. Magrab (Ed.), *Psychological management of pediatric problems*. Baltimore: University Park Press, 1978.

Wright, L. Pediatric psychologist: A role model. *American Psychologist*, 1967, *22*, 323–325.

Wright, L. Behavioral tactics for reinstating natural breathing in tracheostomy addicted infants. *Pediatric Research*, 1969, *3*, 275–278. (a)

Wright, L. Conditioning children when refusal of oral medication is life threatening. *Pediatrics*, 1969, *44*, 969–972. (b)

Wright, L. A diet exercise and behavioral conditioning program for obesity. *Professional Psychology*, 1976, *7*, 417–419.

Wright, L. Suicide. In L. Wright, A. Schaefer, & G. Solomans (Eds.), *Encyclopedia of pediatric psychology*. Baltimore: University Park Press, in press.

Wright, L., & Thalassinos, P. Success with electroshock in habitual vomiting. *Clinical Pediatrics*, 1973, *12*, 594–597.

Wright, L., & Walker, C. Treating the encopretic child. *Clinical Pediatrics*, 1977, *16*, 1042–1045.

Yates, A. *Behavior therapy*. New York: Wiley, 1970.

Young, G. A staggered-awakening procedure in the treatment of enuresis. *Medical Officer*, 1964, *111*, 142–143.

10

Behavioral Medicine in the Occupational Setting

MARGARET A. CHESNEY AND MICHAEL FEUERSTEIN

INTRODUCTION

Industry has recently become a site for intervention and research in behavioral medicine and is becoming recognized as a setting particularly conducive to work in this field. This chapter discusses the characteristics of the occupational setting that facilitate behavioral approaches to health, reviews relevant programs, and describes measurement issues and future directions for behavioral medicine in the work environment.

Applications from a behavioral perspective in the work place are not new. Prior to the introduction of behavioral medicine to this setting, procedures drawn from behavior modification were utilized to promote employee behavior change. One such program demonstrated significant improvement in both work productivity and absenteeism in a group of employees who were given behavioral feedback regarding job performance (Latham & Kinne, 1974). Among applications of behavior modification in occupational settings, the majority have been directed toward improving job performance, job training, and management procedures (Glaser & Klaus, 1966; Goldstein & Sorcher, 1973, 1974; Jablonsley & DeVries, 1972; Nord, 1969; Porter, 1973; Sorcher, 1971).

The distinction between these behavioral programs and those within the scope of behavioral medicine rests in the specific behavior under consideration. While both types of programs have in common the occupational setting and its resources, one is

MARGARET A. CHESNEY • Center for Research on Stress and Health, Stanford Research Institute, Menlo Park, California 94025.   MICHAEL FEUERSTEIN • Department of Psychology, McGill University, Montreal, Quebec, Canada.

directed at work-related behavior while the other is focused on behaviors associated with health.

The characteristics of the work setting that are resources for the study and practice of behavioral medicine are discussed in the first section of this chapter. The second section describes a number of programs in behavioral medicine conducted at the work site. Principles for performing behavioral assessment and evaluation of behavioral medicine programs in the occupational setting are presented in the third section. Finally, possible future directions for behavioral medicine in occupational settings are discussed.

RESOURCES WITHIN THE OCCUPATIONAL SETTING

The occupational setting has a number of resources that make it conducive for both clinical and research programs in behavioral medicine. As in the university environment, the occupational setting is one in which people are accessible. However, the work site offers additional advantages since the stability of the work population is greater than that of the student population. This stability increases the opportunity for longitudinal studies and clinical follow-up (e.g., Gibson, Haynes, & Martin, 1975). In addition, there is typically a broader range of age groups in the work environment, which generates a wide variety of health problems and permits cross-sectional studies.

From both methodological and clinical perspectives, the work setting provides substantial benefits. Methodologically, assessment and treatment are very convenient, as has been demonstrated by cardiovascular screening programs (Alderman & Schoenbaum, 1976; Cathcart, 1977; Davidson, 1974; Felton, 1974; Verdesca, 1974) and psychological counseling programs that have been conducted in this setting (e.g., Kelsey, 1975). In contrast to the clinic, the occupational setting is a more "natural environment." Opportunities for behavioral observation and other assessments in this setting are particularly rich, and although systematic comparative studies have not been performed, the generalizability of these measures to other environments probably exceeds that of measures taken in a typical clinical setting.

Similarly, a particularly salient advantage of behavioral medicine in the work place is that this setting is often both the site of the intervention for behavior change and an environment to which behavioral change is expected to generalize. Also from a clinical perspective, the increased convenience of an on-site behavioral medicine program should improve compliance with treatment programs, since the potential time lost, transportation problems, and inconvenience of typical clinic visits are key variables in the prediction of noncompliance (Chesney, Black, Jordan, & Sevelius, 1978).

Alderman and Schoenbaum (1976) pointed out that individuals in a given work place form a cohesive community, a functionally meaningful group, with existing channels of communication. These characteristics can be utilized by the behavioral practitioner in the design of interventions. For example, information regarding programs can be disseminated through the existing communication channels, and peers can be solicited to perform roles as observers or reinforcers for participants in specific behavioral programs.

In addition, the practitioner in the work setting has the potential to direct greater control over environmental stimuli and contingencies of reinforcement than the practitioner in a clinic setting. For example, in an industrial smoking-cessation program, smoking can be restricted to less desirable locations, cigarette machines can be eliminated, and pay incentives can be offered to employees not smoking on the job.

Some occupational settings have organizational features that are potential resources for behavioral medicine. Many larger industries have health departments that are staffed by industrial physicians and nurses. This staff can serve as agents for on-site intervention and medical consultation (Shelnutt, 1977; Wolter, 1975). In some cases this staff also includes psychologists engaged in counseling outreach in the occupational setting (Felton & Swinger, 1973; Kelsey, 1975).

A second organizational feature that is important to the delivery of services in behavioral medicine is the role that industry, management, unions, and employee organizations play in the health of the employees (Gibson *et al.*, 1975). The increasing number of clinical and research programs in behavioral medicine in the work place appears to reflect the growing concern of management, unions, and other employee groups in efforts directed toward decreasing risk of illness and enhancing employee health. Industries are becoming more aware of the importance of health behavior, preventive medicine, and rehabilitation as the financial burdens associated with illness, including the costs of medical care, absenteeism, job replacement, disability and life insurance, and workmen's compensation, increase (Garbus, Pore, Troendle, Wheeler, & Garbus, 1975; "Kimberly-Clark Health Management . . . ," 1977; Slobogin, 1977; Wood, 1975). To complement this interest, there is some preliminary evidence that providing health programs at the work site is cost-effective (Alderman & Davis, 1976).

RESEARCH AT THE WORK PLACE

In this section, programs utilizing the work site as a laboratory to study issues relevant to behavioral medicine are described. At present, job stress has been the research area that has received the greatest attention. However, smoking and the behavioral aspects of injury and the associated pain have also been investigated. Given the limited number of problem areas related to occupational behavioral medicine that have actually been studied at the work site, the need for additional research in this area is evident.

Occupational Stress

While the specific mechanisms linking physical illnesses (e.g., essential hypertension and coronary heart disease) to stress have not been delineated, it has long been thought that psychosocial factors, such as job stress, play a significant role. Reflecting this assumption, the Occupational Safety and Health Act of 1970 presented a research directive "to evaluate the effects of job stresses on the potential for illness, disease or loss of functional capacity in adults" (Cohen, 1974).

Research conducted in the occupational setting has provided evidence of a link between job stress and illness. Caplan, Cobb, French, Harrison, and Pinneau (1975) conducted a study of 2,010 men in 23 job categories representing a wide range of job stresses and in blue- and white-collar jobs associated with high rates of illness. The following hypotheses were tested through both questionnaire and physiological data: (1) job stress results in psychological and physiological strain in the worker; (2) the worker's characteristics influence these strain measures; and (c) psychological and physiological strain influences rates of illness.

Caplan *et al.* reported that certain job stressors are related to psychological distress. These job stressors included job dissatisfaction, underutilization of skills and abilities, simple and repetitive work, job insecurity, and poor social support from supervisor and co-workers. On the other hand, physiological strain (i.e., blood pressure, heart rate, serum cholesterol, thyroid hormone, serum uric acid, and serum cortisol) were *not* related to job stress. Characteristics of the worker (e.g., personality and psychological "needs") were not related to psychological or physiological strain. With regard to the relationship between job stress and illness, Caplan reported an association between anxiety and gastrointestinal problems, including diarrhea, constipation, colitis, gall bladder disturbances, nervous stomach, and peptic ulcers. The fact that Caplan *et al.* did not observe a relationship between stress and physiological strain suggests the need for further research in this area, given the importance of identifying the physiological mechanisms through which occupational stress leads to illness.

In a more recent study, using a homogeneous population of 1,540 white-collar workers (84% male) in a large financial institution, Weiman (1977) examined Selye's hypothesis that both overstimulation or overutilization and understimulation or underutilization are sources of stress and are associated with a higher level of disease or risk. Weiman confirmed this hypothesis, observing a U-shaped relationship between stimulation (measured by an index of workload, role conflict, task ambiguity, and responsibility) and an index of disease or risk (including smoking, hypertriglyceridemia, hypercholesterolemia, artherosclerotic heart disease, essential hypertension, exogenous obesity, and peptic ulcer). Both the group of officers reporting a lack of stimulation and those reporting an excess had significantly higher indices of disease or risk. It is of considerable interest that both over- and understimulation can result in an increase in stress-related disorders and behaviors associated with health risk. Research on the health of occupational groups whose jobs are characterized by understimulation, such as blue-collar assembly line workers, would serve to further establish this interesting U-shaped relationship between environment and disease.

Similarly, Zorn, Harrington, and Goethe (1977), in a study of West German sea pilots, observed excess cardiac mortality in this occupational group compared to the cardiac death rate of the male population of Hamburg. Although studies report a relationship between stress and heart disease, the mechanism linking these two factors remains unknown. To explore the hypothesis that an increased catecholamine level contributes to the relationship between stress on the job and cardiac death, Zorn and his colleagues measured urinary catecholamines in five sea pilots before, immediately after, and 24 hours following a stressful river-piloting operation. Significant differences were observed between the three assessments. Specifically, a significant elevation in catecholamines between the pre- and posttrip collections and a subsequent drop in catecholamines over the 24 hours following the operation were found.

Also studying the possible link between catecholamines and job stress, Dutton, Smolensky, Leach, Lorimor, and Bartholomew (1978) compared a group of paramedics with a group of fire fighters. While both groups had similar scores on the Schedule of Recent Life Events (Holmes & Rahe, 1967), the paramedics scored significantly higher than the fire fighters on a job stress questionnaire designed for this study. The paramedics also had significantly higher levels of epinephrine and elevated levels of norepinephrine on workdays as contrasted with days off. While it appears from these studies that catecholamines are associated with job stress and that environmentally induced sympathetic arousal may play a role in cardiovascular disease, it is important to consider that catecholamines are significantly influenced by activity alone (Frankenhaeuser, 1975). This consideration is substantiated in the Dutton *et al.* (1978) study, in which the fire fighters demonstrated higher levels of catecholamines on *days off* than on workdays during which they spent the majority of their time sitting at their stations.

While the research discussed above has suggested an association between environmental stress and disease, certain behavior characteristics of the employee may *interact* with characteristics of the environment and influence this association. For example, in the area of coronary heart disease, research by Rosenman and others (cf. Jenkins, 1976a,b; Rosenman, Brand, Jenkins, Friedman, Straus, & Wurm, 1975) has suggested that a set of behaviors known as the Type A behavior pattern (competitive, ambitious, aggressive, and impatient) is associated with a higher incidence of coronary heart disease. The specific relationship among these factors requires clarification.

Currently, Chadwick, Chesney, Black, Rosenman, and Sevelius (1979) are attempting to define the relationship among job and life stressors, personality characteristics and behavior patterns, job and home environments, physiological strain variables, and coronary heart disease risk and status. Three hundred and ninety-seven male salaried workers have been given examinations at their work site assessing these variables over a period of a year and a half. While the data analysis is still in progress, interesting relationships among the variables are emerging. As Zorn *et al.* (1977) noted, higher levels of catecholamines are found to correlate with job stress as measured by the work pressure subscale of the Work Environment Scale (Moos, Insel, & Humphrey, 1974). In addition, urinary epinephrine was also related to impulsiveness as measured by the Eysenck Personality Inventory (Eysenck & Eysenck, 1968). Impulsiveness was also significantly related to the Type A behavior pattern.

Cholesterol was among the coronary heart disease (CHD) risk factors measured at each subject's work site. The high density lipid (HDL) fraction of cholesterol, recently recognized as a protective factor in heart disease (Hulley, Cohen, & Widdowson, 1977), shows a pattern of relationships among the variables that is opposite that observed for catecholamines. Specifically, Chadwick *et al.* (1979) have observed a significant negative association between HDL and the CHD correlates, including high blood pressure, dyspnea, and triglycerides. On the other hand, HDL was related to high scores on personality scales measuring order and nurturance and to low scores on scales measuring autonomy and exhibition. When examined as a whole, the preliminary analyses of this study suggest that the relationship between CHD risk and job stress is more complex than early literature implies. Rather than their having a clear, direct relationship, the evidence from this research appears to indicate that both characteristics of the person and the work setting play a role in increasing health risk.

While the white-collar workers studied by Chadwick *et al.* may be subject to stress in their work setting, certain work conditions may be sources of stress for blue-collar workers also. One such condition that has been the subject of considerable research is shift work. A number of health complaints and problems have been associated with shift-work schedules. The most common complaint of shift workers is reduction in sleep hours (e.g., Carpentier & Cazamian, 1977). Other common complaints and disorders related to shift work include problems with the digestive system, such as peptic ulcer and colitis (e.g., Thiis-Evensen, 1958; Walker & De La Mare, 1971). There is some evidence that these and other health correlates of shift work occur more frequently for a short time after the shift change and among workers who rotate frequently from one shift to another, and that these health problems decrease as a shift becomes permanent (Tasto & Colligan, 1978). Disruptions in circadian rhythms brought about by shift changes have been proposed as an explanation of this pattern (e.g., Maurice, 1975). Wojtezak-Jaroszowa (1978) conducted a laboratory study to examine the physiological effects of disrupting these rhythms and observed that "work capacity" (measured by such factors as oxygen capacity and carbon monoxide production), sensory acuity, and neuromuscular activity were impaired during the night hours.

Research in the health correlates of stressors, such as shift work, may lead to recommendations for industry that will reduce or prevent health problems. For example, Tasto and Colligan (1978) studied 2,400 workers and found job satisfaction to be an intervening variable in the relationship between shift work and health. In light of this finding, they proposed that workers' preferences for particular shifts be taken into account in their job assignment.

In shift work, as in other aspects of occupational stress, further research is necessary to clarify the physiological, behavioral, and psychosocial impact of specific schedules on different types of people. This research would then identify potential areas for behavioral medicine interventions, including stress management, the development of behavioral as well as self-report criteria for more effective shift assignment, and perhaps even modification of the work environment by adjusting work schedules to minimize health risk.

Because the majority of these job stress studies have been naturalistic, they have contributed to our understanding of disease and occupational stress. However, a number of methodological inadequacies characterize this literature and will need to be addressed before any definitive conclusions can be arrived at. Research in occupational stress and disease should consider including dynamic and situational analyses, *behavioral* measures of stress and its psychological variables, and repeated measures of indices of both stress and strain. A current investigation of air traffic controllers by Rose, Jenkins, and Hurst (1978) exemplifies such a research strategy and its methodological characteristics warrant attention by the serious researcher in the area of occupational stress.

Industrial Injury: Low Back Pain—An Illustrative Problem

A second area of attention for research in behavioral medicine at the work site is industrial injury. Primary among occupational disabilities is chronic low back pain. It is estimated that more than 15% of all industrial injuries and more than 20% of all compensation payments made in any given year are related to low back problems (Sternbach, Wolf, Murphy, & Akeson, 1973). The cost of this problem is staggering. For example, in 1971, low back pain cost the State of California $200 million (Bonica, 1974). It has also been estimated that 6.5 million men and women are under treatment for back pain and its associated problems each day. Further, 600,000–700,000 workers are absent from work yearly as a result of back injury. This situation costs United States employers approximately $1 billion annually (Addison, 1976). In the pursuit of preventing these problems, research has been directed toward the identification of the conditions under which they occur.

Magura (1970a,b), for example, confirmed the widely held opinion that there is a markedly higher incidence of low back problems in certain occupational groups. Of 3,316 workers interviewed in a cross section of occupational groups including clerks, bus drivers, police, nurses, and farmers in both light and heavy industry, 429 complained of low back pain. Further study of this sample of workers with low back pain indicated that the *type* of work in which a person is engaged plays an important role in influencing this pain problem. Specifically, Magura identified the weight lifting and bending characteristic of heavy industry, rather than trauma, as the factors most frequently causing this condition. Coughing and standing for long lengths of time were noted as predominant aggravating factors.

Also studying lifting, Chaffin and Park (1973) examined 411 employees in 103 jobs rated for the extent to which lifting was required. Again, a higher incidence of low back pain was correlated with the amount of lifting. Turning the focus to the employee, Chaffin and Park isolated the following five personal risk factors indicative of increased risk of injury: age, weight, stature, previous history of low back pain, and inability to demonstrate an isometric lifting strength in medical testing. This testing, conducted in the industrial medical department, involved each worker's demonstrating his or her lifting capability by reaching down and pulling up on a handle connected by a chain to a force meter.

The identification of these job and personal variables from this research has several implications for the prevention and rehabilitation of low back pain. Jobs requiring performance of behaviors such as lifting, which have been associated with back injuries and pain, could be redesigned to minimize reliance on these problematic behaviors. When redesign is difficult, rigorous employee selection, including behavioral screening procedures such as isometric lifting tests, could be performed. Finally, educational programs could be conducted to increase employee knowledge of appropriate work practices to prevent pain and injury. For example, Miller (1976) described such an educational program, which was implemented in a heavy industry to teach employees proper lifting procedures. The Miller program consisted of a five-minute slide and cassette presentation, given at monthly safety meetings, emphasizing proper lifting behavior. However, the effectiveness of this program has not been systematically evaluated.

Research is needed in the development of behaviorally based screening procedures, programs designed to train workers in appropriate work practices (e.g., guided participant modeling of proper lifting procedures), and programs for on-the-job rehabilitation of the injured worker. Longitudinal studies of these behavioral programs' effectiveness in reducing the incidence of job-related injury are also needed.

Smoking Behavior

Smoking and its associated health hazards has received considerable attention in recent years. With regard to the occupational setting, smoking has been estimated to be responsible for 77 million lost workdays annually (Terry, 1971). Furthermore, the effects of such occupational carcinogens as asbestos and smoking have been widely publicized. For example, asbestos workers who smoke have an eight times greater chance of developing cancer than nonsmoking asbestos workers (Selikoff, Hammond, & Churg, 1968). These findings taken as a whole suggest the importance of investigating smoking behavior and its modification in the occupational setting.

Research on smoking and occupational medicine has focused primarily on general epidemiology. In a study using the 1970 Household Interview Survey data (N = 75,827), Sterling and Weinkam (1976) reported that (1) more blacks smoke, but they are much lighter smokers than whites; (2) employed women smoke with prevalence rates approaching those of males in many occupations; and (3) smoking prevalence is generally higher among blue-collar occupations and lowest among professionals, managers, and proprietors. The finding of a higher smoking prevalence in blue-collar workers was also observed in earlier research by Dunn, Linden, and Breslow (1960). These studies may prove useful in identifying target populations for intervention. In addition, they suggest the need for further research on various job and employee characteristics that may account for differences in prevalence of smoking among occupational groups. This research may also be useful in clarifying the potential role that elements of the occupational setting (e.g., social pressure and job stress) play in the maintenance of smoking behavior.

INTERVENTION AT THE WORK PLACE

The industrial setting is an environment particularly well suited to preventive and remedial health programs. In describing a number of these programs, including those addressing employee health in general and those directed toward particular health problems, this section highlights the program elements most relevant to behavioral medicine. It should be emphasized that these programs have been service-oriented, and therefore, the majority have not been subjected to systematic evaluation.

The New York Telephone Company, realizing that costs for health care were rising at the rate of 13–16% per year, implemented a health screening and referral program that included early detection, health education, traditional ambulatory treatment, hospitalization, and rehabilitation (Wood, 1975). Seventy-one percent of the eligible personnel volunteered for this comprehensive health management program, which was designed to increase employee knowledge and practice of various health behaviors, such as diet and exercise. After the initial three months of the program, a lower rate of absenteeism was noted in comparison to that of a cohort group of employees not in the program. An evaluation of the cost effectiveness has not been reported.

A similar comprehensive health system was implemented at Kimberly-Clark corporate headquarters. This program is operated by 15 full-time health care personnel in facilities specifically designed for multiphasic testing and physical fitness. Sixty percent of the eligible employees are participating in the program, which includes an evaluation of health risks and a health prescription. Preventive and remedial health activities are the principle elements of these prescriptions. These prescribed activities typically include participation in health education or counseling for alcohol and drug abuse, obesity, nutrition, stress, and supervised physical exercise ("Kimberly-Clark . . . ," 1977). Individuals participate in the program during nonworking hours.

While these programs represent innovations in preventive medicine and indicate the growing interest in the behavioral aspects of health, there are no available data on the effectiveness of such programs. In addition, by focusing primarily on health education, they do not incorporate the necessary behavioral technology to develop and maintain preventive health behavior. Given the difficulty in producing long-term health behavior change, it would appear that the use of this technology is critical.

Cardiovascular Fitness

To date, the effectiveness of the majority of interventions prescribed in these general health programs has also not been determined. The effectiveness of physical exercise, however, has been evaluated to a limited degree. Koerner (1973), for example, investigated the outcome of the Xerox Company's physical fitness program in modifying parameters of cardiovascular fitness by comparing 20 male executives (age range = 35–51) who had participated in the program with 20 male executives (age range = 34–51) about to enter the program. The executives who participated in the program had greater aerobic capacity on a treadmill stress test and better inotropic and chronotropic mechanisms for adaptation to greater physical exertion.

In a similar investigation, Fogle and Verdesca (1975) evaluated the Western Electric Company's supervised cardiovascular fitness exercise program, in which participants were encouraged to exercise up to three times per week on company time. One hundred and three management personnel (age range = 30–57) were divided into three groups, depending on their number of physical fitness sessions per week. Participants who exercised more than two times a week in the company's program showed significant improvement in cardiovascular fitness as measured by stress testing. Specifically, those in the frequent exercise group displayed significant reductions in weight, resting and exercise heart rates, and diastolic blood pressure during exercise, as well as significant increases in maximum oxygen uptake at all levels of exercise. Less improvement was observed in participants who exercised one to two times per week, while exercising once a week did not lead to a measurable improvement.

Hypertension Control

With prevention of cardiovascular disease (CVD) as a target, the Campbell Soup Company instituted an atherosclerosis prevention program (Wear, Cox, & Lento, 1975). As in the programs discussed above, after physical examinations, subjects with CVD risk were monitored by the nursing staff, who, for example, designed diets for subjects with high lipid levels and presented weight reduction diets low in sugar and alcohol for overweight participants. The major emphasis of this program was increasing employee awareness of hypertension and identifying hypertensive employees and referring them for treatment. At this time, data evaluating the effectiveness of this program in health behavior change and prevention of atherosclerosis have not been presented.

In light of the positive effects that hypertension control exerts on CVD risk and the observation that the amount of industrial medical department time required for this effort need not be excessive (Wear *et al.*, 1975), it is not surprising that this health problem has received considerable attention in the occupational medicine literature. Initially, hypertension control programs at the work site encompassed screening of hypertensives and administration of antihypertensive medication in the work setting (Alderman & Schoenbaum, 1976; Gibson, Haynes, & Martin, 1975).

However, like all treatment programs, the effectiveness of hypertension screening and treatment is a function of the level of patient compliance. Estimates of noncompliance to prescribed antihypertensive medication ranges from a third to one-half of the patients (Stamler, 1974). For example, in a study of male NASA employees checked after screening and referral, 47% of the hypertensives did not have their blood pressure under control at follow-up (Villafana & Mackbee, 1971). Since, in the vast majority of cases, antihypertensive medication will bring blood pressures to within normal limits, an elevated blood pressure in a patient who has been prescribed medication typically implies noncompliance.

Sackett, Haynes, Gibson, Hackett, Taylor, Roberts, and Johnson (1975) attempted to improve compliance or adherence to antihypertensive drug regimens in 230 Canadian steelworkers by augmented convenience (i.e., seeing the physician at work during working hours rather than at a clinic) and education. This worksite–based program included facts on hypertension, its effects on target organs, benefits of antihypertensive treatment, need for compliance, and reminders for pill taking. A comparison of hypertensives having participated in the compliance program with those who had not participated revealed that neither augmented convenience nor the educational program led to a compliance rate, as measured by pill counts, greater than that observed in the control group. In discussing their results, the authors indicated that participation in health education and the acquisition of health knowledge are insufficient to increase compliance.

In a further attempt to increase compliance to antihypertensive therapy in 38 subjects for whom compliance had been a problem, Haynes, Sackett, Gibson, Taylor, Hackett, Roberts, and Johnson (1976) implemented a work site program of behaviorally oriented strategies. These behavioral strategies included home blood pressure self-monitoring, medication charting, and tailoring of regimens to habits and daily rituals. Hypertensives met fortnightly for six months with a paraprofessional who reinforced improvements in compliance and blood pressure with praise and credit toward ownership of the home blood-pressure–monitoring kit. Six months after the end of this program, compliance rates of participants in the program were compared with those of a control group of hypertensives with compliance problems. At this six-month follow-up, average compliance in the behavioral group had increased 21.3%, while compliance had dropped by 1.5% in the control group.

Chadwick, Chesney, and Jordan (1977) have implemented a stepped-up program of education and counseling interventions to increase compliance with hypertension treatments among 600 hypertensive employees at Lockheed Missiles and Space Company. The hypertension literature, as described above, suggests that while approximately 30–50% of hypertensive patients do not adhere to their treatment regimen and could potentially benefit from compliance counseling, the remaining 50–70% do not require this additional assistance. Therefore, in their hypertension control program, Chadwick and his colleagues offer health education tailored to the individual hypertensive's tenure in the hypertension control process as a first, low-cost attempt at increasing compliance. Those who are not compliant following this educational intervention receive behaviorally oriented counseling at the work site, which includes self-monitoring of blood pressures and adherent behavior, stimulus control strategies for compliance with diet restrictions and medication, contingency management, and the tailoring of treatment behavior to daily habits and rituals.

This individualized treatment program is indicative of the manner in which the availability of patients in the work setting is conducive to preventive, remedial, and follow-up health care intervention from screening to one-to-one health counseling. Although this stepped-up hypertension treatment program is currently under way, preliminary results indicate that it is successful from the perspectives of both treatment effectiveness and cost.

In general, programs of educational and "stepped-up" behavioral interventions tailored to patients' needs would appear to be an economical approach to many problems because they reserve the more costly one-to-one interventions for people requiring them. However, such individually tailored approaches required close follow-up of patients for effective assignment to stepped-up interventions. This level of follow-up itself could be prohibitive in terms of cost and time in the traditional clinic setting. For example, in the Chadwick *et al.* study, blood pressures were taken repeatedly, often only weeks apart, as each hypertensive proceeded through the care process from detection to control. Because blood pressures were monitored and compliance counseling was conducted at each hypertensives' work site, costs were minimized. Thus, the work setting, by permitting easy access to patients, facilitates the utilization of more sophisticated, individualized behavioral treatment programs in what is perhaps a more economical manner than conventional care.

Cardiac Rehabilitation

Another area that holds much potential for clinical application at the work site is the rehabilitation of employees following myocardial infarction (MI). At present, individuals returning to work are receiving counseling by the health teams at industrial sites (Plunkett, 1974; Warshaw, 1974). Behavioral prescriptions are written for the employee–patient, including physical exercise programs, modification of job demands to match the employee's capabilities, and elimination or control of such risk factors as smoking and blood pressure in an attempt to prevent future MIs.

While these programs provide a useful service, it seems likely that cardiac rehabilitation could be facilitated if the unique characteristics of the work site were more optimally utilized. Specifically, following hospitalization, the employee can be systematically reintroduced to work with the aid of graduated job tasks determined jointly by the employee and management. This approach could perhaps assist in reducing the anxiety associated with a return to work. In addition, industry-based behavioral programs can be introduced for the reduction of cardiovascular risk factors (refer to the sections on smoking cessation, cardiovascular fitness, and stress management). The systematic use of social and monetary incentives for modifying various risk factors in conjunction with specific behavioral procedures can be readily incorporated into industry-based programs. Given the incidence of MI in the work force and the difficulties experienced in returning to work, development and evaluation of such programs is certainly warranted.

Stress Management

Stress in the work setting was the target of an intervention program at the Converse Rubber Company conducted by Peters, Benson, and Porter (1977). One hundred twenty-six volunteers at the corporate offices of this manufacturing firm participated in an investigation of the effects of two 15-minute relaxation breaks during each workday. The volunteers were divided into three groups: one group was taught the relaxation response, the second group was instructed to sit quietly, and the third group received no instructions. The first two groups were asked to take two 15-minute relaxation breaks daily. After a period of eight weeks, the group taught the relaxation response showed significantly greater improvements in measures of symptoms, illness days, and performance and sociability than the group given no instruction to relax (Peters, Benson, & Peters, 1977).

A corollary study was conducted on these same subjects to determine whether the relaxation response would lower blood pressure in this predominantly normotensive population. Mean decreases in blood pressure in the relaxation group were 6.7 mm Hg systolic and 5.2 mm Hg diastolic blood pressure. The decreases were significantly greater than the blood pressure changes observed in the group instructed to sit quietly and in the no-treatment control group.

Stress management programs teaching employees techniques of identifying their stress responses and of reducing or coping with job-related stressors, such as job-abolishment, are increasing (Manuso, 1977; Slobogin, 1977). These programs are frequently in the form of workshops that are based superficially on the stress literature and are not systematically evaluated. The research programs that have demonstrated the albeit short-term effectiveness of relaxation or exercise in reducing selected cardiovascular disease risk factors suggest that systematic research-based stress-management and comprehensive CHD-risk interventions could make significant inroads in health management.

As previously mentioned, the work site offers considerable potential for comprehensive stress-management programs. To illustrate the manner in which a stress-management program could be conducted in an occupational setting, a hypothetical program will be described. Such a program could include screening to identify individuals under stress using a variety of behavioral assessment techniques (refer to section on behavioral assessment). Stress management could be conducted in groups with the following components: behavioral assessment, stress-management skills training, and maintenance of stress management strategies.

In the behavioral assessment phase, program participants would identify stimuli that are stressful, including both environmental stressors such as the telephone and internal stressors such as fear of failure. The participants would, by self-monitoring, record these stressors and the subjective and physiological responses they elicit (e.g., anger, impatience, muscle tension, increases in heart rate). Colleagues of the participating employees can assist in identifying stressors by direct behavioral observation.

Employees participating in this program would then be instructed in a variety of stress management skills, including relaxation, exercise, and environmental management. Environmental management would emphasize the employee's ability to circumvent or avoid stressors by environmental change, such as scheduling appointments realistically, minimizing interruptions, and establishing priorities.

Once the employees have acquired the appropriate stress-management skills, they would design individual stress-management plans, which might incorporate contracting for applying relaxation in stressful situations, taking relaxation breaks, managing stressors in the environment, or exercising. Stress management contracts could be self-contracts or contracts between the employee and other participants in the program or management.

An advantage of conducting stress management programs at the work site rests in the access the stress management trainer has to the major natural environment in which most participants experience stress—the work site itself. Thus, once the participant has a stress management plan, the trainer may observe and supervise the participant while practicing stress management in the presence of the actual stressors.

Following the successful implementation of the stress management plan, the focus is placed on the maintenance of stress management skills. In the occupational setting, participants are more accessible for follow-up. Participants could be easily sent, through the company's mailing system, prompts to practice stress management or additional suggestions for stress management. Also, employees could be reconvened periodically for "booster" sessions. The fact that participants are available for follow-up sessions implies that they are also available for follow-up evaluations, which might include self-report stress-measures, assessment of coronary heart disease risk factors, behavioral observation, and physiological monitoring under naturalistic stress situations.

Smoking Cessation

While industry provides a setting conducive to behavioral medicine interventions, the majority of these programs have only begun to utilize unique resources the setting provides. Smoking cessation programs, on the other hand, are more representative of the potential for behavioral medicine in the occupational setting.

The on-site smoking cessation program, similar to other industry-based interventions, reduces the employee lost time, the transportation problems, and the inconvenience often involved in clinic-based programs. The industrial setting also provides an opportunity for more careful health monitoring and follow-up, a characteristic of some importance, given the problems associated with long-term maintenance of smoking cessation (Schwartz & Rider, 1977). With regard to behavioral medicine interventions, a unique feature of the work setting is that it is a relatively closed system in which financial and social reinforcers can be systematically distributed contingent upon appropriate modification in smoking behaviors. While a number of industry- or company-based smoking cessation programs have been established, data on the effects of these programs have rarely been published in the scientific literature, and therefore, systematic evaluation of these programs is not possible.

In general, the industry-based smoking cessation programs include (1) mass communication campaigns using local media to create initial interest in the program; (2) educational materials from various health organizations; (3) continuous reporting of program progress through the firm's communication system; and (4) incentive programs. These specific incentive programs vary in the amount and frequency of the incentives used to maintain smoking abstinence. Certain companies reinforce workers on weekly schedules, while others provide incentives on a monthly, quarterly, or yearly basis.

Intermatic Incorporated of Detroit, for example, has developed a no-smoking pari-mutuel window where employees bet up to $100 on their ability to stop smoking for a year. The company has also contributed $1,000 to be divided among those who succeed. For those not remaining abstinent at the end of the year, the $100 bet is donated to the American Cancer Society. The Aluminaire Standard Glass Company in Phoenix has established a program in which an amount equivalent to what ex-smokers spent on cigarettes is deducted from their paychecks, and at the end of one year, the company matches the paycheck deduction and pays the entire amount to those workers, provided they are not smoking.

The most comprehensive cessation program to date was sponsored by the Dow Chemical Company in Freeport, Texas, and the Texas branch of the American Cancer Society. The program package included education, incentives, and social support as major change agents. The Dow incentive program's rewards for abstinence were determined by employee reports at weekly, monthly, and quarterly intervals. The weekly incentive was a dollar contingent on weekly abstinence. For each month employees reported abstinence, their names were placed in a lottery for a boat and motor. These incentives, combined with chances to win $50 quarterly, were designed to ensure a continued interest in the program as well as incentives to remain abstinent. Exsmokers were used to recruit quitters. For each quitter who did not smoke for a one-month period, the recruiter's name was placed in a separate lottery for a similar boat and motor. This recruiter incentive component provided a source of social mobilization considered useful in the modification of smoking (Janis & Hoffman, 1970).

The program enrolled 395 members as "quitters" and at program termination reported that only 26% of the participants continued to smoke. The 74% abstinence rate observed during the year-long program is promising; however, inadequate follow-up precludes comment on the long-term effects of the program. In addition, the use of self-report as the primary measure of smoking behavior is questionable, particularly in incentive-based programs. The need for more objective measures of smoking behavior (e.g., carboxyhemoglobin and serum thiocyanate) is apparent. Despite these considerations, the Dow program indicated the utility of an *ongoing* industry-based incentive program in facilitating smoking cessation.

While it is reasonable to assume that providing reduced fees and easy access to a proprietary smoking cessation program would facilitate recruitment for and attendance at meetings, this effect was not observed when such a program was offered to hospital personnel (Kanzler, Zeidenberg, & Jaffe, 1976). The investigators reported that when given the opportunity to participate in a "Smokenders" program at the work site at a reduced fee, only 4% of all smokers surveyed actually participated. In addition, when free follow-up group sessions were held, attendance was poor. At termination of the program, the smoking cessation success rate was 67%, which is approximately equivalent to the immediate effects of most programs (Schwartz & Rider, 1977). The Kanzler *et al.* (1976) study suggests that simply offering a program for smoking cessation at the work site is insufficient. While these authors utilized the communication system of the work site, recruitment was voluntary and few employees were interested. It appears that simple recruitment via letters and information is inadequate for motivating large numbers of individuals to participate in smoking cessation programs, and the incentive–peer pressure approach, such as that used by the Dow Chemical program, may be needed. The 24% enrollment figure reported in the Dow program supports this hypothesis. The need for innovative, empirically based recruitment procedures, however, is apparent.

While the recruitment process is a critical problem in smoking cessation and could perhaps be assisted by appropriate environmental modifications, (e.g., use of lotteries), long-term maintenance may also be facilitated through an industry-based program. It is well recognized that a variety of interventions result in short-term cessation; however, three to four months following treatment, cessation rates fall to 30–40% (Schwartz & Rider, 1977). Although the authors are not aware of any systematic analysis of long-term cessation programs in industry, extrapolating from other intervention programs, the work place could potentially be mobilized to facilitate maintenance. For example, co-workers could participate in a "buddy" system, providing a form of social support for continued cessation. In addition, workers could call the occupational health clinic, and a nurse could provide immediate assistance and problem solving. Incentives, as in the Dow program, could be established for weekly maintenance. While all these procedures can be implemented outside the work place, coordination of and access to such programs would be more convenient if they were based at the work site. The clinical advantages of such programs remain to be evaluated.

Pain Control

Behavioral intervention programs have also been designed for patients with low back pain (Addison, 1976; Gottlieb, Strite, Koller, Madorsky, Hockersmith, Kleeman, & Wagner, 1977; Seres & Newman, 1976). These interventions, while not performed in the work enviroment, suggest the potential for behavioral interventions for this prevalent occupational health problem. In these programs, patients typically enroll as inpatients for approximately four weeks and participate in relaxation training and electromyographic biofeedback, reward programs for healthy behavior (e.g., productive activity directed toward goal achievement), and physical reconditioning. Seres and Newman (1976) evaluated these interventions with 100 consecutive patients with low back pain, the majority of whom were injured workers. They reported significant increases in functional capacity and decreases in pain medication following treatment in an inpatient pain clinic. The potential for research directed toward the application of these behavioral procedures for *on-the-job* rehabilitation of patients with low back pain or employees with other disabilities, utilizing the work setting's resources in the treatment design, appears quite substantial. A hypothetical program that illustrates this effect is described below.

A program could be developed in which colleagues and managers of a worker with a pain problem would be instructed to systematically ignore various pain-related behaviors and to socially reinforce nonpain behaviors, including attendance at work. In addition, financial incentives could be systematically implemented for work attendance and gradually reduced as the worker's attendance improved. The employee with chronic pain could also be placed on a fixed-interval schedule of pain medication, conveniently dispensed by the occupational health nurse. Various pain control techniques, such as relaxation, biofeedback, and hypnosis, could be taught to groups of employees experiencing pain problems. Medication could be gradually reduced as the individuals began to learn and effectively implement these pain relief strategies.

As with cardiac rehabilitation, specific exercise programs could be introduced with incentive systems to ensure the maintenance of various target behaviors. It is not unreasonable to assume that an industry-based program could facilitate reductions in medication, pain behavior, and depression; increases in activity level; and attainment of other treatment goals through the proper structuring of the work environment and the teaching of pain control skills. While such pain rehabilitation programs require empirical verification, their potential is great, given the social and economic costs of chronic pain.

BEHAVIORAL ASSESSMENT AND PROGRAM EVALUATION

While industry-based primary health care has increased in recent years, the implementation of behavioral interventions for health problems in this setting is in its developmental stages. As a consequence of the experimental nature of applying behavioral intervention to the problems relevant to occupational medicine, the need for careful, systematic assessment of problem areas and program evaluation should be apparent.

Behavioral assessment has been a topic of much theoretical, empirical, and clinical concern for years. Excellent volumes (Ciminero, Calhoun, & Adams, 1977; Hersen & Bellack, 1976) have been published in the area. The reader interested in a more in-depth analysis of behavioral assessment should refer to these materials. The present intent is to provide a general description of the behavioral assessment with its various components and to discuss the application of this analytic approach to health behavior change within the context of the industrial setting. The goal is to provide a practical framework for determining where to intervene and how to evaluate a program, once it is initiated.

For purposes of clinical utility, the behavior of an individual is conceptualized in a behavioral analysis as influenced by antecedent stimuli, or a variety of precipitating events; organismic variables, or conditions within the individual, such as internal physiological state, thoughts, and feelings; and the consequences of certain actions. The acronym most frequently referred to in the behavioral assessment literature for this conceptualization is S-O-R-C or stimulus–organism–response–consequence. The goal of a behavioral analysis, therefore, is to identify the various components of the SORC model. That is, for each target behavior or group of behaviors requiring change, and analysis of the following elements is completed in order to develop an understanding of the problem behavior and to generate intervention strategies to modify it: (1) the factors that appear to set the occasion for the behavior; (2) the thoughts, feelings, and physiological state of the individual preceding and subsequent to the execution of the behavior; and (3) the actual consequences of the given behavior.

The behavioral assessment is the key to any successful intervention. The data-gathering phase of the assessment requires considerable effort on the part of the health care provider as well as the patient. However, this initial effort is often well justified. In addition to providing specific information on the problem area, the data collected during the initial assessment and planning stages provide a baseline from which to continuously evaluate treatment progress. Given the emphasis on cost effectiveness and accountability, this additional aspect of the preintervention evaluation far outweighs the initial effort of collecting the data for the behavioral analysis.

A variety of techniques are used to gather the information required for a behavioral analysis of a given problem area. The approaches most frequently implemented in behavioral assessment that are applicable to the occupational setting include the behavioral interview, behavioral observation, self-monitoring, physiological monitoring, and self-report. The behavioral interview consists of a systematic probing for information regarding the development and maintenance of the target behavior. Through a series of properly timed questions, the interviewer can develop hypotheses within a social learning framework as to the nature of the problem. Information is gathered in order to support or refute these hypotheses. A second approach by which clinical data are obtained is direct observation of the behaviors of interest. Employee self-monitoring or recording of target behaviors and antecedent events that influence the target behaviors has also been used. The monitoring of physiological indices when relevant to the target problem(s) has also been used to assist in the conceptualization and identification of a given problem. Another frequent assessment technique is the use of self-report schedules and inventories.

Assessment in the occupational setting is distinguished from assessment in the clinic by the fact that most of the assessment can actually occur in the naturalistic or work setting. Although the specific benefits of such an assessment strategy in the work setting remain to be determined, the use of behavioral assessment (particularly, behavioral observation) in other naturalistic settings (e.g., classroom and home) has provided significant insight into relevant target behaviors. Most of the approaches to behavioral assessment outlined above have been utilized to some degree in behavioral medicine programs at the work place.

In a high-blood-pressure education program, Chadwick, Chesney, and Jordan (1977) implemented the behavioral interview strategy. Patients were interviewed as to specific problem areas. Following these interviews, treatment goals were delineated, and behaviorally based intervention programs were designed. In addition, self-monitoring and physiological monitoring of target behaviors have been implemented in the area of hypertension treatment compliance (Chadwick et al., 1977; Haynes et al., 1976) and stress assessment and management (e.g., Peters, Benson, & Peters, 1977; Peters, Benson, & Porter, 1977; Zorn et al., 1977). While these procedures are also useful in smoking assessment and cessation at the work place, the use of physiological monitoring has not as yet appeared in the work-site–related literature. The potential application of a variety of self-report inventories to assess job-associated health problems is apparent. For example, inventories have been used extensively in research on occupational stress and may in the future provide a useful index of changes in job-related target behaviors.

In general, given the *in vivo* nature of the work setting, when feasible behavior can be evaluated under the stimulus conditions that are assumed to contribute to the target problem(s), perhaps providing a more valid index of the problem. It is this major factor that provides unprecedented opportunities for the behavioral health care provider in the areas of both assessment and intervention. That is, evaluation and modification of target problems can be undertaken in the environment in which the problem generally occurs. This characteristic of occupational behavioral medicine should facilitate our understanding of basic health and disease processes and provide meaningful clinical data to assist in our intervention efforts.

As was previously indicated, one key aspect of the behavioral analysis is the identification of well-defined target behaviors. Fortunately, most of the targets of behavioral interventions for health problems have clearly measurable behavioral or physical characteristics (e.g., decrease in blood pressure, increase in pill taking, decrease in time away from work because of disability, decrease in smoking via reductions in carboxyhemoglobin). While perhaps apparent to most behavioral clinicians and investigators, it must be emphasized that the major indicator of change for any intervention in behavioral medicine is whether the individual is no longer presenting with the problems he or she originally entered treatment for. This goal may be somewhat optimistic with certain individuals or specific problems; however, a change in the self-report of a given individual or a "clinical impression" is hardly sufficient grounds for the continuation of a given program. Evaluation of change in observable behavior should be implemented when possible.

Program evaluation at the work site can occur at both the individual and the group level. At the individual level, continuous monitoring of target behavior(s) permits evaluation of the treatment's impact in an uncontrolled manner; however, if the objective is to track changes in the target behavior(s) following treatment, this type of data can provide some degree of useful information. If the goal of evaluation is to more systematically evaluate the specific effects of a given intervention on an individual basis, a number of useful experimental single-subject design options are available (Barlow, Blanchard, Hayes, & Epstein, 1977; Hersen & Barlow, 1976). In a setting where funds for evaluation are minimal, the single-subject approach can effectively integrate clinical procedure with evaluation without detracting from either. When evaluation on a group basis is of interest, the standard research designs, with their specific assets and limitations, are available (Paul, 1969).

FUTURE DIRECTIONS

A number of factors appear to have contributed to the increased emphasis on behavioral medicine at the work place, including greater attention to disease prevention, financial considerations, and convenience. This increased activity can provide limitless opportunities for research and intervention at the work place. The programs that have been discussed and the potential programs described point to three future directions for behavioral medicine in the work environment.

First, as research in behavioral medicine continues to focus on increasingly complex questions, such as the mechanisms by which behavior is linked to disease processes, greater attention may be directed to utilizing the work site as a laboratory. This new setting can provide a "real-life" extension of the traditional research laboratory.

Considering the growing number of workmen's compensation claims for disorders (e.g., cardiovascular disease and pain) related to psychosocial factors in the worker's environment, the need to accurately evaluate the impact of such factors is substantial. A second direction that behavioral medicine may take is the development of assessment procedures that permit identification of the role these psychosocial factors actually play in a given individual's compensation claim. A case in point is the American Heart Association's attempt to develop guidelines that take into account such factors as physical and emotional stressors for the evaluation of claims related to stress, strain, and heart disease (Scherlis, 1976). While this type of evaluation is certainly a formidable task, given the current state of our knowledge, it illustrates the potential and critical need for research and clinical activity in this area.

As knowledge in behavioral medicine increases, our ability to intervene at the environmental level in an attempt to prevent illness and enhance health will also increase. Thus, a third direction that behavioral medicine in the work place may take is research followed by interventions in the systematic design of environments reflecting the impact that psychosocial factors exert on health. As with enviromental design to reduce worker exposure to various health hazards, such as suspected carcinogens, modifications of the work environment could be initiated to change working conditions associated with health risks and health problems.

The potential for behavioral medicine at the work site rests on an optimal utilization of the unique characteristics of this setting for both research and intervention. As a research laboratory, the occupational setting provides an opportunity for furthering our understanding of person $\times$ environment interactions in the etiology and treatment of a number of health problems. However, the widespread application of most interventions in occupation–behavioral medicine must await well-controlled clinical evaluation that uses the industrial setting as the location for delivery. Indeed, the work site may provide an environment with a number of problems for the delivery of behavioral health care services that differ from those found in the standard outpatient clinic. Given the resources of the occupational setting, it is inviting to assume that clinic-based interventions, still in their developmental stages, will be applicable to this new setting. It must be empirical verification of industry-based research and intervention that determine the future of behavioral medicine in the occupational setting.

SUMMARY

The application of behavioral medicine at the work place has increased in recent years. Researchers and clinicians are becoming aware of the unique opportunities of the work site as a setting for basic research and interventions for environmentally related or modifiable health problems. The work site as a closed system also provides a setting conducive to facilitating change in health behavior through the appropriate management of the environment.

A number of research programs, particularly in the areas of occupational stress and occupationally related pain, have been implemented at the work site. This use of the work site as a laboratory provides a setting that facilitates the analyses of person $\times$ environment interactions in disease processes.

In regard to intervention at the work site, programs have been developed to reduce cardiovascular risk, modify stress, eliminate cigarette smoking, and prevent back injury. While the design and evaluation of these programs have been limited, management and employees are interested in such programs, and the development of more sophisticated analyses of program impact is possible. Given the developmental status of these intervention programs, the need for effective assessment and program evaluation strategies is apparent. This chapter briefly describes behavioral assessment and its application to the work site. Program evaluation is also discussed.

Behavioral medicine applied to the work setting holds much potential. Future programs can be developed to more effectively reduce job-related stress and cardiovascular risk. The ultimate goal of several rehabilitation programs is to return the individual to a "socially productive" status. Programs directed at a gradual reentry to work that utilize the occupational health facilities and the unique aspects of the work environment to facilitate this transition could provide viable service. The contribution of occupational behavioral medicine depends upon the effective utilization of the unique opportunities of the work environment.

REFERENCES

Addison, R. G. Behavior modification can cure back pain. *Occupational Health and Safety*, 1976, *45*(1) 28–29.

Alderman, M. H., & Davis, T. K. Hypertension control at the work site. *Journal of Occupational Medicine*, 1976, *18*(12), 793–796.

Alderman, M. H., & Schoenbaum, E. E. Hypertension at the work site. *New England Journal of Medicine*, 1975, *293*(2), 65–68.

Alderman, M. H., & Schoenbaum, E. E. Hypertension control among employed persons in New York City: 1973–1975. *Occupational Health and Society*, 1976(Summer), 667–377.

Barlow, D. H., Blanchard, E. B., Hayes, S. C., & Epstein, L. H. Single-case designs and clinical biofeedback experimentation. *Biofeedback and Self-Regulation*, 1977, *2*, 221–240.

Bonica, J. J. (Ed.). *Advances in neurology*, Vol. 4. New York: Raven, 1974.

Caplan, R. D., Cobb, S., French, J. R. P., Harrison, R. V., & Pinnean, S. R. Job demands and worker health. DHEW Pub. No. (NIOSH) 75–160, 1975.

Carpentier, T., & Cazamian, P. *Night work*. Geneva: International Labour Office, 1977.

Cathcart, L. M. A four year study of executive health risk. *Journal of Occupational Medicine*, 1977, *19*(5), 354–357.

Chadwick, J. H., Chesney, M. A., Black, G. W., Rosenman, R. H., & Sevelius, G. G. *Psychological job stress and coronary heart disease*. Cincinnati: NIOSH, 1979.

Chadwick, J. H., Chesney, M. A., & Jordan, S. C. *High blood pressure education in an industrial setting*. Paper presented at the Annual High Blood Pressure Education Research Program Meeting. Washington, D.C., May 18–19, 1977.

Chaffin, D. B., & Park, K. S. A longitudinal study of low-back pain as associated with occupational weight lifting factors. *American Industrial Hygiene Association Journal*, 1973, *34*, 513–525.

Chesney, M. A., Black, G. W., Jordan, S. C., & Sevelius, G. G. *Unexpected predictors of compliance among newly referred hypertensives*. Paper presented at the National Conference of High Blood Pressure Control, Los Angeles, Calif., Apr. 2–4, 1978.

Ciminero, A. R., Calhoun, K. S., & Adams, H. E. (Eds.). *The handbook of behavioral assessment*. New York: Wiley-Interscience, 1977.

Cohen, A. NIOSH behavioral research programs. In C. Xintaras, B. L. Johnson, & I. de Groot (Eds.), *Behavioral toxicology*. Cincinnati: NIOSH, 1974.

Davidson, W. L. Hypertension: The silent hazard. *International Journal of Health and Safety*, 1974, *43*, 21–23.

Dunn, J. E., Linden, G., & Breslow, L. Lung cancer mortality experience in certain occupations in California. *American Journal of Public Health*, 1960, *50*, 1475–1487.

Dutton, L. M., Smolensky, M. H., Leach, C. S. Lorimor, R., & Bartholomew, P. H. Stress level of ambulance paramedics and fire fighters. *Journal of Occupational Medicine*, 1978, *20*(2), 111–115.

Eysenck, H. J., & Eysenck, S. B. G. *Eysenck Personality Inventory*. San Diego: Educational and Testing Service, 1968.

Felton, J. S. How to pinpoint future heart disease. *Occupational Health and Safety*, 1974, *43*, 26–29.

Felton, J. S., & Swinger, H. Mental health outreach of an occupational health service in a government setting. *American Journal of Public Health*, 1973, *63*(12), 1058–1063.

Fogle, R. K., & Verdesca, A. S. The cardiovascular conditioning effects of a supervised exercise program. *Journal of Occupational Medicine*, 1975, *17*(4), 240–246.

Frankenhaeuser, M. Sympathetic-adrenomedullary activity, behaviour and the psychosocial environment. In P. H. Venables & M. J. Christie (Eds.), *Research in psychophysiology*. New York: Wiley, 1975.

Garbus, S. B., Pore, M., Troendle, D., Wheeler, M., & Garbus, S. Catch employee hypertension and cut absenteeism rate. *Occupational Health and Safety*, 1975, *44*, 48–50.

Gibson, E. S., Haynes, R. B., & Martin, R. H. Vascular diseases in employed males: A perspective on preventive and remedial programs in industry. *Journal of Occupational Medicine*, 1975, *17*(7), 425–429.

Glaser, R., & Klaus, D. J. A reinforcement analysis of group performance. *Psychological Monographs: General and Applied*, 1966, *80*, 1–23.

Goldstein, A. P., & Sorcher, M. Changing managerial behavior by applied learning techniques. *Training Rehabilitative Medicine*, *1974*, *6*, 81–88.

Goldstein, A. P., & Sorcher, M. *Changing supervisor behavior*. New York: Pergamon, 1974.

Gottlieb, H., Strite, L. C., Koller, R., Madorsky, A., Hockersmith, V., Kleeman, M., & Wagner, J. Comprehensive rehabilitation of patients having chronic low back pain. *Archives of Physical and Medical Rehabilitation*, 1977, *58*, 101–108.

Haynes, R. B., Sackett, D. L., Gibson, E. S., Taylor, D. W., Hackett, B. C., Roberts, R. S., & Johnson, A. J. Improvement of medication compliance in uncontrolled hypertension. *Lancet*, 1976, *1*, 1265–1268.

Hersen, M., & Barlow, D. H. *Single case experimental designs: Strategies for studying behavior change*. New York: Pergamon, 1976.

Hersen, M., & Bellack, A. S. (Eds.). *Behavioral assessment: A practical handbook*. Oxford, England: Pergamon, 1976.

Holmes, T. H., & Rahe, R. H. The social readjustment scale. *Journal of Psychosomatic Research*, 1967, *11*, 213–218.

Hulley, S. B., Cohen, R., & Widdowson, G. Plasma high-density lipoprotein cholesterol level. *Journal of the American Medical Association*, 1977, *238*, 2269–2271.

Jablonsley, S. F., & DeVries, D. L. Operant conditioning principles extrapolated to the theory of management. *Organizational Behavior and Human Performance*, 1972, *1*, 258–340.

Janis, I. L., & Hoffman, D. Facilitating effects on daily contact between partners who make a decision to cut down on smoking. *Journal of Personality and Social Psychology*, 1970, *17*, 25–35.

Jenkins, C. D. Recent evidence supporting psychologic and social risk factors for coronary disease: First of two parts. *New England Journal of Medicine*, 1976, *294*(18), 987–994. (a)

Jenkins, C. D. Recent evidence supporting psychologic and social risk factors for coronary disease: Second of two parts. *New England Journal of Medicine*, 1976, *294*(19), 1033–1038. (b)

Kanzler, M., Zeidenberg, P., & Jaffe, J. H. Response of medical personnel to an on-site smoking cessation program. *Journal of Clinical Psychology*, 1976, *32*, 670–674.

Kelsey, J. E. Professional counseling in a company with a broad dispersion of work locations. *Journal of Occupational Medicine*, 1975, *17*(11), 702–705.

Kimberly-Clark health management program aimed at prevention, *International Journal of Occupational Safety and Health*, 1977, *46*, 25–27.

Koerner, D. R. Cardiovascular benefits from an industrial physical fitness program. *Journal of Occupational Medicine*, 1973, *15*(9), 700–707.

Latham, G., & Kinne, S. B. Improving job performance through training in goal setting. *Journal of Applied Psychology*, 1974, *59*, 187–191.

Magura, A. Investigation of the relation between low back pain and occupation: 1. Age, sex, community, education and other factors. *Industrial Medicine and Surgery*, 1970, *39*, 465. (a)

Magura, A. Investigation of the relation between low back pain and occupation: 2. Work history. *Industrial Medicine and Surgery*, 1970, *39*, 504. (b)

Magura, A. Investigation of the relation between low back pain and occupation. *Scandinavian Journal of Rehabilitative Medicine*, 1974, *6*, 81–88.

Manuso, J. S. J. Coping with job abolishment. *Journal of Occupational Medicine*, 1977, *19*(9), 598–602.

Maurice, M. *Shift work*. Geneva: International Labour Office, 1975.

Miller, R. L. When you lift, bend your knees. *International Journal of Occupational Health and Safety*, 1976, *45*, 46.

Moos, R. H., Insel, P. M., & Humphrey, B. *Work environment scale*. Palo Alto, Calif.: Consulting Psychologists, 1974.

Nord, W. R. Beyond the teaching machine: The neglected area of operant conditioning in the theory and practice of management. *Organizational Behavior and Human Performance*, 1969, *4*, 375–401.

Paul, G. L. Behavior modification research: Design and tactics. In C. M. Franks (Ed.), *Behavior therapy: Appraisal and status*. New York: McGraw-Hill, 1969.

Peters, R. K., Benson, H., & Peters, J. M. Daily relaxation response breaks in a working population: II. Effects on blood pressure. *American Journal of Public Health*, 1977, *67*(10), 954–959.

Peters, R. K., Benson, H., & Porter, D. Daily relaxation response breaks in a working population: 1. Effects on self-reported measures of health, performance and well-being. *American Journal of Public Health*, 1977, *67*(10), 946–953.

Plunkett, E. R. Cardiac at work: Practical aspects of heart disease on the job. *Occupational Health and Safety*, 1974, *43*, 20–22.

Porter, L. W. Turning work into nonwork: The rewarding environment. In M. D. Dunnette (Ed.), *Work and nonwork in the year 2001*. Monterey, Calif.: Brooks/Cole, 1973.

Rose, R. M., Jenkins, C. D., & Hurst, M. W. Health changes in air traffic controllers: A prospective study 1. Background and description. *Psychosomatic Medicine*, 1978, *40*, 142–165.

Rosenman, R. H., Brand, R. J., Jenkins, C. D., Friedman, M., Straus, R., & Wurm, M. Coronary heart disease in the western collaborative group study: Final follow-up experience of 8½ years. *Journal of the American Medical Association*, 1975, *233*(8), 872–877.

Sackett, D. L., Haynes, R. B., Gibson, E. S., Hackett, B. C., Taylor, D. W., Roberts, R. S., & Johnson, A. L. Randomized clinical trial of strategies for improving medication compliance in primary hypertension. *Lancet*, 1975, *1*, 1205–1207.

Scherlis, S. (Chairman). Report of the committee on stress, strain and heart disease. *News from the American Heart Association*. Dallas: American Heart Association, 1976.

Schwartz, J. L., & Rider, G. Smoking cessation methods for the United States and Canada: 1969–1974. In J. Steinfield, W. Griffiths, K. Ball, & R. M. Taylor (Eds.), *Proceedings of the Third World Conference on Smoking and Health*. DHEW Pub. No. (NIH) 77–1413, 1977.

Selikoff, I. J., Hammond, E. C., & Churg, J. Asbestos exposure, smoking and neoplastia. *Journal of American Medical Association*, 1968, *204*, 106–112.

Seres, J. L., & Newman, R. I. Results of treatment of chonic low-back pain at the Portland Pain Center. *Journal of Neurosurgery*, 1976, *45*(1), 32–36.

Shelnutt, E. OHN's can spot hypertensive symptoms, maintain treatment. *International Journal of Occupational Health and Safety*, 1977, *46*, 18–19.

Slobogin, K. Stress. *New York Times Magazine*, November 20, 1977, pp. 48–50, 95, 98, 100, 102, 104, 106, 108, 110, 112, 114.

Sorcher, M. A behavior modification approach to supervisor training. *Professional Psychology*, 1971, *2*, 401–402.

Stamler, J. The problem and the challenge. In *Hypertension Handbook*. Rahway, N.J.: Merck, Sharp, & Dohme, 1974.

Sterling, T. D., & Weinkam, J. J. Smoking characteristics by type of employment. *Journal of Occupational Medicine*, 1976, *18*, 743–754.

Sternbach, R. A., Wolf, S. R., Murphy, R. W., & Akeson, W. H. Aspects of chronic low back pain. *Psychosomatics*, 1973, *14*, 52–56.

Tasto, D. L., & Colligan, M. J. Health consequences of shift work. DHEW (NIOSH), U.S. Government Publication, 1978.

Terry, L. The future of an illusion. *American Journal of Public Health*, 1971, *61*, 233–240.

Thiis-Evensen, E. Shift work and health. *Industrial Medicine and Surgery*, 1958, *27*, 493–497.

Verdesca, A. S. Hypertension screening and follow-up. *Journal of Occupational Medicine*, 1974, *16*(6), 395–401.

Villafana, C., & Mackbee, J. The value of continued followup in a preventive medicine program. *Industrial Medicine and Surgery*, 1971, *40*(4), 11–15.

Walker, J., & De La Mare, G. Absence from shift work in relation to length and distribution of shift hours. *British Journal of Industrial Medicine*, 1971, *28*, 36–44.

Warshaw, L. J. Placing and managing the cardiac patient. *Occupational Health and Safety*, 1974, 16–19.

Wear, R. F., Cox, M. E., & Lento, H. G. An atherosclerosis prevention program: Evaluation of the first six years. *Journal of Occupational Medicine*, 1975, *17*(5), 295–303.

Weiman, C. G. A study of occupational stressor and the incidence of disease/risk. *Journal of Occupational Medicine*, 1977, *19*(2), 119–122.

Wojtezak-Jaroszowa, J. Physiological and psychological aspects of night and shift work. DHEW (NIOSH) Publication, Library of Congress No. 77-600069. Washington, D.C.: U.S. Government Printing Office, 1978.

Wolter, M. J. The nurse's expanding nursing role. *Occupational Health and Safety*, 1975, *44*, 22–25.

Wood, L. W. The Bronx study: A trial of health care management. *Journal of Occupational Medicine*, 1975, *17*(10), 648–651.

Zorn, E. W., Harrington, J. M., & Goethe, H. Ischemic heart disease and work stress in West German sea pilots. *Journal of Occupational Medicine*, 1977, *19*(11), 762–765.

Author Index

Subject Index

Abdominal pain, 241–242
Abused drug, 166, 175, 177, 183
Academic underachievement, 254
Academy of Behavioral Medicine Research, xi, xii, 7
Acetylcholine, 167, 183
Adherence. *See* Compliance
Agoraphobia, 174
Alcohol, 164, 165, 166, 167, 168, 175, 176, 177, 178, 179, 183
    abuse, 149
Alpha biofeedback
    and alcoholism, 149
    and chronic pain, 149
    and drug abuse, 149
    and hypnotic training, 149
Altered states of consciousness, 165, 167, 177
American Psychological Association, 38, 60
Amobarbital, 167, 180
Amphetamine, 167, 176, 178, 179, 180, 183
Analgesic, 177, 179, 181, 182
Anger, 207
    and stress-coping control, 207, 208
Anorexia nervosa, 120, 121, 255
Antabuse treatment compliance, 25–26
Antecedent stimuli, 102, 103, 104
Anxiety
    and effectiveness of stress-coping technique, 208, 209
    and faulty coping, 216
    and helplessness, 215
    and hospitalization, 216
    interpersonal anxiety, 208
    and relaxation technique, 215
    speech anxiety, 208
    and stress inoculation training, 206
    test, 208–209

Apomorphine, 183
Appointment keeping
    behavioral analysis report and, 20
    contracting and, 20–21
    dental coupon incentive and, 17, 20
    importance of, 18
    personal contact and, 18
    personalized medical care and, 20
    scheduling systems and, 20
    telephone reminder and, 18–19
    written reminder and, 18
Assertive training, 242, 255, 257
Assessment, 35, 46, 47, 48, 49, 50, 52, 54, 55, 56, 57, 58, 59
    methodological issues in, 124–125
    psychological, 232, 241
Assessment questionnaires, 113–116
Asthma, 76, 82, 89, 91
    chronic, 215
    coping style, 215
    treatment of, 149–150
        airway resistance feedback, 149
        with biofeedback, 204–205
        with EMG feedback, 150
        relaxation training, 150
Attribution effect, 158
Aversive conditioning, 183

Baseline measurements, 106–108, 122
Behavior, experimental analysis of, 44, 46, 47, 56, 58
Behavior modification. *See* Behavior therapy
Behavior rehearsal, 257
Behavior therapy, 1, 2, 3, 4, 5
    cognitive, 157
Behavioral assessment, 268, 279, 283, 284
    basic principles of, 105–108

303